Nutrition for Sport and Exercise

A Practical Guide

To *Pops*,
In loving memory

Companion website

This book is accompanied by a website:

www.wiley.com/go/daries/nutrition

The website features:

- Student exercise and answers

Nutrition for Sport and Exercise

A Practical Guide

Hayley Daries MSc (Med) R.D. (SA) (UK)

Consultant Dietitian, Sport & Clinical Nutrition
Hayley Daries Nutrition Consultancy
Durbanville, Cape
South Africa

WILEY-BLACKWELL

A John Wiley & Sons, Ltd., Publication

Registered office: John Wiley & Sons, Ltd, The Atrium, Southern Gate, Chichester, West Sussex, PO19 8SQ, UK

Editorial offices: 9600 Garsington Road, Oxford, OX4 2DQ, UK
The Atrium, Southern Gate, Chichester, West Sussex, PO19 8SQ, UK
2121 State Avenue, Ames, Iowa 50014-8300, USA

For details of our global editorial offices, for customer services and for information about how to apply for permission to reuse the copyright material in this book please see our website at www.wiley.com/wiley-blackwell.

Library of Congress Cataloging-in-Publication Data

Daries, Hayley.
  Nutrition for sport and exercise : a practical guide / Hayley Daries.
       p.   ;   cm.
  Includes bibliographical references and index.
  ISBN 978-1-4051-5354-6 (pbk. : alk. paper)
  I. Title.
  [DNLM: 1. Nutritional Physiological Phenomena.   2. Sports–physiology.   3. Diet.
4. Exercise–physiology. QT 260]
  613.7–dc23

                                                                      2012014814

A catalogue record for this book is available from the British Library.

Cover image: © iStockphoto: © François Pilon (large background image); left to right: © micron, © GMVozd, © Jim Parkin, © Georgina Palmer, © Hshen Lim

Cover design by Meadan Creative

Set in 9.5/13 pt Meridien by Aptara® Inc., New Delhi, India
Printed in Singapore by Ho Printing Singapore Pte Ltd

1   2012

Contents

Companion website

This book is accompanied by a website:

www.wiley.com/go/daries/nutrition

The website features:

- Student exercise and answers

Preface

I am a teacher at heart, and for this purpose I have been absorbing knowledge from a very young age. My first inspiration came from my father, Winston Warren Daries (*Pops*), who taught me in primary school. He had a gift for teaching and inspired his students with his enthusiasm for Geography. Later life brought me other great teachers in the field of nutrition and sport, like Professor Edelweiss Wentzel-Viljoen (dietetics) and Professor Timothy Noakes (sport and exercise medicine), and my previous colleague and author, the late Mary Barasi (nutrition) who are all great examples of Excellence in their respective fields.

Hence, the idea of this book first came about while lecturing Sport and Exercise Nutrition at the University of Wales Institute, Cardiff (now Cardiff Metropolitan University) and Cardiff University. There Mary Barasi recognized my dedication to sport and teaching and recommended me to Blackwell's Nigel Balmforth. I will never forget my nerves and excitement on the day of our first meeting, and I am so grateful for the opportunity to impart what I know and have experienced in this field.

This book is for the many students, athletes and teachers who share my passion for sport and exercise nutrition. While it has a sound scientific underpinning, it presents the fundamental principles in an easy-to-read format. The subject is rapidly expanding and athletes and students want to know about the latest scientific research, the dietary habits of other athletes, and the spec on the most fashionable supplement. A book that can combine the science of sport and exercise nutrition with application of knowledge (as student exercises) and real food choices (as recipes) seems to achieve more than one objective. The students want to know 'why?' and the athletes want to know 'who to?' It is the 'hands on' part that will make it all stick in the end; this I have learnt through my work with students and athletes in the field.

Hayley Daries
2012

Acknowledgments

I would like to thank the team at Wiley-Blackwell, including Nigel Balmforth, Katrina Hulme-Cross and Rupert Cousens. It is also with a grateful heart that I thank Sara Crowley-Vigneau for her support, encouragement and profound professionalism in the final leg of the manuscript. I have had the privilege of expert guidance and advice from Rebecca Huxley, and also thank Amit Malik for his contribution.

I have been very lucky to find Rene Petersen who helped with the recipes and did an excellent job, and Cheryl Wolfe whose optimistic assistance I could rely on day and night and who has exceptional organizational and technical skills.

I thank my husband Rupert, *triathlete par excellence,* with whom I share my love for exercise, and who has always been there with little and big rewards along the way. I am blessed with a wonderful family, also my cheerleading squad who always believed in me and saw me through all the seasons of my manuscript.

Natalie, Vanessa, Michelle, your families and Mom, Thank You So Much.

Last but not least, I thank all the athletes and students who have always been at the forefront of inspiration for me to complete this incredible journey.

Foreword

It is a special privilege to write the foreword for the book by a former student. For it is in the writing of a book that one acquires the wisdom that no teacher can ever impart. Teachers can provide the tools and perhaps the spark, but never the desire nor the commitment to expend the thousands of hours that are required to produce a work of substance as is this book.

I know Hayley Daries as an inquisitive, independent, self-directed but impatient thinker who is dissatisfied with the way things are. She is driven to understand what is beyond the horizon of our knowledge. The research for her Masters degree sought to answer the question: How much do athletes really need to drink during exercise? At a time when the global standard was 'drink as much as tolerable', she was one of the first courageous enough to question whether drinking according to the dictates of thirst might be better. Her findings were amongst the first to question the value of drinking at high rates during exercise.

Hayley's gentle nature belies a steely strength and firm resolve to make a difference in all that she undertakes – as a teacher, clinician, researcher, writer, wife and mother. She does not need nor does she seek external affirmation; she alone is the best judge of the quality of the work she undertakes in all the different components of her life. Her standard is perfection. She told me about this book only after most of it had been written and then only to seek my advice about a specific section. She knows that she knows better than others on exactly what it is she needs to write. And this knowledge has been earned at the coalface – advising athletes what they need to eat and then putting that practical information together in lectures and articles, an ongoing process that will continue for as long as she practices her calling.

Hayley describes that her passion is to write a book that provides a practical resource for athletes, based on a sound analysis of the science of sports nutrition. Students, she says, want to know 'why' and the athletes want to know 'how to'. In fact, both really want to understand both the practical 'how' and the scientific 'why'. Hayley has succeeded admirably in describing both the art and the science of sports nutrition in a friendly and easily accessible format. She has succeeded in her goal of producing the practical information that she believes is often missing from the purely scientific texts. It is this information that she thinks will in the end 'make it all stick'. And so her book will find a special place in the discipline because it resonates with the goodness, the honesty, the practicality and the intellectual integrity of its author.

Hayley knows that the abiding principle she learnt from me is that, at its core, science is about disproving that which we hold the most dear. She is aware of the maxim that 50% of what we teach is wrong but the problem is that we do not know which 50% that is. The core belief in sports nutrition mirrors that of the nutritional sciences both of which are founded on the belief that carbohydrate is the crucial macronutrient for both health and for competitive sport. Fat on the other hand is branded as unhealthy and a poor choice for those who are active. But the nature of our knowledge is that it is, and must always be, in flux.

Prior to the 1960s the worldview of nutrition was altogether different. Then it was believed that fat and protein are the healthy choices for athletes whereas carbohydrates are fattening. Athletes were also advised not to drink during exercise. The advice on fluid replacement was clearly wrong. But are we absolutely certain that our understanding of the ideal macronutrient composition of both the healthy and the athletic diet is beyond question?

I pose this question to remind us all that our eternal search is for the truth. And truth as one scientist wrote is like a mirage; the closer we approach it, the more likely it is to disappear.

Until we have that final truth, there is much in the nutritional sciences, especially as they apply to sport and health, which remains an art.

We must never forget that.

Professor Timothy Noakes OMS, MBChB, MD, DSc, PhD (hc),
FACSM, (hon) FFSEM (UK)
Discovery Health Professor of Exercise and Sports Science
University of Cape Town
Sports Science Institute of South Africa

CHAPTER 1

Introduction

Key terms

Energy balance	Practical food skills
Positive energy balance	Travel fatigue
Negative energy balance	Body composition
Nutrition knowledge	Estimated average requirement (EAR)
Dietary goals	Performance analysis techniques
Food group models	Physical demands of exercise
Dietary reference values (DRV)	Preceding diet
Guideline daily amount (GDA)	Training adaptations
Dietary extremism	

The importance of an adequate diet for athletes

It has been clearly demonstrated that the nutritional composition and adequacy of an athlete's diet has an impact on performance and overall well-being. The consumption of food and fluid as fuel and hydration, before, during and after training and competition, can affect the athlete's nutritional and immune status, health, body mass and composition, energy stores and nutrient availability, exercise performance and recovery.

Participation in all types of exercise, ranging from recreational exercise to competitive sport increases the physical demands on the body. Their increased energy expenditure requires athletes to consume higher energy intakes and specific amounts of nutrients from food and fluids, in the pursuit of meeting the demands of sport and exercise. Therefore, an important goal of an adequate diet for athletes is achieving and maintaining energy balance, which aims to restore energy reserves and leads to greater fulfilment of health and performance goals. While positive energy balance (when energy intake is higher than energy expenditure) encourages weight gain,

---

Nutrition for Sport and Exercise: A Practical Guide, First Edition. Hayley Daries.
© 2012 Blackwell Publishing Ltd. Published 2012 by Blackwell Publishing Ltd.

negative energy balance (when energy intake is lower than energy expenditure) can result in weight loss. However, there are consequences to both positive and negative energy balance that need to be considered in the long term. Positive energy balance may lead to over-fatness and chronic illness, and negative energy balance may result in an increased risk of muscle tissue loss, fatigue, injury and illness.

An adequate diet involves more than just energy balance, as key nutrients and fluid replacement have a role in preparation, support and enhancement of the athlete's exercise and sports performance. An adequate sports diet also prevents some negative effects associated with prolonged exercise, such as nutrient fatigue. The nutrients, namely, carbohydrates, proteins and fats provide energy for exercising muscles. The proportion of these nutrients required are dependent on factors such as the athlete's body weight, age, gender, intensity and duration of exercise and timing of meals (i.e. eating before, during and after training or competition). While many athletes believe they are eating a high-carbohydrate, low-fat eating plan, on closer inspection or analysis of the diet it is often revealed that the diet is in fact a high-fat, low-carbohydrate plan, and not much different to the average western diet. Participation in exercise may also increase the need for certain vitamins and minerals, those that have specific functions in exercise metabolism and the immune system.

All athletes start out with recreational exercise. Some may continue this level of exercise participation indefinitely. However, for many athletes, participation in sport can become highly competitive and this environment requires that athletes train and compete at their maximum capacity. The need for an adequate sports diet can help athletes sustain strenuous activities that may be of varying intensity, duration, frequency and skill.

To help an athlete achieve an adequate sports diet, the goals set out in the following text can be applied to all athletes participating at any level of sport. These goals form the foundation of the athlete's everyday diet, which can then be tailored to suit the individual needs of an athlete as their demand for food and fluid change through various stages of training, competition and recovery.

Goals of an adequate sports diet

- To follow the basic healthy eating guidelines
- To meet energy and nutrient requirements
- To maintain health and well-being in both short term and long term
- To reach and maintain a healthy body mass, appropriate body composition levels, including body fat and body muscle tissue, and body water, as well as other health indices (i.e. waist circumference).
- To plan and implement training and competition nutrition strategies

- To ensure optimal hydration before, during and after exercise
- To treat suboptimal nutrient levels and any known nutritional deficiencies
- To treat and manage any ailments or diseases (i.e. diabetes) while eating for sport
- To determine if or when nutritional supplements may be of benefit to the diet and exercise performance

Barriers to achieving an adequate sports diet and best food practice

Although athletes are constantly seeking ways to improve exercise performance, there may be a number of reasons that may prevent athletes from choosing or adhering to an adequate sports diet or adjusting their dietary behaviour to achieve optimum performance. The following will be discussed in the subsequent text:
- Athletes' source of information (i.e. the media) and misconceptions about optimal sports nutrition practices
- Poor nutrition knowledge
- Dietary extremism
- Poor practical food skills
- Frequent travel

Athletes' primary source of information and misconceptions

There is a plethora of information available through the media, and surveys on athletes have found that many athletes rely on the media as the primary source of nutrition information (Jacobson and Aldana, 1992). Thus at the time, TV, commercials, magazines, advertisements, books, popular magazines and newspapers appeared to be a source of nutritional information for athletes. Another media forum, the Internet, has become accessible and affordable to athletes. Various social networking websites allow users to exchange information by chat-room forums, email and instant messaging, some allowing content to be distributed in 'real-time' as it is uploaded. Facebook, Bebo and Twitter are among the popular online social networks.

However, not all forms of information are credible or substantiated by scientific evidence (also referred to as *evidence-based information*), and may lead to confusion for many athletes. This confusion may be one reason why athletes lack understanding in this specialised science of sport and exercise nutrition. It is advisable that athletes educate themselves about sources of valid and reliable information, try to access nutritional support programmes that are available to them or seek the advice or counselling of a qualified sports dietitian or sports and exercise nutritionist if they require specialist dietary advice.

Poor nutrition knowledge

Since knowledge, attitudes and beliefs may act to encourage or discourage behaviour change (Thompson and Byers, 1994; Main and Wise, 2002), lack of knowledge about sports nutrition may be a barrier for athletes who wish to follow an adequate sports diet and make favourable dietary choices. It seems that while some athletes may perceive themselves to have an understanding of nutrition for athletes, their perception may not match their performance in a knowledge survey. With the rise in over-drinking during exercise, a recent survey examined how 'beliefs about hydration and physiology drive drinking behaviours in runners'. Winger et al (2011) found that most runners relied on personal experience of 'trial and error' as a factor influencing their drinking behaviour. However, the survey revealed this group of athletes' inadequate understanding of physiological principles underlying hydration practices, putting them at risk over-hydration and its consequences.

Some athletes may have a general nutrition knowledge base, but fair poorly when asked questions specifically about the diet for athletes. Most athletes in recent surveys have been unable to identify the role of sport-specific nutrients such as carbohydrates and its role in exercise (Dunn et al, 2007), and/or proteins as a fuel for exercise. The latter misconception, that protein is a primary source of energy for muscle contraction, is a common finding among athletes surveyed (Zawila et al, 2003; Condon et al, 2007; Rash et al, 2008). It is, therefore, not surprising when athletes regard protein supplementation as necessary for exercise performance (Rosenbloom et al, 2002; Rash et al, 2008).

Not all athletes have poor nutrition knowledge, as certain groups of athletes appear to have a higher level of knowledge in nutrition. Apart from having a few misconceptions, elite athletes competing at national level, scored higher on nutrition-related multiple-choice, general knowledge and sport-specific questions than their age-matched non-athletes (Cupisti et al, 2002). Similarly, Raymond-Barker et al (2007) found that competitive endurance athletes' level of knowledge of general nutrition was significantly higher than non-athletes of the same age group and gender.

What knowledge would benefit athletes?

Athletes need to understand the concepts in energy and fluid balance. In general these include, but are not exclusively:

- energy and its terms, i.e. kilocalorie, kilojoule;
- their individual energy expenditure and energy intake, and the relationship between dietary intake and physical performance;

- proportion of nutrients in the diet, i.e. percentage of carbohydrate, protein and fat. That is, do athletes know what a 60% carbohydrate-rich diet means?
- the nutrient carbohydrate, and glycaemic index and sport;
- the nutrient protein, amino acids and the required amount and effects of excessive intake;
- the nutrient fat and requirements for sport, fat adaptation diets and their effects;
- the nutrient water and the fine balance between dehydration and over-hydration in sport and the consequences thereof;
- the nutrient alcohol and its impact on sports performance and recovery;
- vitamins, minerals, dietary allowances and their role in health and exercise; and
- antioxidants, muscle soreness and requirements for athletes of various sports.

Athletes may not be able to practically apply their nutrition knowledge to make favourable food choices, due to the following reasons:

- Some may have a misunderstanding of food groups, or pictorial food guides like the Eatwell Plate (UK), MyPlate (USA) or the food pyramid guides, and its basic dietary guidelines. For example, the athletes surveyed by Dunn et al (2007) had problems translating nutrition knowledge into food choices as only half the questions about food choices were correctly answered. Furthermore, with a mean score of 36 points (out of 67) for the section on food groups, merely a third of athletes knew *how many* servings of fruits and vegetables are recommended daily. It is like having a few pieces of the puzzle but not being able to see the whole picture.
- Other studies have also shown that while athletes may have the knowledge, or know what advisable eating behaviour is, favourable dietary practices may not be applied (Nichols et al, 2005; Robins and Hetherington, 2005).
- An inability to understand the profile of foods within food groups, i.e. those foods within one food group have a similar, not identical nutrient make-up. For example, pasta, potatoes and bread are all starch that contain carbohydrates and have a similar nutrient profile when it comes to macronutrients (carbohydrate, protein and fat content). However, when it comes to micronutrients, a potato is rich in Vitamin C, potassium and copper, while pasta is a good source of Vitamin B_2 (riboflavin) and manganese and copper. Brown and wholemeal bread contains Vitamin B_1 (thiamin) and B_2 (niacin), and minerals iron, magnesium, copper and others. Therefore, while each serving of pasta, potato and bread yields similar amounts of carbohydrate, protein, fat and likely copper, the rest of the micronutrient contribution is quite different. That is why it makes

sense to have a variety of foods within a food group. If a person just eats pasta and avoids potatoes and bread, they miss out on these foods that are rich in iron, magnesium, manganese and fibre. If the pattern persists over weeks or months, they can be at risk of suboptimal nutrient levels that can eventually lead to nutrient deficiencies.
- An inability to read food labels and choose the most appropriate packaged food or supplement as part of an adequate sports diet. In urban areas where there is no lack of access to processed and packaged food, athletes are bombarded with branding, nutritional claims, symbols of endorsement, ingredient lists and nutritional information. If they are not guided by what to look for to meet their individual health and exercise performance goals, they may fall prey to clever marketing and advertising of food companies, retailers and anecdotes of other athletes.
- Not knowing how to interpret and use dietary reference values (DRV), like recommended nutrient intakes (RNI), or guideline daily amounts (GDA) in their individual diets.

Athletes may not be able to convert scientific sports nutrition principles into achievable dietary practices because they do not know:
- about their body weight loss (through sweat) or gain (through overdrinking) during exercise and its impact on their health and performance;
- about ergogenic aids (performance-enhancing aids) and its uses;
- about pre-, during and post-competition nutrition strategies;
- about sport-specific nutritional needs, i.e. fluid strategies to use in endurance sports.

Dietary extremism

Athletes who have misconceptions about nutrition and sports performance may be trapped by dietary extremism, which can limit the variety of foods they consume in their diet. Dietary extremism includes the following:
- Obsessive behaviour around food
- Disordered eating, i.e. food restriction, binge eating
- Excessive use of supplements, either nutritional or ergogenic aids
- Consuming very low (calorie) energy diets leading to underweight and low body fat levels
- Very low-fat diets
- Vegan diets, or extreme fibre intake
- Exclusion of one or more food groups
- Regularly skipping meals
- Fad diets
- Detoxification, 'cleansing' diets or excessive, inappropriate use of laxatives for weight loss

While vegetarianism is not an extreme dietary regimen, athletes need to pay special attention to their diet and ensure suitable plant proteins are consumed if eggs, dairy and/or fish are not consumed in their diet.

Poor practical food skills

The pattern of consumption and food selection may be influenced by athletes' food preference (choosing one food over another) (Jonnalagadda et al, 2004). Athletes may lack the practical food skills or motivation in preparing appropriate meals. The following factors may have an effect on athletes' food preference and affect whether they achieve an adequate sports diet and best food practice:

- Limited food and nutrition knowledge
- An inability to cook
- Lack of cooking facilities
- Limited access to food or healthy recipes
- Recipes with unknown ingredients or that seem long and complicated
- Poor food selection
- Overuse of highly processed foods (i.e. processed cheese, luncheon meats, sausage and/ or bangers, which are high in fat, salt and have a high calorie, low nutrient value).
- Overuse of take-out foods
- Lack of motivation to prepare fresh food
- Inability to recognise nutrient quality of meals
- Inability to convert scientific nutrition principles into real food choices
- Limited time to prepare food to fuel and sustain their performance, such as in the case of athletes who have a heavy training load with little time between exercise sessions, or who have a busy lifestyle involving other responsibilities and commitments.

Frequent travel

The need for travel has increased in both recreational and competitive sport, attracting all levels of athletes to train and compete abroad (Waterhouse et al, 2004). Long distance travel can lead to travel fatigue, a temporary condition that can be overcome by appropriate preparation and precautions, before and during a flight. However, when travel involves a long distance flight across several time zones, athletes may experience jet lag for several days thereafter. Various methods have been proposed to counter the effects of jet lag, and to adjust the body clock as quickly as possible. Although there is insufficient evidence available for the 'feeding hypothesis', and the Argonne diet for athletes, Waterhouse et al (2004) suggests ways to minimise the effects of jet lag, including melatonin ingestion, bright-light-exposure-avoidance and management of sleep.

If local travel is involved, athletes travelling to a new venue may not be adequately prepared for training and competition due to the following reasons:

- Lack of preparation of foods and fluids
- Having an insufficient supply of foods and fluids for the duration of the event
- Feeling compelled to consume *all* the foods and fluids they have brought along
- Insufficient funds to purchase food or fluids
- Trying new foods or supplements for the first time during competition

Although this may seem trivial to athletes, athletes' performance is often affected when they are not prepared or not able to get a particular food or drink at the new venue, one that they previously used during training. They then have to try a new food or drink, not known to them and with no idea of how it may affect their performance. If partaking in an endurance or team event, it may be that the event organisers have done well to provide beverages and race snacks for the athletes, although an athlete should never count on this. Rather be pleasantly surprised by the events' food and fluid supply than disappointed or distraught by lack of supply. In the end it seems a clear choice to make, that is, to come to an event in the best possible shape by being prepared with foods and fluids suited to individual taste, considering the number of hours and numerous sacrifices athletes make on a daily basis for their sport. Since sport and exercise performance is multi-factorial, why spend all that time concentrating on the exercise component and then throwing it away by lack of preparation around nutrition.

Foreign travel poses another challenge for athletes, and depending on their level of performance, may be frequent (several times a year or season) or infrequent (once a year or less). Since there are restrictions with regards to what one may be able to take on board an aircraft, it limits the athletes' nutrition preparation strategies. It is best then for them to familiarise themselves with the destination country, city and venue as much as possible by obtaining information prior to departure. This will depend heavily on their accommodation of choice, facilities that are available there and the surrounding area or sporting venue. At athletes' villages they may be restricted and not allowed to bring in any food, fluid or supplementation.

They may be exposed to different foods than their home country, unknown brands of food, foreign language food labels and cultural staple foods. If venturing out and about, at worse, they may be exposed to unsafe foods or water. Athletes at a high level of performance, i.e. professional athletes or those representing their country may have a team of people to coordinate their trip and manage these challenges. Other athletes may not be so lucky and the result is that their nutritional intake and performance will depend on their resourcefulness.

Rationale for following sport and exercise nutrition principles

While talent and ability contribute to overall sports performance, nutrition knowledge and good food practices can make a difference between winning and losing. The rationale for adhering to sport and exercise nutrition principles has been provided through years of scientific research and observation of athletes, both in laboratory settings, and in the field, i.e. in real life competitions. The literature reported in this book demonstrates that partaking in sport and exercise places energy and nutrient demands on the human body, in addition to those required for basic bodily functions, survival, prevention of disease and promotion of health. Thus, from a nutrition standpoint, understanding energy and nutrient requirements for sport and exercise participation, and applying these principles is of key importance to achieve and maintain a healthy body and achieve optimal sports performance.

The following factors influence energy and nutrient requirements:
- The athlete's body composition (fat mass and lean body mass (muscle mass), weight (body mass) and height).
- Type of sport participation, i.e. intermittent-, power- or endurance-type exercise affecting intensity and duration of exercise, and subsequent fuel use during the activity.
- Environment, i.e. preceding diet, will affect fluid and nutrient requirements.

Other factors such as genetics, or natural ability, and training adaptations will affect, or change the athlete's physiology that in turn affects the energy and nutrients they require, and how efficient their bodies are at using these resources.

Body composition affects dietary needs

All athletes are individuals with different dietary needs and exercise demands that depend on type, duration and intensity of exercise, age, gender, weight and body composition and lifestyle. Body composition (body fatness and lean body mass) is estimated using physical body measurements (anthropometry) including weight (body mass), height, waist circumference, mid-arm muscle circumference, body frame size, body mass index (BMI) and skinfold thickness. These measurements, as well as age and gender are used for determining the estimated average requirements (EAR), which will be discussed in Chapter 2.

Factors affecting fuel use during exercise

At a competitive level of sport, high demands are placed on athletes' energy and nutrient stores. Performance analysis techniques are a way to assess these demands so that the knowledge can be applied in training and competition performance, and used toward the dietary plan. It is used by researchers and in high-performance laboratories and provides useful information that tracks and measures athletes' activities during sport participation, especially in sport that relies on a high number of activities and requires a high level of skill, such as squash or football. For example, football is a high-intensity intermittent type of exercise and players need to be agile and fast as well as being skilled. Although running rates as one of the most energy-demanding activities, other activities such as tackling, jumping, accelerating, turning and getting up from the ground place physical demands on players and test the athletes' perpetual and motor skills performance. The analysis of football players' activities shows the physical capacity differences in playing position. Studies indicate that male midfield players have the highest aerobic power compared with attackers and defenders (Bangsbo et al, 1991; Bangsbo, 1994). Male footballers cover an average distance of 11 km (6.8 miles) during a 90-minute match. This corresponds to a mean speed of 7.2 km/h (4.5 miles/h). How far a player runs is just one measure of the physical demands of the game. One thousand metres (1100 yd) are covered in high-intensity running that comprises of 20 very short, fast sprints. Elite female players cover similar distances and high-intensity runs as male players. Players can change activities every 3.7 seconds of the game, yielding 1459 activity changes (Mohr et al, 2004).

Environmental factors

The preceding diet and amount of stored nutrient that is available affect energy and nutrient requirements of the athlete.

Nutrients derived from ingested food and fluid is converted to fuel during exercise. The body also stores nutrients in organs and tissues, which goes a long way to sustaining a given exercise intensity and duration. An optimal diet will provide the athlete with sufficient fuel stores, and with nutrients that are essential for energy metabolism and vital bodily functions. For example, nutritional factors such as antioxidants affect the strength of an athlete's immune system and their ability to recover between sessions. These will be discussed in greater detail in Chapter 7.

Another factor that affects energy and nutrient requirements is training adaptations. Exercise training combined with the optimum diet has the ability to change and adapt the athletes' physiology, causing an altered exercise metabolism that may favour sports performance. The greatest impact on exercise performance through enhanced physiological and biochemical adaptations may be in the application of specific nutritional principles to support athletes' intensive training demands (Maughan, 2002). Spriet and Gibala (2004) emphasised existing and new developments in nutritional practices that may influence adaptations to training. These are:

1 caffeine ingestion and its ergogenic effect;
2 creatine ingestion and its ability to increase muscle fibre size;
3 using intramuscular triacylglycerol (IMTG) as a fuel during exercise, and its repletion; and
4 gene and protein expression in muscles and the role of nutrition.

The authors stress that research in these areas will alter nutritional recommendations given to athletes, which will improve the adaptive response to training. Chapter 9 will explore the performance-enhancing (ergogenic) effects of caffeine and creatine.

Endurance training increases fat oxidation that allows more fat to be used as a source of fuel during exercise. Increased oxidation of circulating fatty acids and triglycerides (or triacylglycerol) in the muscle (Kiens et al, 1993; Phillips et al, 1996) occurs as a result of training duration. There are ample stores of fat in the body. IMTG is the small amount of fat (a few hundred grams) in muscle found between muscle fibres and as fat droplets within muscle cells. Even in the leanest endurance runner there are several thousand grams of fat from adipose tissue (fat under the skin and in the abdomen between the organs). 'Fat-loading' diets have been used by trained and untrained endurance athletes to improve fat oxidation and spare carbohydrate during exercise. Jacobs et al (2004) observed that even previously untrained males who cycle trained for 10 days and consumed a high-fat diet, increased their rate at which fat was burned during 90 minutes of exercise, thus sparing carbohydrate. However, although carbohydrate was spared, performance did not improve after 90 minutes. Fat as a fuel for exercise will be explored further in Chapter 6.

Furthermore, trained athletes become adapted to higher oxidative stress by producing more antioxidant enzymes that enhances the enzymatic antioxidant system, and hence, endurance trained athletes have an enhanced endogenous antioxidant defence system (Kanter, 1998).

Furthermore, when protein is metabolised, nitrogen is excreted by urine, faeces, sweat and other secretions such as skin, hair and nails. Training adaptations may improve protein retention to a greater extent than that of the average healthy person. Chapters 5 and 6 provide further information regarding training adaptations.

It is imperative that athletes formulate their own individual goals and identify the barriers that limit the fulfilment of these aspirations. They can equip themselves with evidence-based knowledge and practical food skills to make better (informed) choices. The factors influencing athletes' energy and nutrient requirements and how to address it will be discussed in detail in the subsequent chapters.

Chapter summary

- The nutritional composition of an athlete's diet affects their nutritional status and health, body mass and composition, nutrient availability, exercise performance and recovery.
- The goals of an adequate sports diet can be used to establish a nutritional foundation for any athlete, participating in any sport at every level of exercise.
- The barriers that may prevent athletes from choosing an adequate sports diet, or adjusting their dietary behaviour to achieve optimum performance are, their own misconceptions about optimal sports nutrition practices, poor nutrition knowledge, dietary extremism, poor practical food skills and frequent travel.
- Of key importance is that athletes need to understand energy and nutrient requirements for sport and exercise participation, and apply these principles to achieve and maintain a healthy body and optimal sports performance.
- Athletes need to be aware of the physical demands of their sport so that they can use this knowledge to consume an energy- and nutrient-rich diet for sport that will support their training and competition.
- The preceding diet plays an important role in energy metabolism during exercise.
- Trained athletes develop adaptations that enhances their ability to perform, and recover between exercise sessions.

CHAPTER 2

The Athlete's Energy Needs

Key terms

Energy	Anthropometric measurements
Kilocalorie	Nutritional assessment
Kilojoule	Weight
Dietary carbohydrate	Height
Glucose	Weight-for-height indices
Glycogen	Body mass index (BMI)
Protein	Waist circumference
Amino acids	Waist–hip ratio
Fats	Frame size
Fatty acids	Skinfold thickness
Triglyceride	Dietary reference values (DRV)
Alcohol	Reference nutrient intake (RNI)
Adenosine triphosphate (ATP)	Basal metabolic rate (BMR)
Adenosine triphosphatase (ATPase)	Basic energy expenditure (BEE)
Adenosine monophosphate (AMP)	Harris-Benedict equation
Adenosine diphosphate (ADP)	Schofield equation
Substrate partitioning	Estimated energy requirements (EAR)
The 'crossover' concept	Physical activity levels (PAL)
Aerobic metabolism	Thermic effect of food
Anaerobic metabolism	Estimated energy cost of activity

Energy

All energy originates from the sun and various forms of energy exist to do work in the body including light, chemical, mechanical, osmotic, electrical and heat (thermal) energy. Plant and animal foods provide energy and nutrients such as carbohydrate, protein and fat.

Nutrition for Sport and Exercise: A Practical Guide, First Edition. Hayley Daries.
© 2012 Blackwell Publishing Ltd. Published 2012 by Blackwell Publishing Ltd.

Energy is measured in kilocalories (kcal) or kilojoules (kJ) where,

1 kcal = 4.184 kJ
1000 kcal = 4.184 megajoules (MJ)
1 kJ = 0.239 kcal
1 MJ (1000 kJ) = 239 kcal

(Thomas and Bishop, 2007)

The nutrients providing energy

Dietary carbohydrate (CHO) is the major energy source in the diet, and is a critical source of fuel for the contracting muscles during exercise, especially during high-intensity exercise. The simplest form of carbohydrate is glucose, and all carbohydrate-rich foods are converted to glucose. Carbohydrate is stored as glycogen in the liver and muscles. The liver supplies the blood with glucose, which maintains the brain's essential glucose supply. Very low levels of blood glucose or hypoglycaemia (<3 mmol/L) can starve the brain of glucose, leading to a comatose state or brain damage.

1 g of CHO = 4 kcal (16 kJ)

The total carbohydrate stores in the body (liver and muscle glycogen and blood glucose) of a ~70 kg man is ~480 g with a caloric value of ~1920 kcal and roughly enough to run for 100 minutes or ~20 miles (Newsholme and Leech, 1983; Noakes, 2001; Maughan, 2002). Carbohydrate supplies fast energy during intense exercise (when compared with other nutrients protein and fat) and is the preferred energy source. Since exercise at a higher intensity or for a prolonged time rapidly depletes the body's carbohydrate stores, it is essential to maintain carbohydrate intake through the day before, during and after training. Grains and cereals, fruits and vegetables, sugary and glucose-based food, snacks and drinks are carbohydrate rich. Excess carbohydrate in the diet can be converted to fat.

Water is an essential nutrient that has many life-giving functions. It is stored with glycogen, ~3 g of water is stored with each gram of glycogen. During exercise water is lost when carbohydrate is used, and as sweat to dissipate heat that is built up through energy metabolism. The requirements for water increase during exercise.

Protein builds and maintains tissues and has a minimal role as a source of energy during exercise, providing 2–8% of energy supply for muscle contraction. Protein has a larger role after exercise and during recovery in the repair of damaged muscles fibres resulting from exercise, such as for ultra-endurance athletes who have the highest needs for post-exercise protein. The building blocks of protein are amino acids. Protein is stored in lean (muscle) tissue and during starvation, when not enough energy is available protein has the potential to convert to glucose and free fatty acids (FFAs) as an alternative energy supply.

1 g of protein = 4.1 kcal (17 kJ)

A 70 kg man with 12% body protein has 8.5 kg protein mass equal to 34,000 kcal of energy (Jeukendrup and Gleeson, 2004). Protein-rich foods include fish, poultry, meat and alternatives like eggs, beans, legumes and nuts.

Fat is the most concentrated source of energy and supplies some fuel for exercise, which increases depending on the duration and intensity of exercise. The basic units of fat are glycerol and FFAs and in this form they can be used by the muscle during exercise. The body stores fat as triglyceride in adipose tissue (around the organs and under the skin) as intramuscular fat known as triacylglycerol droplets in muscle, and a small amount in the plasma. Some endurance athletes have training adaptations that allow them to store more fat droplets in their muscles, for use during exercise.

1 g of fat = 9.4 kcal (37 kJ)

A 70 kg healthy adult male has roughly 10,000 g (10 kg) of fat equal to ~90,000 kcal enough to run for 4700 minutes (Newsholme and Leech, 1983; Noakes, 2001; Maughan, 2002; Jeukendrup and Gleeson, 2004). There is more than enough energy from fat to run slowly and continuously for more than 3 days, or for 1000 miles at 100 kcal per mile. Fats are found in a number of foods but the highest quantities of natural fats are found in vegetable oils, fish oils, butter, nuts and seeds.

Alcohol is not suitable before, during or after exercise as it can cause dehydration, leads to poor fuel sources, impaired skills and increase in heat losses. Alcohol causes vasodilation and impairs the recovery and repair phase that is essential after exercise. High alcoholic beverages increase urinary losses that may prevent athletes from achieving optimal rehydration after exercise. Refer to Chapter 3 for further information about alcohol and sensible consumption.

1 g of alcohol = 7 kcal (29 kJ)

Not all nutrients have an energy value, that is, vitamins, minerals and water do not contain energy but have vital roles in health and exercise.

Energy and nutrients as fuel for exercise

ATP

Every cell requires and consumes oxygen so that it can convert chemical energy (fuel) from the food we eat into mechanical energy. A

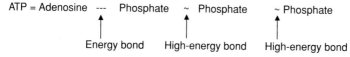

Figure 2.1 Basic formula of adenosine triphosphate (ATP).

high-energy compound is produced called adenosine triphosphate (ATP) that is required for cellular work. During exercise, contracting muscle cells have high demands for ATP (the 'energy currency') that provides kinetic energy for skeletal muscle to do mechanical work. Heat is also produced in the process and is lost through the lungs through breathing and the skin in the form of sweat (loss).

Figure 2.1 provides a schematic drawing of ATP. High-energy bonds exist between the phosphate groups and are symbolised by ~. Each high-energy bond stores 8000 kcal of energy. When the third phosphate group is released from adenosine by the enzyme adenosine triphosphatase (ATPase), energy is released and adenosine diphosphate (ADP) is formed. Subsequently, the second phosphate group is released for energy and forms adenosine monophosphate (AMP). Figure 2.2 illustrates the release of energy for muscle contraction by the breakdown of ATP, first to ADP and then to AMP. Figure 2.3 shows how the potential energy from plant and animal food sources ensures that a constant supply of energy is available.

The body has the ability to select the most appropriate fuel for a specific exercise. There are various factors that influence which nutrient will be used as fuel during exercise including intensity and duration of exercise.

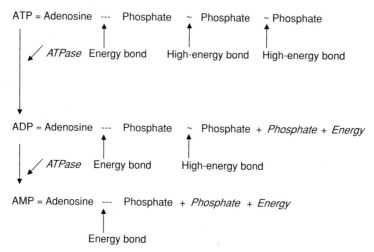

Figure 2.2 Adenosine triphosphate (ATP) becomes adenosine diphosphate (ADP) and adenosine monophosphate (AMP).

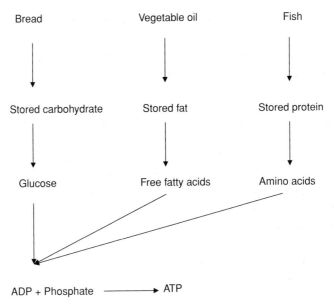

Figure 2.3 Energy from food ensures a supply of adenosine triphosphate (ATP).

Effect of intensity of exercise on fuel use

The intensity of exercise pays a role in the choice of fuel or nutrient that will be used during exercise. The balance of carbohydrate and fat oxidation, called substrate partitioning is for the most part influenced by exercise intensity (Brookes and Mercier, 1994).

Figure 2.4 demonstrates how increasing exercise intensity (measured by maximal oxygen uptake or VO_2max) affects energy demand, and carbohydrate use (as muscle glycogen and blood glucose) during running. During low exercise intensity (<50% VO_2max) blood carries sufficient oxygen (aerobic metabolism) to the muscles and fat is the predominant fuel, equal to more than half of the energy production during exercise. At this low intensity of exercise, carbohydrate supplies about one-third of energy. The 'crossover' concept by Brookes and Mercier (1994) suggests that the greater the intensity of exercise, the greater the reliance on carbohydrate as an energy source. As exercise intensity increases over 50% VO_2max, carbohydrate becomes the major fuel for the contracting muscles as energy from fat cannot be released fast enough above 60–65% VO_2max. During prolonged exercise at moderate intensity of 70–75% VO_2max, carbohydrate provides about 50–60% of energy, and fat 40–50% of energy. Most of the energy will be derived from muscle glycogen. At very high exercise intensity over 75% VO_2max (equal to running at a marathon speed of ~18 km/h in the aforementioned example), rapid energy is needed. At this point, carbohydrate mainly from muscle glycogen can be used to fuel the

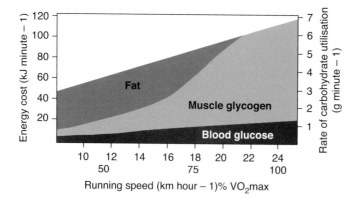

Fuel sources change as exercise intensity increases. This chart shows that as
VO_2max increases more energy is used and more carbohydrate is needed.

Figure 2.4   Effect of intensity of exercise on the change in fuel sources. (With
permission from Timothy D. Noakes.)

contracting muscles as it is the only fuel that can rapidly be converted
(anaerobic metabolism, without oxygen) to provide energy (Noakes,
1985).

Carbohydrate ingestion is critical and maintains blood glucose, especially
during the last stages of endurance-type exercise. Nutrient-related fatigue
occurs after 3 hours in the fasted state because blood glucose decreases,
and its contribution to energy decreases below 30%.

Effect of duration of exercise on fuel use

The duration of exercise also affects which fuel or nutrient will be used
during exercise. Duration implies for how long the athletes exercises, and
can be a measure of time, in days, hours, minutes or seconds. Figure 2.5
shows how fuel sources change over the period of time during a prolonged
exercise bout of 120 minutes. In this example, the intensity of exercise was
50% VO_2max. As exercise time increases, the glycogen in the working
muscles decreases, that is, the contribution of muscle glycogen to energy
supply decreases over time, with more reliance on blood glucose toward
the end of prolonged exercise. However, blood glucose can by no means
sustain prolonged exercise, and beyond 90 minutes its contribution toward
energy supply decreases. Energy production then relies on fatty acids that
contribute predominantly to the energy demand of exercise in these late
stages. In practice, this implies that endurance athletes can continue exercising, but must reduce their pace or intensity and slow down. This is due
to fat metabolism that takes place at a much slower rate than carbohydrate,
i.e. it does not yield ATP as fast. It takes 2–3 hours of exercise at 60–80%
VO_2max before glycogen becomes depleted. Bosch et al (1993) found

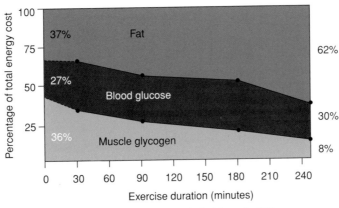

Fuel sources change over a period of time. (In this example the exercise intensity was 50% VO_2 max).

Figure 2.5 Effect of duration of exercise on change in fuel sources. (With permission from Timothy D. Noakes.)

increased oxidation rates of fat from 6% to 43% of total energy when and exercising at 70% VO_2max for 3 hours. Their subjects only ingested water during the trials. Training adaptations helps athletes enhance and prolong the use of fatty acids, sparing glycogen, thus helping to improve exercise performance.

Nutritional assessment of the athlete

In order to calculate the energy and nutrient requirements of an athlete, certain measurements must be taken on the body, known as anthropometric measurements. These are measurements of body weight, lengths, circumferences and thicknesses of parts of the body (Wardlaw et al, 2004). A summary of the anthropometric measurements of body composition (fat mass, lean body mass and water) is provided in Table 2.1.

Table 2.1 Anthropometric measurements of body composition.

Protein status	Fat stores	Body water
Mid-arm muscle circumference (MAMC)	Triceps skinfold thickness	Bioelectrical impedance
Grip strength	Body mass index (BMI)	Biochemistry
Nitrogen balance		Fluid balance charts
Plasma proteins		Rapid weight change
Plasma urea		Girth (ascites)
		Pitting oedema

Source: Thomas (2001).

Anthropometric measurements are part of the overall nutritional assessment that may include dietary assessment (taking a diet history, or food frequency questions and analysing the food records) as well as other investigations such as biochemical assessment and a physical examination. This information can then be used to determine the athlete's energy and nutrient requirements and individual dietary plan, menus and recipes.

Anthropometry

Weight

Body weight or mass is one of the most important measurements in nutritional assessment of any person. It is an important variable for calculations of energy expenditure equations in both the clinical setting, and to determine the energy and nutrient needs of athletes. Weight includes measurement of lean tissue, fat and fluid. Short-term fluid balance, therefore, will affect weight result.

Tools of the trade: It is preferable to use an electronic scale. For non-ambulatory persons, a bed or chair scale is often used. Other calculations of weight can be made from the following measurements: knee height, calf circumference, mid-arm circumference and subscapular skinfolds.

Height

Stature or standing height is measured from 2 to 3 years of age and older.

Tools of the trade: A stadiometer or wall-mounted measuring board is used in children and adults, height in centimetres for children and metres for adults. In non-ambulatory persons arm span or demi-span is used. This measurement is roughly equal to the height (within 10% of the actual height/stature) for both males and females. Alternatively, knee height can be used to determine stature, a measurement taken on the left side using a large broad-blade sliding calliper.

Weight-for-height indices

Height-for-weight tables have been replaced by weight-for-height indices, since the latter are used by dietitians and doctors to better predict health risks associated with chronic disease or poor nutrition. The preferred weight-for-height index should be maximally correlated with weight and minimally correlated with stature/height. In other words, it should be equally good at indicating body mass, no matter how tall or short a person is. The Quetelet index is named after a Belgian astronomer who used statistics of populations to observe that the weight of adults of differing heights is nearly the square of stature/height. The Quetelet index is commonly known as body mass index (BMI) and is the most widely used height-for-weight index. In practice, BMI is often used to assess degree of obesity (body fatness), as it is closely associated with estimates of body fat content. It is over-fatness not overweight that determines health risk, i.e. development of diseases associated with lifestyle, like type 2 diabetes, cardiovascular disease, high blood pressure and certain cancers. BMI is calculated as follows, using *metric measurements*:

$$BMI(kg/m^2) = \frac{\text{Body Mass in kilograms (kg)}}{\text{Height in metres (m)} \times \text{Height in metres (m)}}$$

or

$$BMI(kg/m^2) = \frac{weight(kg)}{height^2(m)}$$

For example, if an athlete weighs 62 kg and is 1.68 m tall, BMI will be 22 kg/m^2

$$BMI = \frac{62 \text{ kg}}{1.68 \text{ m} \times 1.68 \text{ m}}$$

$$BMI = \frac{62 \text{ kg}}{2.82 \text{ m}^2}$$

BMI = 21.98, rounded off to 22 kg/m^2

A BMI of 22 is considered within the healthy range (see Interpretation of BMI results).

Alternatively, BMI can be calculated in *imperial measurements* as follows:

$$BMI(kg/m^2) = \frac{\text{weight (in pounds)} \times 703.1}{height^2(\text{in inches})}$$

Interpretation of BMI results

Severely underweight: <16 kg/m^2
Underweight: 16–19 kg/m^2
Normal range: 20–25 kg/m^2
Overweight: 26–30 kg/m^2
Obese: 31–40 kg/m^2
Morbidly obese: >40 kg/m^2

(Thomas, 2001)

The limitations of BMI

BMI may be convenient to use in clinical settings as charts applicable to both males and females. BMI is both a convenient and reliable indicator of obesity since it correlates well with estimates of body composition, but in certain individuals, BMI should be used with caution as an indicator of obesity as seen in the following text.

Interpretation of BMI differs between age groups. While BMI may be used for adults aged 20–65 years of age, it is inapplicable for use in children, adolescents and elderly people as their proportion of lean body mass is changing. Although, in some countries, BMI guidelines are adapted for use by pregnant women (to advise weight gain during pregnancy), and special BMI charts exist for use in children and adolescents' growth monitoring.

There are still some areas where BMI may be misinterpreted in adults, and therefore, are to be used with caution in the following groups of people:

- In patients with oedema or dehydration, who have distorted fluid balance
- In athletes or body builders/power lifters, who have a high proportion of lean body (muscle) mass
- In persons who are tetraplegic, who has enforced immobility

At best, BMI can be used as a simple first step screening tool for overweight, and ideally other additional measurements need to be used to confirm *over-fatness*.

Waist circumference

A measurement that determines over-fatness is waist circumference taken in centimetres or inches using a tape measure, which gives an indication of body fat distribution. A high waist circumference indicates that fat that is stored viscerally or in the abdominal area, and is associated with higher health risks. Healthy waist circumference is $\leq$80 cm ($31\frac{1}{2}$ in.) for women and $\leq$94 cm (37 in.) for men. A waist circumference of >88 cm ($34\frac{1}{2}$ in.) in women and >102 cm (40 in.) in men substantially increases health risk. Chapter 6 provides further information about body fat distribution, health risks and guidelines for body fat loss.

Waist–hip ratio

Waist–hip ratio (WHR) was defined as the waist circumference divided by the hip circumference, i.e. waist girth (cm)/hip girth (cm). WHR is a measure of deposition of abdominal fat, i.e. central or upper body obesity. Unlike BMI, there is no consensus to define a cut-off point for WHR, although reviews consistently use the same cut-off values. A raised WHR has been taken to be 0.95 or more in men and 0.85 or more in women.

Body frame size

There are several methods to estimate body frame size, i.e. ankle girth, wrist circumference, frame index 2 and elbow breadth. Elbow breadth is less affected by degree of adiposity (fatness). Since it measures skeletal breadth, it can be used an as indicator of frame size.

Tools of the trade: Elbow breadth frame gauge, calliper blades. Measurements are in centimetres or inches.

Skinfold measurement

A skinfold thickness measurement is a double fold of skin and subcutaneous adipose tissue, grasped by the thumb and index finger of the left hand and large enough to form approximately parallel sides. Care should be taken to elevate only skin and adipose (fat) tissue. It is often used to estimate body fatness in athletes and should be done by a skilled professional for reliability and accuracy.

Tools of the trade: Skinfold calliper is used for the measurements, taken in millimetres to determine the sum of skinfolds. Standard (generic or population-specific) equations and tables are used for reference, although specific equations have been developed for different sports modalities. Measurement can include the following sites: tricep, bicep, subscapular, suprailiac, calf, thigh, abdominal.

Limitations of skinfold measurements and equations

The use of generic equations in estimating or tracking changes in body composition from skinfold thicknesses may be criticised in highly trained athletes involved in certain sports. Equations by Jackson and Pollock, or Evans could not accurately measure percent fat mass and other indices of body composition in elite judo athletes (Silva et al, 2009). In professional soccer (football) players, Reilly et al, 2009 found that the equation of Withers used to estimate percent body fat by skinfold thicknesses has the lowest bias and highest agreement with referenced values by Dual energy X-ray absorptiometry (DEXA). When compared with DEXA and 16 different equations, Durnin's equation best estimated percent fat from skinfold thicknesses in elite sport climbers (Romero et al, 2009).

Differences in skinfold compressibility in men and women could account for variability in repeated measurements by the same skinfold technician or by different technicians taking the same skinfold measurements (McRae, 2010).

Considering the aforementioned limitations, skinfold thickness measurements may also be misinterpreted in the following instances:

• In adults of older age who have changes in body fat deposits and distribution
• In very obese people with excessive subcutaneous fat
• Skinfolds taken by untrained persons or inexperienced technicians

Dietary assessment

Athletes' habitual energy and nutrient intake

Many studies have surveyed athletes' dietary intakes including surveys of teams, basketball players, cyclists, dancers, field hockey players, American football players, soccer players, gymnasts, ice skaters, rowers, runners, soccer players, swimmers, triathletes, volleyball players and wrestlers (for review see Hawley et al, 1995; Marquart et al, 1997). It is clear that differences exist between the dietary needs of non-athletes and recreational exercisers, and that of elite or high-performance athletes, who have higher training demands for sport. Information from surveys is useful for knowledge of the habitual intake and dietary practices of athletes by age group, or sport can highlight the nutrition issues for certain athletes and sports.

Recreational athletes

On average, non-elite, recreational athletes have daily energy intakes close to 2200 kcal for females and 2500 kcal for males. Carbohydrate intake is lower than the recommended intake for athletes. Females consume around 290 g CHO/day, and males consume over 300 g but less than 400 g CHO/day (Worme et al, 1990). At these levels, males and females consume a ~55% carbohydrate-rich diet, and intake of around ~4–5 g CHO/kg BW/day. Protein intake in recreational athletes is reportedly higher than Recommended Dietary Allowance (RDA) (reference nutrient intake (RNI)) at around 1.2–1.4 g/kg BW/day. Fat intake is moderate at around 1.0–1.2 g/kg BW, although athletes sometimes consume slightly more than the 30% of energy from fat that is recommended (Worme et al, 1990; Hinton et al, 2004).

Elite athletes

To date, few studies have assessed elite or high-performance athletes' nutritional intake using a large sample and representing various different sports like the classic study by Van Erp-Baart et al (1989). Recent evidence provides updated dietary intake data showing the trend in energy and nutrient intake, and dietary supplement use by elite athletes.

Lun et al (2009) assessed the nutritional intake of 324 high-performance athletes. The athletes' average daily energy intake was 2918 kcal for males and 2304 kcal for females. The proportion of total daily energy intake from carbohydrates was 53%, or 5.1 g/kg BW/day. Athletes had a 19% protein-rich diet, or 1.8 g/kg BW/day. Fat intake was 28% of total daily energy intake. Micronutrient intake from both food sources and supplement use was higher than recommended levels. Supplementation appeared to significantly increase athletes' energy and nutrient intake. Increased dietary supplement use by elite athletes has been reported previously (Huang et al, 2006) although recently a follow-up study (between 2002 and 2009) found a downward trend in supplement use by Olympic athletes (Heikkinen et al, 2011).

Six hundred and fifteen elite (professional) athletes' dietary intake was assessed and compared to data (of non-athletes) from a nationwide dietary survey. Male athletes' average energy intake was 3513 kcal/day of which carbohydrate contributed less than 50% of total daily energy intake, and fat energy, 35%. Female athletes had lower energy intakes but a similar proportion of nutrients in their diets. However, dietary iron intake was compromised in female athletes. Similar to Lun et al (2009), elite athletes in this study had higher than recommended micronutrient intakes (Gábor et al, 2010).

The athletic world has always been fascinated by the skill, endurance and the relentless tenacity of elite Kenyan runners. A 'tribe of runners', of Kalenjin ethnicity, have dominated many prestigious running events across the world and many are revered world-class Olympians and world champions in the middle- and long-distance races. Reasons for their running dominance have included favourable genes, (high-)altitude training and dietary intake.

During the summer season, as athletes train and prepare to compete, average energy expenditure of these runners is 3605 kcal/day, and is lower than their average energy intake of 2987 kcal. Most runners obtain their energy from carbohydrate sources, which make up 76.5% of daily energy intake. Their staple foods consist mainly of vegetarian foods such as bread, boiled potatoes, boiled rice, porridge, cabbage, kidney beans and a stiff maize meal paste called *ugali*, that make up 86% of daily energy intake. Energy from animal sources contributes the remainder 14% of their total energy intake, in the form of milk (11%) and meat (1%, mostly beef). Kenyan runners of this ethnicity consume 10.1% protein energy, and of the 75 g protein/day (1.3 g protein/kg BW) they eat only 33% in the form of animal sources, the rest (67%) they get from vegetable sources. Fat intake is very low, only 13.4% of daily energy intake, making up 46 g of fat energy, mainly from animal sources. It appears that no specific hydration strategies are employed by Kenyan runners. In this group of runners, training for 8 km or 12 km cross-country events or the 1500 m event, no fluid is ingested before and during training, with some runners ingesting only modest amounts of water after training. The average total water intake for the day is 1113 mL, with the rest of fluid intake coming from tea consumption. An average of 1243 mL of tea is consumed throughout the day (Onywera et al, 2004).

Further evidence of the drinking habits of Kenyan runners has been reported since the 2004 study. Fudge et al (2008) measured fluid intake and markers of hydration status in elite Kenyan endurance runners during a crucial 5-day training period before the national trials for the 2005 IAAF Athletics World Championships. The runners remained well hydrated with *ad libitum* fluid intake, and showed no signs or symptoms of heat strain at any time.

Overall, dietary intake data indicate the need for adequate energy and nutrients and better food quality in athletes' diets, especially as demands for energy and nutrients increase during participation in high-performance sport.

Nutritional analysis by hand

Standard food tables provide the nutritional value of foods (energy, nutrients) of commonly consumed foods. McCance and Widdowson's The Composition of Foods Sixth Summary Edition (Food Standards Agency, 2002) provides comprehensive nutrient data for over 1200 of the most commonly consumed foods in the UK. It covers all food groups and includes updated information on key foods such as milk, cheese, bread, breakfast cereals and meat and meat products. It is an essential handbook for students and professionals in all food and health disciplines.

Nutritional analysis by computer

Several nutritional analysis software packages are used by professionals in education, the National Health Service, industry and in the private practices. These software packages have programmes that analyse dietary intake, recipes and menus, as well as a few other nutrition-related functions.

Determining the athlete's energy requirements

Recreational exercisers or moderately active adults

The energy needs of adults (aged 19–50 years) involved in exercise of less than 1 hour a day (habitual and structured exercise) will be met by the dietary reference values for food energy and nutrients in the United Kingdom (DH, 1991). Dietary reference values (DRV) for energy is 2200–2900 kcal for women and men, respectively. The RNI for carbohydrate could be met by a 50–55% energy contribution or an intake of 400 g/day (men) and 300 g (women). A protein intake equivalent to 12–15% of energy or 70 g (men) and 60 g (women) is recommended and based on 1.0 g protein/kg BW/day. Fat should be no more than 30–35% of daily energy intake or 95 g (men) and 72 g (women). Even alcohol, within sensible limits (<5% of energy intake), may be considered in the general diet of moderately active persons.

As duration and intensity of exercise increases, the athlete's energy needs increase and so does their dependence on individual nutrients. Recommendations for most athletes are:

- ~60% or more energy from carbohydrate;
- 10–15% energy from protein; and
- 20–25% energy from fat.

However, the nutrient needs of athletes are often expressed as g/kg BW/day for both carbohydrate and protein, especially for athletes who compete at high levels and need to reach nutrient targets. Low-energy diets may not provide sufficient protein for training and recovery, or carbohydrate to maintain and restore glycogen stores. Therefore, it is more useful to express energy needs in g/kg BW/day. A carbohydrate intake of 5–10 g/kg BW/day appears to meet the needs of the majority of athletes (Coyle, 1991; Rodriguez et al, 2009), but intensity and duration of training should be considered as carbohydrates needs may be met by intakes as low as 3 g/kg BW/day or with 12 g/kg BW/day (Burke et al, 2004; Castell et al, 2010). A protein intake of 1–1.7 g/kg BW/day is sufficient, but the demand varies between individual athletes and also depends on type of sport (Lemon, 1995; Tarnopolsky, 1999; Tipton and Wolfe, 2004; Rodriguez et al, 2009).

However, these guidelines should never replace the work involved in determining the athlete's *individual* energy and nutrient needs, although it is useful as a reference guide for assessing dietary intake and evaluating nutritional goals of the athlete.

Determining the athlete's individual energy and nutrient needs

Basal metabolic rate

Energy balance is when the sum of energy intake from food, fluids and supplements is equal to energy expended through exercise, basal metabolism and the thermic effect of food (TIF; Swinburn and Ravussin, 1993).

Standard equations (i.e. Harris-Benedict or Schofield) or modified standard equations estimate a person's basic energy expenditure (BEE) or basal metabolic rate (BMR). For the general (healthy) population including most physically active individuals in the United Kingdom, energy requirements can be determined from the BMR reference tables by weight, age and gender (see Appendix Reference values for estimated energy expenditure).

Activity factors

Estimated Average Requirements (EAR) for adults is calculated taking into account the BMR and the total cost of activity or physical activity levels (PAL) for adults, which is the ratio of overall daily energy expenditure (from occupational and non-occupational activities) to BMR.

EAR for energy $= \mathrm{BMR} \times \mathrm{PAL}$

Where PAL is indicated as,
Inactive men and women: factor 1.4
Moderately active women: factor 1.6
Moderately active men: factor 1.7
Highly active women: factor 1.8
Highly active men: factor 1.9

(Thomas and Bishop, 2007)

Finally, a combined factor for the TIF and the estimated energy cost of activity also now known as the thermic effect of exercise (TEE) is added to determine total daily energy expenditure.

Energy cost of exercise

Energy expenditure is a measurement of power produced per unit of time and is measured in kcal/min (and kJ/min). Standard tables exist for measured intensity of activity. They provide the estimated energy cost of any physically related activity or sport relative to body weight.

For example, for a 70 kg athlete, the estimated energy cost of the following activities will be as follows:

- Badminton (6.8 kcal/min)
- Boxing (sparring) (15.5 kcal/min)
- Cricket (average of batting & bowling) (6 kcal/min)
- Cycling (racing) (11.8 kcal/min)
- Gymnastics (4.6 kcal/min)
- Hockey (field game, competition, structured) (9.8 kcal/min)
- Running (marathon, 7 min per mile) (14.6 kcal/min)
- Soccer (football) (12.2 kcal/min)
- Squash (14.8 kcal/min)
- Tennis (10.2 kcal/min)
- Water polo (competition) (13.5 kcal/min)

McArdle et al (1991, 2010)

Energy values are at best averages, as individual variability does exist. For example, Chapter 1 showed the physical demands of playing football. Although the approximate energy expended by a 70 kg person playing football may be 9.8 kcal/min or 882 kcal (3704 kJ) for a 90-minute game, variation could exist depending on body weight of the athlete, position played and performance level or skill of the player. Competitive football players have high-energy needs, around 6700 kJ (1595 kcal), which is the estimated energy cost of a competitive match (Bangsbo, 1994). This is equivalent to a rate of 17.7 kcal of energy expended per minute. Refer to Table 2.2 for calculations of athlete's individual energy expenditure.

It is clear that athletes are unique with individual energy and nutrient requirements. Many athletes are focused on meeting their nutritional goals and want to make informed food choices. They can use their energy allowance to choose foods that provide sufficient fuel, and health-enhancing nutrients for optimal nutritional status and exercise performance. Many have developed, to their benefit, well-tuned eating habits to assist in exercise and sport performance. However, some are lured by the unproven claims of performance-enhancing (ergogenic) aids, often at the expense of a good diet. The use of jargon or fashionable supplements and products are impressionable factors and are common among athletes of all

Table 2.2 Calculating athlete's individual energy needs.

Although the energy cost of training can be as high as more than a third of the total daily energy expenditure, during competition athletes compete at peak levels of what they can physically, physiologically and mentally sustain, hence the cost of exercise will be much greater.

Option 1
How to estimate an athlete's daily energy needs using prediction equations
1 Determine basal metabolic rate (BMR) by using the ready reference table for adults (refer to Appendix).
2 Multiply by the relevant physical activity level (PAL) (refer to *activity factors*).
3 Add the estimated energy cost of activity, taking into account body weight and the intensity, duration and frequency of exercise (refer to *energy cost of exercise*).

Example
In the week before a marathon race, a 70 kg male runner trains for 6.5 hours at a 4-min/km pace. This 38-year-old man is moderately active (PAL = 1.7).

Step 1. Calculate daily energy expenditure.
- BMR × activity level factor = 1678 × 1.7 = 2853 kcal

Step 2. Calculate weekly exercise (duration (time) × (cost of activity). Divide by 7 to obtain daily energy expenditure (for exercise).
- Running at marathon pace = 14.6 kcal/min (see *energy cost of exercise*)
- Convert minutes to hours to determine cost of 6.5 hours of running per week, and then divide by 7 for daily cost of activity
- 14.6 × 60 × 6.5 = 5694 ÷ 7 = 813 kcal

Step 3. Determine your total daily energy expenditure by adding the figures from daily energy expenditure and cost of activity.
- 2853 + 813 = 3666 kcal

Step 4. Determine individual nutrient needs by percentage contribution to total energy intake.
- Carbohydrate, contributing 60% of total energy intake:
  3666 kcal × 60% ÷ 4 = 550 g
- Protein, contributing 12% of energy:
  3666 kcal × 12% ÷ 4 = 110 g
To determine amount of fat, all nutrients must make up 100% (In this example, energy from alcohol was not included).
Therefore,
60%(carbohydrate) + 12%(protein) = 72%
100% − 72% = 28% of energy remaining for fat
- Fat, contribution 28%:
  3666 kcal × 28% ÷ 9 = 114 g
Therefore, the runner's daily energy and nutrient requirements are:
  Energy: 3666 kcal (15,397 kJ)
  Carbohydrate: 550 g
  Protein: 110 g
  Fat: 114 g

(continued)

Table 2.2 (Continued)

There is another way of expressing nutrient needs of athletes. This is useful for athletes who have low energy (and low carbohydrate and protein) intakes or vegetarian athletes whose protein intake may be compromised. It is also useful for athletes with very high carbohydrate and protein needs, such as ultra-distance endurance athletes. In this event, it is important to meet the individual nutrient targets, especially carbohydrate and protein, so that performance and recovery are not compromised. Expressed as gram of nutrient per kilogram body weight per day (g/kg BW/day) and using the aforementioned example, the 70 kg runner will have the following nutrient requirements:

Carbohydrates: 550 g ÷ 70k g = 7.8 g/kg BW/day

Protein: 110 g ÷ 70 kg = 1.5 g/kg BW/day

Fat: 114 g ÷ 70 kg = 1.6 g/kg BW/day (for prudency, fat is usually just expressed as g/day)

The chapters that follow will provide food guides, basic dietary guidelines, food portion lists and other practical tools that assist in helping the athlete convert the scientific calculations of energy and nutrient requirements into real food choices.

calibres. Thus, they risk losing the grounding of a healthy diet, balanced in energy and nutrients and one that promotes health and well-being.

Laying the foundation of a good diet involves applying basic nutrition principles and the use of practical nutrition strategies to change and/or improve an athlete's current diet, a kind of fine tuning that has been used successfully and safely by many athletes who achieve their best performances.

Chapter summary

- Plant and animal foods provide energy and nutrients such as carbohydrate, protein and fat.
- Energy is measured in kilocalories (kcal) or kilojoules (kJ).
- Dietary carbohydrate (CHO) is the major energy source in the diet and is stored in the liver and muscles. The energy value of 1 g of CHO is 4 kcal.
- Water is an essential nutrient required for many physiological functions.
- Protein builds and maintains tissues and is stored in lean tissue. 1 g of protein is equal to 4.1 kcal.
- Fat is an abundant source of energy and the average healthy male has ~90,000 kcal of fat energy. 1 g of fat equals 9.4 kcal.
- Alcohol has 7 kcal/g and can lead to harmful effects.
- During exercise, contracting muscle cells have high demands for the high-energy compound called adenosine triphosphate (ATP) that provides kinetic energy for skeletal muscle to do mechanical work.
- The greater the intensity of exercise, the greater the reliance on carbohydrate as an energy source during exercise.

- As duration of exercise increases, the glycogen in the working muscles decreases, and there is more reliance on blood glucose toward the end of prolonged exercise, but beyond 90 minutes its contribution toward energy supply decreases. Energy production from fatty acids contributes predominantly to the energy demand of exercise in the late stages of prolonged exercise.

- Anthropometric measurements are measurements of body weight, lengths, circumferences and thicknesses of parts of the body that are part of the overall nutritional assessment of the athlete.

- Body mass index (BMI) is the most widely used height-for-weight index and is often used in practice to assess degree of obesity (body fatness) as it is closely associated with estimates of body fat content. A BMI of 20–25 kg/m^2 is considered healthy.

- Healthy waist circumference is ≤80 cm (31$\frac{1}{2}$ in.) for women and ≤94 cm (37 in.) for men.

- A skinfold thickness measurement is often used to estimate body fatness in athletes using skinfold callipers and should be done by a skilled professional for reliability and accuracy.

- Dietary reference values (DRV) and reference nutrient intake (RNI) for adults (aged 19–50 years) will be sufficient to meet the energy and nutrient requirements of recreational exercisers or moderately active individuals that are involved in exercise of less than 1 hour a day (habitual and structured exercise).

- A carbohydrate intake of 5–10 g/kg BW/day appears to meet the needs of the majority of athletes, as does a protein intake of 1.0–1.7 g/kg BW/day, which is sufficient, although the demand varies between individual athletes and also depends on type of sport.

- Using equations or references tables for the basal metabolic rate (BMR) is the starting point for estimating the athlete's average energy requirement (EAR).

- Physical activity levels (PAL) for adults is the ratio of overall daily energy expenditure (from occupational and non-occupational activities) to BMR.

- Energy expenditure is a measurement of power produced per unit of time and is measured in kcal/min. Standard tables assist in providing the estimated energy cost of any physically related activity or sport relative to body weight.

- It is useful to know the dietary intakes of recreational and competitive athletes by age group or sport, as it can highlight the nutrition issues for certain athletes and sports.

CHAPTER 3

Laying the Foundation of a Good Diet

There is rigorous science behind the principles of sport nutrition and its application in training and competition settings. However, the cornerstone of a good training diet starts with laying the foundation of healthy eating by following key messages and better dietary practices. Recreational or elite athletes partaking in sport and exercise will be presented with nutritional challenges. For example, athletes need to meet high energy demands placed by high-intensity exercise, prolonged strenuous exercise, or repeated bouts of exercise, require practical skills regarding food preparation, plan for multiple competitions and know what to eat when travelling to unfamiliar destinations. Strategies that can achieve a number of nutritional goals at the same time are most useful to help athletes integrate separate issues and save time and resources. The ultimate aim of any sports and exercise nutrition professional would be to convey their knowledge of nutritional science into real food and fluid choices for the athlete. Athletes want accessible and appetising food and fluid options. Determining menus and recipes for athletes is one method to make sure of appropriate food selection, while planning an individualised supplement programme may

Nutrition for Sport and Exercise: A Practical Guide, First Edition. Hayley Daries.
© 2012 Blackwell Publishing Ltd. Published 2012 by Blackwell Publishing Ltd.

help athletes to weed out the plethora of expensive and non-beneficial supplements that bombard the sports market.

The training or foundation diet holds the key to overall exercise performance. The nutritional goals of the athlete's foundation diet are to meet their basic energy and nutrient requirements, to promote immediate and long-term health and longevity, to achieve and maintain a healthy body mass and acceptable level of body fat and lean body mass, to promote optimal performance and recovery and to accommodate appropriate and beneficial experimentation with competition nutrition strategies.

Food group illustrations

Many countries have developed their own set of nutritional guidelines for the general population. As a practical illustration of nutritional science, and to help people identify their daily nutritional needs in the form of real food choices and in some food groups to identify the minimum portions required, food group models have been designed. A food group model may take many forms and most countries have their own model, and others adopt and adapt another's, in line with their unique public health policy. The plate model is a pictorial food guide that has become a recognised visual tool to assist people in making healthier food and beverage choices. In the United Kingdom, *the eatwell plate* (Figure 3.1) is used and described as a healthy eating policy tool of the government. It aims to help the public choose healthier diets, and the government's strategy to achieve this is outlined in the 2010 public health white paper entitled 'Healthy Lives, Healthy People'.

The eatwell plate visually displays different food groups of a healthy balanced diet. Each segment represents a food group and the balance that is required in a healthy diet. It does not represent one meal, rather it emphasises the overall diet that is healthy and well balanced. It may be easier to achieve the balance over a longer term, i.e. weekly rather than trying to balance the diet every day of every week. Additional healthy eating messages support *the eatwell plate* visual tool and should be used along with the government's eight tips for making healthier choices.

The eatwell plate's five segments represent the five food groups and how much of each should be eaten in the diet as follows:
- 33% from bread, rice, potatoes, pasta and other starchy foods (eat plenty and choose wholegrain varieties).
- 33% from fruit and vegetables (eat plenty, at least five portions of a variety of fruit and vegetables daily).
- 15% from milk and dairy foods (eat some, choose lower fat alternative whenever possible).

The eatwell plate

Use the eatwell plate to help you get the balance right. It shows how
much of what you eat should come from each food group.

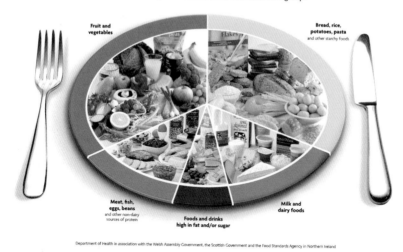

Department of Health in association with the Welsh Assembly Government, the Scottish Government and the Food Standards Agency in Northern Ireland

Figure 3.1 The *eatwell plate*. (Crown copyright material is reproduced from the
Department of Health in association with the Welsh Assembly Government, the
Scottish Government and the Food Standards Agency in Northern Ireland.)

- 12% from meat, fish, eggs, beans and other non-dairy sources of protein
  (eat some, choose lower fat alternatives whenever possible; eat at least
  two portions of fish a week, including a portion of oily fish).
- 8% from foods and drinks high in fat and/or sugar (eat just a small
  amount).

  The government's eight tips for making healthy choices (DoH, 2011):

1 Base your meals on starchy foods.
2 Eat lots of fruits and vegetables.
3 Eat more fish – including a portion of oily fish each week.
4 Cut down on saturated fat and sugar.
5 Try to eat less salt – no more than 6 g/day.
6 Get active and try to be a healthy weight.
7 Drink plenty of water.
8 Do not skip breakfast.

Accessibility of *the eatwell plate,* and healthy eating tips

- *Age*: Persons over the age of 5 can use *the eatwell plate,* although children
  aged 2–5 years should gradually move to eating the same foods as the
  rest of the family and in proportions displayed on *the eatwell plate.*

- *Ethnicity*: People of different ethnic origins and cultural practices can use it.
- *Body weight*: Persons of a healthy weight as well as those who are overweight can use it.
- *Food choice*: Meat eaters as well as non-meat eaters (e.g. vegetarians) can use it.

Limitations of *the eatwell plate*

- *Special dietary needs*: While *the eatwell plate* is a useful tool for most adults, limitations exist because of individual requirements and specialised dietary needs. The frequency of servings and recommended portion sizes are not included in *the eatwell plate,* and certain individuals (under medical care, or with special dietary needs) are advised to seek the advice of a general practitioner or a registered dietitian about the individual suitability of *the eatwell plate*.

  Clearly, these restrictions assist in protecting individuals from misuse or misinterpretation of *the eatwell plate* and its supporting messages.

From food pyramid to food plate

The Food Pyramid Guide is another food model that has been in use in other countries and by different cultures (i.e. the adapted Indian and Mediterranean food pyramid guides). Launched in the United States in 1992, the pyramid displayed four food groups stacked in the shape of a pyramid. Recommendations with regard to the number of servings from each food group flanked the pyramid. Even though the pyramid was revised in 2005, expanding the number of food groups and incorporating exercise, the underlying message may have been poorly received (or understood and applied) as the prevalence of obesity continued to rise.

In June 2011, the US Department of Agriculture (USDA) announced *MyPlate*, a new visual tool for communicating the USDA's key nutrition messages that promote healthy eating, including the following:

- Balancing calories by eating smaller portions.
- Make at least half the plate fruits and vegetables and half of grains and wholegrain.
- Switch to fat-free or low-fat milk.
- Reduce sodium-rich foods.
- Rather than sugary drinks, drink water instead.

MyPlate has four different coloured and sized segments of the plate representing the proportion of fruits, vegetables, grains and protein in the diet, with a smaller circle on the side of the plate for dairy products.

These guides educate the public and guide them to a healthier lifestyle for optimum health. It is as important for athletes as for the general public to apply these key messages to lay a good foundation for a healthy diet. Only then can they add specialised sport nutrition strategies that achieve the nutritional advantages accompanying a trained athlete. It is the same strategy used when laying the foundation of a good training programme, or base, which takes time and dedication, yet gradually prepares the athlete so that they reach their best physical form in pursuit of achieving accolades in sports performance.

Incorporating dietary guidelines in the athlete's diet

How can the average recreational athlete or the seasoned professional who has little knowledge of nutrition and who is looking for a simple and practical guide for health and optimum performance use a dietary tool like *the eatwell plate* and the government's healthy eating messages?

Food is meant to nourish and to be enjoyed, but many athletes worry about the adequacy of their diets. The foods, fluids and any supplements that the athlete chooses should be enjoyable, and not merely because it is prescribed or is based on an anecdote from a well-known competitor or a performance-enhancing theory. If food items are chosen merely for its performance-enhancing abilities, it may introduce a restricted diet that is not very accessible, and may be dull and unappetising. Compliance to such an eating plan may be low, and in the long-term health could suffer. As with the general population, it is advisable that athletes eat a variety of foods, with suggestions provided in Table 3.1, a food guide for sport and exercise. Each food group has a range of nutrients, some with a known role in sport and exercise. Eating daily portions from each group will help fulfil the daily recommended nutrient intake levels for optimal nutritional status, health and exercise performance.

Some athletes may be focused solely on a certain food, fluid or supplement that aids their performance; in that case they tend to be reluctant to disturb their pattern of eating. This practice may limit their intake of a variety of nutrients across the spectrum of food groups, especially if certain foods are restricted or avoided. It is especially true in the case of faddy eaters, or athletes with intolerances that may often exclude an entire food group. For example, in the case of lactose (milk sugar) intolerance, milk and dairy products are avoided. Often, and without professional dietary advice, no substitute will be used for the essential vitamins and minerals that are obtained from a food group. Nutrient deficiencies may arise if a food or group is avoided for a lengthy period of time without choosing alternative dietary sources or supplementation.

Table 3.1 Food guide for sport.

Food or drinks group	Major nutrients	Suggestions for portions for athletes	Examples of food and drink in this group with approximate servings	Recommendations for athletes
Fluid and non-alcoholic drinks	Water Sodium carbohydrate, i.e. glucose, sucrose, fructose, maltose	6–8 glasses water per day Add an extra ~400 mL of fluid for every 1 h of exercise	<1 h of exercise: Water >1 h of exercise: Diluted fruit squash; carbohydrate-based energy (or sports) drinks Other beverages: Herbal teas rich in antioxidants, e.g. red bush (rooibos) tea	~400 mL/h (smaller athletes) and up to 800 mL/h (heavier athletes) of a 5–10% carbohydrate drink (providing 30–70 g carbohydrates per hour of exercise). Take sodium as required, it can be taken in drinks or as salted snacks (Refer to Chapter 8).
Vegetables	Vitamins A and C, folate, magnesium, potassium fibre[a], Carbohydrate	3–5	*~5 g carbohydrate per serving:* 1 cup raw salad, or 2 Tbsp vegetables, or 150 mL vegetable juice	Eat a variety of colours Limit adding fat or creamy sauces Limit adding excess sugar or syrup
Fruit	Carbohydrate, fibre, vitamins A and C, folate, magnesium, potassium	2–4	*~15 g carbohydrate per serving:* 1 medium fresh fruit, or 2 small fruits, or 1 slice melon/pineapple, or 12 grapes, or 7–10 strawberries, or 125 mL pure fruit juice, or 3 Tbsp tinned or stewed fruit, or 1 small matchbox size dried fruit (Refer to Chapter 4 for fruits with larger carbohydrate servings (25 g CHO)	Eat a variety of colours Avoid adding rich creams Limit adding sugar or syrup Always eat the skin where possible (e.g. apple skin) Choose fresh fruit juice instead of sweetened varieties
Breads, cereals, pasta, rice, potatoes	Carbohydrate, B vitamins, magnesium, iron, calcium, zinc	5–14	*~50 g carbohydrate per serving:* 3–4 slices bread, or 2 cups Breakfast cereal, or 2 cups pasta/rice, or large (250–300 g) baked potato (Refer to Chapter 4 for foods with smaller carbohydrate servings (25 g CHO)	Choose high-fibre types Limit fried, roasted potatoes Avoid fried rice/noodles Avoid adding rich sauces or creamy dressings to pasta

(continued)

37

Table 3.1 (Continued)

Food or drinks group	Major nutrients	Suggestions for portions for athletes	Examples of food and drink in this group with approximate servings	Recommendations for athletes
Fish, poultry, meat and alternatives	Protein, some essential fats, B vitamins, folate, magnesium, phosphorous, iron, zinc	2–3[b]	*~20 g protein, ~3–10 g fat per serving:* ~90 g (three slices or equal to the size of a pack of playing cards) lean meat, chicken, turkey or fish, or two eggs *~10 g protein per serving:* 200 g baked beans or 60 g nuts/seeds or peanut butter *(high in plant fats)*	Choose lean cuts of meat only Cut off visible fat before cooking, remove skin of poultry Eat oily fish one or more times per week (sardines, salmon, pilchards, mackerel, and herring) Choose fish without batter, not deep-fried Strictly limit/avoid high-fat processed meats Beans and pulses are very low in fat
Milk and milk products	Calcium, phosphorous, protein, carbohydrate, vitamins A and D, magnesium, zinc, vitamin B12, riboflavin, pro-biotics (yoghurt)	2–3	*~12 g carbohydrates, ~8 g protein per serving:* 200 mL milk/calcium-rich soya milk (soya milk has less protein and carbohydrate per serve), or 1 (150 g) pot yoghurt/fromage frais, or *<2 g carbohydrates, ~8 g protein per serving:* 50 g cottage cheese or 1 matchbox size (30 g) cheese	Choose lowest fat versions Use reduced-fat cheese or cottage cheese Choose yoghurt with live cultures (source of pro-biotics)
Fats, oils and sugars	Fat, vitamins and essential fatty acids (from fats and oils), Carbohydrates (from sugars)	Prudent intake is recommended	*~15 g fat per serving:* 1 Tbsp olive, vegetable, nut oil 1 Tbsp olive oil margarine ($\frac{1}{2}$ avocado[c]) *~15 g carbohydrate per serving:* 1 Tbsp glucose/sugar/honey	Use pure oils (not blended oils) Use low fat spreads Limit/avoid hard fats like butter, lard, ghee and other foods high in saturated fats (pastries, pies, fatty cuts of meat, hard cheeses) Allow some optional calories from energy drinks, sweets and bars

Source: Material from Hayley Daries Practice.

1 Tablespoon (Tbsp) = 15 mL; 1 teaspoon (tsp) = 5 mL.

[a]Fibre is known as non-starch polysaccharide (NSP).

[b]The protein requirement will depend on the individual athlete's body weight.

[c]Avocado is a fruit but has a high content of monounsaturated fat.

The recommended diet for athletes has the same basic principles, although in addition, there are specialised sport nutrition strategies with respect to certain foods and fluids and how they are used by the body *during exercise.* For example, foods and drinks high in sugar are recommended in small amounts on *the eatwell plate,* since they are usually high in calories and can contribute to weight gain for most individuals. In the athlete's diet, sugary foods and drinks that have a high glycaemic index (GI) have a place in their eating plan providing quick fuel during exercise and facilitating recovery of fuel stores after exercise. This is one example of many that demonstrates that while the healthy eating fundamentals remain a cornerstone of the athlete's diet, the application of specific exercise and sport nutrition principles need to be considered. Meeting their immediate high energy requirements and nutrient demands that are specific to sport and exercise are important targets for any athlete, in addition to their long-term health and well-being. The guidelines below in the first instance serve the health of the athlete, and secondly provide a good foundation for the training diet. These fundamentals will ultimately aid performance and recovery in sport, and in conjunction with the food guide for sport (Table 3.1), could be a reference guide for athletes to keep their diets on track all through the year.

Starchy foods are ideal fuel for exercise

The carbohydrate needs of athletes are high as it is the preferred source of energy during exercise and sport. Breads, rice, potatoes, pasta and other starchy foods are a good source of carbohydrate, B vitamins, magnesium, iron, calcium and zinc. Wholegrain (bread, pitta, chapatti and cereals), wholemeal (bread, pitta and chapatti) and whole-wheat (pasta and brown rice) varieties of these grains, oats and starchy vegetables like corn, pumpkin, peas and butternut are ideal starches that are packed with energy, nutrients and fibre. Fibre is the indigestible part of food that is important for regular and healthy bowel movements and also for prevention of certain cancers. The recommended fibre intake for adults is 18 g/day. Foods rich in fibre include wholemeal bread, wholegrain breakfast cereals, porridge oats, brown rice, whole-wheat pasta, fruit and vegetables, and pulses like beans and lentils. According to dietary surveys, very few athletes meet their daily fibre needs (Tilgner and Schiller 1989); hence, it is an issue that needs to be addressed when laying the foundation of a healthy sports diet. Chapter 4 provides further details of the importance of carbohydrates in the athlete's diet.

Make fruit and vegetables a major part of the diet

Portion for portion, fruit and vegetables have a lower energy value than other foods (energy is mainly from carbohydrates and protein). However, it contains high quantities of fibre, vitamins, minerals and antioxidants like phytochemicals (health-enhancing nutrients that protect the body against harmful radicals). The minimum recommended intake of fruit and vegetables for adults are 5 portions a day, where 1 portion equals 80 g of fruit or vegetable. The Department of Health provides a list of 80 g edible portion equivalents, e.g. *each* of the following portions weighs 80 g:

- 1 medium fresh apple.
- 2 spears of broccoli.
- 150 mL fruit juice.
- 1/3 cereal bowl of fresh carrots, sliced.
- 1 heaped tablespoon of tomato purée.

Dietary surveys in the United Kingdom show many people do not meet this 5-a-day requirement, and athletes are no different. In theory, exercise may increase the need for certain vitamins and minerals, resulting in a high turnover and subsequent losses of these micronutrients. Further discussion of the evidence is presented in Chapter 7.

Athletic groups who are at risk of compromised micronutrient status are athletes who:

- consume very low-energy diets;
- consume too little fruit and vegetables;
- follow a very low-fat diet;
- eliminate one or more food groups from the diet;
- consume a high proportion of low nutrient-dense foods and drinks;
- experience menstrual dysfunction (female athletes);
- follow a vegetarian or vegan diet.

Recommendations based on current dietary reference values[1] (DRVs) and reference nutrient intakes[2] (RNIs) for healthy people in the United Kingdom are as appropriate for the athletic population for a number of reasons. For example, a training adaptation allows endurance-trained athletes to have an enhanced endogenous antioxidant defence system (Kanter, 1998). Thus, for majority of trained athletes, there appears no need to supplement with antioxidants in addition to RNIs provided they consume recommended intakes of micronutrients from dietary sources and have a replete antioxidant vitamin and mineral status.

Athletes with a known deficiency (e.g. iron deficiency) or low stores, have a good motivation to supplement, although the best effort must be made to increase dietary sources of the vitamin, mineral or antioxidant that is deficient. The most common mineral deficiency observed in athletes is iron deficiency. In particular, athletes participating in endurance sports require additional iron and can obtain it from supplementation (Córdova et al, 2002). Other surveys on nutritional intake of athletes show that one or more of the following vitamins and minerals fall short of recommended intakes: calcium, some B vitamins, iron, folate, zinc and magnesium (Worme et al, 1990; Felder et al, 1998; Hinton et al, 2004).

Despite some athletes' real need for supplementation above dietary intake, the rise in supplementation sales may indicate that athletes are at risk of misusing nutritional supplements, which can be a dangerous practice. The convenience of 'pill-popping' often appears to outweigh the nutritional challenges many athletes face, i.e. time constraints for food purchase and preparation, high energy and nutrients demands, and athletes' lack of cooking skills. Poor dietary practices or lack of nutritional knowledge are not sound reasons for athletes to use supplements.

Fish is rich in protein and heart-healthy fat

Protein is required by athletes to maintain and increase lean body mass, strength and power, to provide an added fuel source during endurance exercise, to aid fluid retention and for various other functions that underpin metabolic processes and recovery from exercise. Protein is lost in sweat, as much as 18 g/day, although training adaptations may improve athletes' protein retention. Other losses occur in urine, faeces, and skin, hair, nail secretions.

In the United Kingdom, the RNI for protein is 0.75 g of protein/kg BW/day, equivalent to 55.5 g protein/day for men aged 19–50 years, and 45.0 g protein/day for same-aged women (Department of Health, 1991). The habitual diets of British adults reveal a diet high in protein (Henderson et al, 2003) and sufficient to cover the needs of a vast majority of athletes. However, dietary surveys of athletes show high protein intakes, often more than twice the recommended intake and up to 3 g/kg BW/day in certain groups (Van Erp-Baart et al, 1989; Kleiner et al, 1990; Coetzer et al, 1993; Onywera et al, 2004). For athletes with increased energy demands, as long as energy expenditure is matched by adequate energy intake, protein intake is sufficient and there is no need to supplement the diet with additional protein. However, food sources of protein in the diet and factors such as the biologic value of protein, the type and content of fat and overall nutritional quality of the protein are important considerations for athletes. Fish is an excellent source of protein, and lower in calories and fat than meat and chicken. It is a good source of B vitamins and contains vitamin E, iron and zinc. This makes it a healthy choice for athletes, as well as easy to prepare. Some varieties can be eaten raw, many others are tinned and ready to eat, and most fresh varieties cook fairly rapidly by poaching, steaming, grilling, or baking in a traditional or microwave oven, or on the barbecue. Two portions per week are recommended for healthy eating, including at least one portion of oily fish, found in herring, kippers, mackerel, pilchards, sardines, salmon, trout and fresh tuna. Oil-rich fish is rich in vitamins A and D, but it is the polyunsaturated fat, namely omega-3 fatty acids that makes it a heart-healthy substitute for red meat (which contains more saturated fat). Omega-3 fatty acids protect against blood clot formation, help lower blood pressure and reduce risk of heart attacks and strokes. Furthermore, omega-3 fatty acids can improve an entire range of depressive symptoms (Servan-Schreiber, 2004).

Making sense of food labels. A portion of fish is about 140 g.

Make room for healthier fats in the diet

There is a large supply of stored fats (triglyceride) under the skin and within muscle fibres. Fat stores are beneficial to endurance or ultra-endurance athletes who rely on fat to spare muscle and liver glycogen (stored carbohydrate) and delay nutrient-related fatigue during prolonged exercise.

Fat-loading or fat adaptation is a diet strategy used by well-trained endurance athletes that involves increasing the proportion of fat in their diet for 3–5 days or longer. The effects of a short- and longer-term, high-fat diet for endurance athletes have been well reviewed (Helge, 2002; Yeo et al, 2011).

However, fat is very concentrated in energy and because every gram has double the energy compared with carbohydrates and proteins, a small amount of fat added to a meal will quickly increase the energy content of the meal. Diets high in fat result in weight gain, an increase in fat mass, and a change in body composition.

In general, athletes are advised to look after their long-term health irrespective of what training diet or competition-loading regime they follow. A high-fat diet is linked to obesity and can raise blood lipids, including cholesterol levels, increasing the risk of heart attack and stroke. Choosing the right types of fat is important and certain fatty acids benefit hormonal well-being and brain function. Using more soft fats, or poly- and monounsaturated fatty acids from oils, nuts, seeds, oily fish, and avocado is better than consuming a diet high in hard fats or saturated fatty acids from butter, cream, fatty meats, pies, pastries, cakes and biscuits.

In the athlete's diet, fat is often eaten at the expense of carbohydrate, because high-fat meals are filling and satiable and the athlete may not be able to meet their carbohydrates and protein requirements if their meals are high in fat. This is often the case with athletes who try to follow a carbohydrate-loading regime but who eat creamy pasta meals with rich sauces or three-cheese or meaty pizzas. It is not that pasta or pizza that is high fat; on the contrary, they are excellent sources of carbohydrates that can assist the loading phase before competition. However, if athletes choose these dishes with high-fat toppings or dressings, they may not be getting as much carbohydrate as they require. Table 3.2 provides a few examples of popular carbohydrate-based dishes, and ideas for keeping such meals high in carbohydrates and low in fat. Recipe ideas, which are

Table 3.2 Favourite carbohydrate-based dishes.

Moderate-carbohydrate, high-fat menu items	Choosing high-carbohydrate, low-fat options	Eat in with these recipes (see recipes in Chapters 3, 4, 5, 6 and 7)
Meat entrée	Vegetable entrée without oil or butter, salad or fruit entrée	Greek salad with lemon vinaigrette, avocado and prawn salad, melon and parma ham
Fried rice or noodles	Steamed rice or noodles, or Basmati rice	Sun-dried tomato risotto, sweet and sour pork with noodles
Creamy soups	Minestrone, clear soups with noodles or vegetables, bean- or vegetable-based soups	Classic pea and ham soup, roasted onion and potato soup
Regular meat (beef) lasagne with full fat cheese (cheddar) and rich creamy white sauce	Lean mince or soya mince lasagne with medium fat cheese (mozzarella) and white sauce made with skim milk, or vegetarian lasagne	*Meat-free dishes*: Bean and lentil burgers, tofu and vegetable stir-fry
Pasta and rich creamy sauce (e.g. béchamel, carbonara, regular dressing), Ravioli with meat or cheese	Pasta with tomato-based sauce (e.g. bolognaise, napoletana), or plain with parmesan cheese and salad, pasta or potato salad with reduced-fat dressing, Ravioli with ricotta and spinach	Tomato and basil pasta sauce Warm potato and grilled pepper salad
Pizza with four-cheese topping or with salami, pepperoni	Pizza with mozzarella cheese and tomato, or pizza with vegetables or fruit as a base, may add beans or lean chicken, meat or fish	Gypsy ham and cheese sandwich, spicy chicken wrap, veal steak rolls, turkey burgers
Fried chips, roasted potatoes	Baked potato with light mayonnaise, or with baked beans/bean salad, or salsa dressing.	Jacket potato with tuna and mayo filling, Haricot bean mash
Cream-based dessert (tiramisu), cheesecake, pastry	Fresh fruit, sorbet, low-fat dessert, jelly, baked or stewed fruit, frozen yoghurt	Strawberry fruit salad, Oven-baked nectarines with walnut and ricotta
Garlic bread	Plain, crusty bread, pitta, chapatti or naan bread without butter	

Source: Recipes added to material from Hayley Daries Practice.

provided in this book, are given as eat-in suggestions. The importance of fat as a fuel during exercise and high-fat diets for athletes is discussed in further detail in Chapter 6.

Making sense of food labels. Foods containing a lot of fat have 20 g fat or more per 100 g product, and/or 5 g saturates fat or more per 100 g. Foods with a little fat contains 3 g fat or less per 100 g, and/or 1 g saturates or less per 100 g (Food Standards Agency, 2006).

A little sugary food and fluid fuels exercise

Compared with the general population, athletes have higher energy expenditure and requirements and simple carbohydrates (or sugars) provide quick energy to refuel and recover during and after exercise. Sugary foods and drinks may include amongst others, sucrose (sugar), glucose, fructose, maltose, dextrose or another simple carbohydrate. As part of a training diet and pre-competition diet the use of some simple sugars is beneficial as it rapidly increases carbohydrate stores that will help to improve prolonged exercise.

The GI is a ranking of carbohydrate-rich food that is a useful tool for the general public and is used in weight management and for diabetics. The GI is a nutrition tool that assists patients in controlling fluctuating glucose levels in the blood, improve satiety, delay hunger and reduce blood cholesterol. While low and moderate GI foods should provide the basis of most healthy diets, it is also the foundation of the training diet for athletes. Frequent consumption of high GI foods and fluids are not recommended for the general population, due to the rapid rise in blood glucose levels following its intake, and some foods' low-nutrient content. But the latter advice could confuse athletes, especially as high GI foods and fluids play a role in the athletes training, competition and recovery diet, helping to maintain glucose levels *during* exercise (Walton and Rhodes, 1997) by providing rapid energy to sustain duration and intensity of exercise. *After* exercise, a high GI diet improves the storage of glucose in the muscles, as much as 30% increase when compared with a low GI diet (Burke et al, 1993). GI is discussed in further detail in Chapter 4.

Making sense of food labels. Foods containing a lot of sugar have 10 g sugars or more per 100 g product, while foods containing a little sugar have 2 g sugars or less per 100 g (Food Standards Agency, 2006).

Sodium (salt) and water balance

Athletes lose sodium in sweat, and it is the amount of sodium (and potassium) in the body that determines the amount of water (or water balance) (Noakes, 2001). Foods and drinks with sodium stimulate thirst and encourage drinking, therefore preventing dehydration. However, the average diet is high in sodium as most British adults consume about 9 g salt/day. According to Noakes (2001), the average runner's daily salt intake is enough to cover the salt needs of a marathon a day. So, although sodium replacement is not essential during exercise, overdrinking during exercise can cause serum sodium concentration to become diluted and can lead to exercise-associated hyponatremia (EAH) and the life-threatening condition known as exercise-associated hyponatremic encephalopathy (EAHE). While it is not clear whether sports drinks with *low sodium content* (~20 mmol/L) can minimise EAH (Noakes, 2007), salt-rich snacks and drinks with a higher sodium content may be lifesaving to those athletes at risk of hyponatremia. Refer to Chapter 8 for further discussion on fluid balance and sodium.

Athletes, as the public, need to be guided by recommendations for salt intake as high salt intake can lead to high blood pressure, a risk factor for stroke, heart disease, kidney disease and gallstones. High salt intake can also promote calcium loss from the body especially if the body has low levels of calcium. In the United Kingdom, the recommended salt intake is 6 g (2.4 g sodium/day) for adults aged 19–50 years. Foods high in salt include bacon, ham and tinned meat, processed meats, ready-to-eat or convenience foods, cheese, smoked meats and fish, tinned and packaged legumes, soups and tinned vegetables, most savoury and salted snacks, stock powders and meat extracts.

Making sense of food labels. Foods containing a lot of salt have 1.25 g salt (0.5 g sodium) or more per 100 g product, whereas foods containing a little salt have 0.25 g salt (0.1 g sodium) or less per 100 g (Food Standards Agency, 2006).

Maintain a healthy weight

Overweight and obesity is excess fat accumulation in adipose tissue, resulting from consuming more energy than is expended. Scientific studies, surveys of athletes and high-performance laboratories collect data about elite athlete's weight and body composition, helping to identify well-matched levels for sport performance. An excess fatness can negatively affect exercise performance since extra fat weight does not improve strength, agility, mobility or muscular appearance, neither does it increase speed, power or endurance. For example, a marathon runner requires endurance and speed both of which will be reduced by excess fat or 'dead' weight. A powerlifter requires strength, and aims to have a higher muscle mass to fat ratio.

Furthermore, there are several health risks of obesity for all people including athletes. The risk of disease increases, including diabetes, heart disease, stroke and certain cancers. Body mass index (BMI) charts provide an indication for adults of the right weight for their height. The ideal BMI for adults is 20–25 kg/m² irrespective of age. BMI is a useful tool for assessing body weight for the general population and some athletes. However, for those athletes who are involved in power sports like weight lifting or sprint events, BMI measurements may be distorted if an athlete has a high proportion of muscle mass, which is not considered in BMI charts. For example, a 100-m-track athlete may present with a high BMI (over 25 kg/m²) due to a large proportion of lean body mass, but have perfectly healthy body fat levels and an ideal waist circumference. The high energy needs of some groups of athletes fluctuate throughout various stages of the athlete's exercise programme and for certain athletes, very active involvement in sport is seasonal. On their less active period, they may maintain a high-energy diet and weight will steadily climb if energy intake increases while energy output through exercise is reduced. Furthermore, a change in body composition will affect the athlete's 'comeback' to the competition season. The less they steer from their ideal weight and body composition profile, the better able they are to enter competition season in the best possible shape. Energy-dense foods containing a high amount of fat, sugar and/or alcohol would have to restricted for optimum health anyway but especially during periods of less activity.

Maintaining hydration

Water is an essential nutrient. In mild climates such as the United Kingdom, drinking 6–8 glasses (1.2 L) of water or other fluids daily is recommended. During exercise, water is lost through sweat (along with sodium, potassium and other minerals), and as water losses exceed fluid intake, dehydration can occur. In certain sports such as ultra-distance-endurance events, finishers with the fastest times are often the most dehydrated, up to 12% body weight loss reported (Sharwood et al, 2004). Drink volumes of 400 mL and up to 800 mL/h is sufficient to meet the hydration needs of most athletes. However, there is also an increase in overdrinking in sport, especially recreational athletes who receive confusing messages about the dangers of dehydration. Drinking too much fluid during exercise can lead to serious health consequences (discussed in Chapter 8).

Consumption of excess alcohol as a binge or regular heavy drinking can lead to weight gain, intoxication and detrimental effects on health and fitness. In the short term, it can be associated with violence and accidents. In the long term, it can raise blood pressure, have damaging effects on the liver, heart and other organs, nervous system, can cause vitamin and mineral deficiencies and increase the risk of certain cancers. Recommended sensible drinking limits are 3–4 units/day for men and

Table 3.3 Unit equivalents of various alcoholic beverages.

Alcoholic beverage	Equivalent of 1 unit (8 g ethanol in United Kingdom)
Beer, lager, cider (standard strength)	One small, half a pint (300 mL)
Wine	One small glass (100 mL)
Fortified wine (sherry, port)	One small glass (50 mL)
Spirits (whisky, vodka, gin, etc.)	One single pub measure/tot (25 mL)

Source: Data from Thomas and BDA (2001).

2–3 units/day for women. Risks associated with age or stages of the life cycle (pregnancy, menopause) are affected by alcohol intake (Thomas and BDA, 2001). Table 3.3 provides estimates of a unit for various alcoholic beverages.

For athletes, drinking alcohol before, during or after exercise is discouraged and can affect sport performance. It affects motor skills and balance during exercise, and in the recovery period following exercise, drinking alcohol can cause vasodilation. This leads to heat and water loss that can worsen dehydration. In the case of a sports injury, vasodilation can increase bleeding, which will prolong recovery from an injury. Dietary surveys show that athletes who take part in team sports are at risk, as this group of athletes commonly consume alcohol. In a dietary survey of Dutch athletes, Van Erp-Baart et al (1989) found that athletes participating in team sports consumed more than 5% of total energy from alcohol. Athletes who regularly consume alcohol after a game or match would be at risk of dehydration and poor recovery of muscle glycogen stores. They often drink alcohol at the expense of eating more carbohydrate- and protein-rich foods, which are essential for recovery from exercise.

Athletes better have breakfast

The first meal of the day is more important to health and performance than most people realise. Maintaining blood sugar levels, boosting the day's energy and nutrient intake, and improving mental and physical performance are some benefits of eating a healthy breakfast. Athletes' levels of stored carbohydrate (glycogen) need to be replenished after an overnight fast, more so if they exercise or compete in the morning. As a guide, athletes can aim to consume around 25% of their day's energy and nutrients from breakfast. Breakfast is the ideal time for a meal rich in carbohydrates, vitamins, minerals, fibre and some protein. A nutritious breakfast may include muesli, fruit and yoghurt, or a vegetable omelette, or beans on toast with a glass of orange juice. These breakfast recipes and a few more follow at the end of the chapter.

While the dietary guidelines form the cornerstone of the athlete's training diet, the next chapters will delve into the detail of individual nutrients required for exercise metabolism and optimal performance.

Chapter summary

- The cornerstone of a good training diet starts with laying the foundation of healthy eating by following key nutrition messages and better dietary practices.
- Food group models may take any form such as a plate model of Food Pyramid Guide, and most countries have their own model, while others adopt and adapt another's in line with their unique public health policy.
- In the United Kingdom, *the eatwell plate* is the government's healthy eating policy tool that aims to help the public choose healthier diets.
- Each segment of *the eatwell plate* visually displays a food group and the balance that is required in a healthy diet. Additional healthy eating messages support *the eatwell plate* and should be used along with the government's eight tips for making healthier choices.
- The Food Pyramid Guide used by the United States since 1992 displayed four food groups stacked in the shape of a pyramid. In June 2011 it was replaced with *MyPlate*, a new visual tool for communicating the USDA's key nutrition messages that promote healthy eating.
- The recommended diet for athletes has the same basic principles, although in addition, there are specialised sport nutrition strategies with respect to certain foods and fluids and how they are used by the body *during exercise*.
- Starchy foods rich in carbohydrates provide an ideal fuel for sport and exercise.
- Making fruits and vegetables a major part of the daily diet is protective and health promoting.
- Athletes can obtain a rich source of protein and heart-healthy fat from at least two servings of fish per week, including one from oily fish.
- Athletes need to consume less saturated fat and make room for healthier monounsaturated and polyunsaturated fats.
- A small amount of sugary foods and fluids, and the use of the glycaemic index (GI) tool, can benefit athlete's training, competition and recovery.
- Electrolytes like sodium (salt) are lost in sweat and have a role in maintaining water balance during exercise.
- Athletes need to eat the right amount for a healthy weight and body composition to meet the physical demands of exercise.
- Water is essential for hydration during exercise, but drinking alcohol before, during or after exercise is discouraged and can affect sport performance.
- Eating breakfast maintains blood sugar levels, helps restore athletes' level of stored carbohydrate (glycogen), boosts the day's energy and nutrient intake and improves mental and physical performance. These are some benefits of eating a healthy breakfast.

Notes

1 Dietary reference values (DRVs) are UK estimates of energy and nutrient requirements for healthy people.
2 Reference nutrient intakes (RNIs) are UK estimates of proteins, vitamins and minerals for healthy people.

Breakfasts and Smoothies

Following an overnight fast, it is important to '*break fast*' as soon as possible after waking. There are several recipes here to start to day, but remember to aim for a breakfast to meet about 25% of your daily calorie needs.

A Muesli & Granola Breakfast

(Makes 975 g)

Ingredients

45 ml (3 Tbsp) sunflower oil	50g (2 oz) raw almonds, roughly chopped
100 ml honey/maple syrup	50 g (2 oz) pecan nuts, roughly chopped
500 g (18 oz) rolled oats	80 g raisins
50 g (2 oz) sunflower seeds	80 g dried apricots, chopped

Method

1 Preheat the oven to 150°C.
2 Melt the honey and oil in the microwave.
3 Add together the oats, seeds and nuts in a large mixing bowl. Drizzle the honey and oil over the mixture and stir until thoroughly mixed.
4 Spoon the mixture into a deep baking tray and spread the mixture until even.
5 Bake for 30 minutes, turning once or twice during baking until crispy and golden brown.
6 Allow the baked muesli–granola to cool down before adding the raisins and apricots.
7 Store in a clean airtight container.

Nutrition analysis per portion

Energy	451 kcal (1896 kJ)
Protein	9.3 g
Carbohydrate	51.5 g
Fat	19.1 g
Cholesterol	0 mg
Fibre	9.1 g

Food note: Oats have a high soluble fibre content that aids digestion and helps lower blood cholesterol levels. Rolled oats has a lower GI and a higher fibre content than instant oats. Sunflower seeds contain polyunsaturated fatty acids and is rich in linoleic acid.

Banana and Peanut Butter Smoothie

(Serves 1/1 Glass)

Ingredients
2 bananas, peeled
45 g (2 oz) peanut butter
200 mL low-fat milk

Method
1 Place all the ingredients into a blender.
2 Process until smooth.

Nutrition analysis per portion

Energy	543 kcal (2282 kJ)
Protein	21 g
Carbohydrate	47 g
Fat	28 g
Cholesterol	18 mg
Fibre	5.3 g

Food note: Bananas are rich in potassium needed to lower blood pressure. Peanut butter contains monounsaturated fat, niacin and magnesium. Choose low salt and low sugar varieties.

Beans and Chickpeas on Toast

(Serves 3)

Ingredients

15 mL sunflower oil

1 small red onion, chopped

3 cloves of garlic, finely chopped

1 × 400 g tin cannellini beans, drained

1 × 400 g tin chickpeas, drained

$\frac{1}{2}$ × 400 g tin whole tomatoes, roughly chopped

30 mL (2 Tbsp) brown sugar

Salt and pepper to taste

Basil for garnishing

6 slices of rye bread, toasted

Method

1 Sauté the onions in the oil for 1 minute.
2 Add the garlic and sauté for another 2 minutes.
3 Add the beans, chickpeas and tomatoes and allow to simmer for 5 minutes.
4 Add the sugar and seasoning. Cook for a further 5 minutes or until the sauce thickens.
5 Sprinkle with the chopped basil.
6 Serve immediately on the still warm toasted rye bread.

Nutrition analysis per portion

Energy	683 kcal (2870 kJ)
Protein	28.5 g
Carbohydrate	97 g
Fat	10.5 g
Cholesterol	0 mg
Fibre	21 g

Food note: Pulses or legumes like chickpeas and cannellini beans are a good source of plant protein, fibre and rich in the B vitamin, *folic acid*.

Berry Smoothie

(Serves 2/2 Glasses)

Ingredients
250 g (9 oz) strawberries and blackberries
30 mL (2 Tbsp) honey
1 cup yoghurt

Method
1 Place all the ingredients into a blender.
2 Process until smooth.

Nutrition analysis per portion
Energy	189 kcal (792 kJ)
Protein	6.4 g
Carbohydrate	31 g
Fat	3 g
Cholesterol	10.6 mg
Fibre	3 g

Food note: Most berries are an excellent source of vitamin C and beta-carotene. Yoghurt contains calcium, and beneficial bacteria known as *probiotics*, which is good for bowel health.

Broccoli Omelette

(Serves 2)

Ingredients

25 mL olive oil

100 g (4 oz) broccoli, cut into
florets and sliced

5 mL (1 tsp) parsley, chopped

3 extra large eggs, (free range,
organic), beaten

Salt and pepper

Method

1 Heat the oil in a frying pan. Sauté the broccoli for 3 minutes. Season with herbs.
2 Season the eggs with salt and pepper.
3 Pour the eggs into the pan and stir into the broccoli. Once the eggs start to set, cover the pan with a lid until thoroughly cooked.
4 Fold the omelette in half and serve immediately.

Nutrition analysis per portion

Energy	417 kcal (1755 kJ)
Protein	20.3 g
Carbohydrate	4.2 g
Fat	35 g
Cholesterol	571 mg
Fibre	2.7 g

Tip for weight reducers: Lower calories and fat by reducing the amount of olive oil used in the omelette.

Food note: Eggs are a high-quality protein (BV of egg white = 100), and rich in vitamins B_{12} and D. Broccoli is an excellent source of vitamin C, soluble fibre and health-enhancing phytochemicals (anticancer functions). *Parsley is* rich in vitamins A, B, C, iron, calcium, potassium and soluble fibre. Chew on a sprig of organic parsley to freshen the breath.

French Toast with Strawberry Fruit Salad

(Serves 2)

Ingredients

2 eggs, beaten

4 slices whole-wheat bread

10 mL sunflower oil

250 mL strawberries, halved

1 banana, peeled and sliced

30 mL honey

125 mL low-fat yoghurt or Crème

Fraîche

Method

1 Heat the oil in a frying pan.

2 Dip the slices of bread into the beaten egg and place in the heated pan.

3 Fry the bread slices on each side until golden brown (adjust heat if necessary).

4 Assemble the entire dish on a plate by placing the fruit on the French toast.

5 Drizzle with honey and yoghurt.

Nutrition analysis per portion

Energy	442 kcal (1857 kJ)
Protein	15.6 g
Carbohydrate	58 g
Fat	13.4 g
Cholesterol	235 mg
Fibre	6.2 g

Tip for weight reducers: Using egg whites (not the yolks) reduces the fat and cholesterol content of the dish.

Food note: Whole wheat is not refined and contains fibre, and plenty of B vitamins – two reasons why it reduces the risks associated with cardiovascular disease and cancer. B vitamins are good for managing stress.

Orange, Carrot and Pineapple Juice

(Makes ±500 mL)

Ingredients
3 oranges, peeled
3 carrots, peeled
$\frac{1}{2}$ pineapple, peeled and cored

Method
1 Cut the fruit into chunks and feed it into the juicer.
2 The juice can either be enjoyed immediately or be refrigerated.

Nutrition analysis per portion
Energy	153 kcal (560 kJ)
Protein	1.75 g
Carbohydrate	24 g
Fat	0.25 g
Cholesterol	0 mg
Fibre	6.75 g

Food note: Carrots are an excellent source of beta-carotene and soluble fibre. There is more beta-carotene in cooked carrots than in its raw form.

Oven-Baked Nectarines with Walnut and Ricotta Filling

(Serves 4)

Ingredients
4 nectarines, halved and cored
150 g (5 oz) ricotta cheese
75 g (3 oz) walnuts, chopped
15 mL (3 tsp) honey
250 g low-fat yoghurt, for serving

Method
1 Preheat the oven to 180°C.
2 Mix the ricotta cheese, walnuts and honey together.
3 Place the nectarines onto a baking tray and spoon the filling into the cored halves.
4 Bake for 15 minutes until done.
5 Serve warm with the yoghurt.

Nutrition analysis per portion

Energy	289 kcal (1215 kJ)
Protein	10 g
Carbohydrate	20 g
Fat	18 g
Cholesterol	23 mg
Fibre	2.3 g

Food note: Walnuts are high in omega-fatty acids and plenty of minerals. All nuts are a good source of protein and vitamin E.

CHAPTER 4

Carbohydrates

<table>
<tr><td colspan="2">Key terms</td></tr>
<tr><td>Carbohydrate</td><td>Fructose</td></tr>
<tr><td>Carbohydrate value</td><td>Glucose polymer</td></tr>
<tr><td>Dietary glucose</td><td>Carbohydrate requirement</td></tr>
<tr><td>Sugars</td><td>Glycaemic index (GI)</td></tr>
<tr><td>Starch</td><td>Glycaemic load (GL)</td></tr>
<tr><td>Blood glucose</td><td>Carbohydrate loading</td></tr>
<tr><td>Muscle glycogen</td><td>Classical super-compensation protocol</td></tr>
<tr><td>Liver glycogen</td><td>Modified carbohydrate-loading regime</td></tr>
<tr><td>Muscle biopsy</td><td>Fibre</td></tr>
<tr><td>Glycogen synthase</td><td></td></tr>
</table>

The following terms are commonly used to describe carbohydrates or characteristics of carbohydrates: sugars or starches, simple and complex 'carbs', glycaemic index (GI) and fibre. A carbohydrate is a nutrient that is a component of food. Carbohydrates, along with proteins, fat and alcohol contain energy. The carbohydrate nutrient is found mainly in vegetables, fruits, cereals, grains, legume-type food, as well as sugary foods and drinks. Compared with fat and alcohol, carbohydrate is not as dense in energy (4 kcal/g or 17 kJ/g). However, it is the primary, most rapid source of fuel for the body, especially to power exercise and sport. Every mechanical and physiological process in the body requires energy, and carbohydrates are the preferred source of fuel for exercise and sport.

The simplest form of carbohydrate is a glucose molecule. This is the only form in which the body, at the cellular and molecular level, can use it. Many other forms of carbohydrate exist, chemical structures that are short or long. These chemical structures are what differentiate sugar from pasta or a simple glucose drink from a glucose polymer drink. The simplicity or

Nutrition for Sport and Exercise: A Practical Guide, First Edition. Hayley Daries.
© 2012 Blackwell Publishing Ltd. Published 2012 by Blackwell Publishing Ltd.

complexity of the carbohydrate structure influences its digestion, absorption and metabolism in the body. However, in the end, all of these short or long chemical structures of carbohydrate are converted to glucose.

From carbohydrate to energy

When an athlete is at rest and going about habitual activities, the energy is derived from carbohydrate and fat. Very little energy is derived from protein because it is used mostly to build and maintain tissues and muscles. As seen in Chapter 2, a healthy person has ample supplies of fat, and less supplies of carbohydrate. Therefore, it makes sense to use fat at rest and during activity or exercise, as there are vast supplies. However, fat makes energy very slowly (within minutes) as compared to carbohydrate that makes energy very quickly (within seconds). The timing of the use of carbohydrate and fat has to do with how much oxygen is available. At rest, a person is breathing normally and enough oxygen is available so that is why fat can be used. In physical activity, exercise or sport, however, carbohydrate is the preferred source of energy because the body converts carbohydrates to energy most rapidly, compared with the other energy-giving nutrients. Carbohydrate in food is broken down to glucose molecules that are stored in the blood, muscles and liver. During activity or exercise that involves any measure of muscular effort, the energy needs increase. Whether oxygen is available or not, the stored glucose provides the most rapid fuel, something that fat cannot do in the absence of oxygen. For example, at very high intensities of exercise such as a short sprint lasting a few seconds, the energy derived is mostly from glucose. Stored glucose is formed into energy compounds, called phosphocreatine (PCr) and adenosine triphosphate (ATP) that are stored in the mitochondria of the cells in the muscle. Energy is also stored in fat droplets in muscles. The mitochondria are the powerhouses where all energy is made and fuels the working muscles and every cell of the body. Carbohydrate is the most important nutrient in the athlete's diet because it supplies rapid energy from its energy reserves (stored glucose, glycogen) for high-energy ATP and PCr.

Foods containing carbohydrates

As mentioned previously, carbohydrates are mostly found in plant foods like fruit, vegetables, in the wheat, corn and rye that are used to make breads, rice and cereals, and legumes and beans. Foods and drinks containing sugar, glucose, fructose (fruit sugar), maltose and dextrose are also a source of carbohydrate. Some animal-derived foods like milk, cheese and yoghurt also contain a significant amount of carbohydrate. All of the aforementioned plant foods including nuts and seeds contain some carbohydrates, and most carbohydrate-rich foods (from plant sources) contain dietary fibre or non-starch polysaccharide (NSP), an indigestible nutrient that aids digestion, helps regulate blood glucose levels and has other important health-promoting benefits. For the general population, all forms of carbohydrate can be consumed and for health reasons, some (i.e. sugars) less than others (i.e. starches). Fruits and vegetables are packed with nutrients essential for health and exercise and should be consumed daily.

Carbohydrate value

Each carbohydrate-rich food has a carbohydrate value, that is, the amount of carbohydrate in one serving of that food. Some foods are rich sources of carbohydrate while others contain only minimal amounts of carbohydrate.

Table 4.1 displays some foods and drinks commonly consumed by athletes in suggested servings providing 25 g of carbohydrate (CHO). The energy value of a typical vegetable serving is 25–30 kcal (105–126 kJ).

Table 4.1 Athlete's carbohydrate selection: snack and drink ideas for fuelling.

Food or drink item	Examples of 25 g CHO servings
Foods containing starch and fibre	
Fresh fruit – bananas, pears, apples	2 small bananas
Dried fruit – raisins, dates, fruit rolls or sticks	3 tablespoons raisins
Fruit juice or fruit squash	200–250 mL pure fruit juice
Whole-grain crackers, oatcakes, rice cakes	6
Muffins, pancakes	1 English muffin
Sandwiches, rolls, bagels with jam, honey or syrup	1 thick slice of bread + 1 teaspoon honey or jam
Sugary foods and drinks	
Energy drinks, 4–10% CHO solution (4–10 g CHO/100 mL)	250 mL (10% CHO) or 625ml[a] (4% CHO); average = 420 mL (*hourly fluid intake during exercise:* ~400 mL)
Sweets – jelly beans, wine gums, fruit pastilles	30 g ($\frac{1}{2}$ of a small 67 g packet)
Cereal bars, energy bars	1 bar (~35 g)
Energy (sports) gel	1 sachet
Sugary chocolate bar	1 bar (~50 g)

Source: material from Hayley Daries Practice.
[a]Drinks and gels that are very concentrated in CHO should be consumed in late stages of exercise.

Compared with other food that has more carbohydrate value, like grains, cereals and fruits, vegetables are lowly ranked in terms of carbohydrate value but are nutrient-dense foods that deliver a powerful package of antioxidants. These antioxidants mop up harmful oxygen radicals that enter the body and accumulate through the environment (pollution, smoke), the foods we eat and the increase in oxygen intake from exercise. The carbohydrate value of a thin slice of bread, for example, is 15 g CHO, 3 g protein and 2–3 g fat. Other non-energy giving nutrients such as select vitamins and minerals are also found in a slice of bread. The latter adds no significant energy value to the bread; they are merely there to help the process of digesting, absorbing and metabolising the bread. For this reason, foods are unique, in that every natural food source has the select nutrient make-up to help its conversion to energy for use in the body.

Stores of carbohydrate in the body

Excess carbohydrate derived from food that is not used for energy is stored in the blood, muscles and liver. It is in the form of glucose in the blood, and glycogen in the liver and muscle. It should be noted that a tiny but essential amount of glucose (about 2 g or 8 kcal) is stored in the brain.

In an 80 kg man, the average liver glycogen is 100 g (400 kcal), and muscle glycogen is 400 g (1600 kcal) (McArdle et al, 2010). The amount of glucose in the blood is minimal, just enough to last a few seconds or less than 1 minute of physical activity. Theoretically, in the aforementioned example, there is enough glycogen in the liver and muscles to last for about 2 hours of continuous exercise. Although muscles hold the most stores of carbohydrate, these stores are vulnerable during exercise. In practice, the glycogen content of the muscle may be depleted after 30–40 minutes of high-intensity exercise or competition, although a 30-second run sprint can deplete one-third of glycogen stores (Nevill et al, 1989). Once glycogen decreases to a certain level, the athlete cannot exercise at the same level, be it time or intensity. This is due to the muscles reduction in contractility.

Measurement of muscle glycogen

The measurement of muscle glycogen has become an important area of study in the respective fields of physiology, biochemistry and sports nutrition. Since most of the body's carbohydrate stores are found in muscle, it makes sense to determine the scope of the muscle's ability to store glycogen, and what influences the storage and remaking of glycogen. Applying these answers can be useful for certain athletes (i.e. endurance athletes

like cyclists, runners, triathletes, swimmers, etc.) whose performance relies heavily on their carbohydrate stores.

Glycogen stores in the muscle are measured by a technique known as
a muscle biopsy using a needle to withdraw a very small piece of muscle
tissue. The tissue is cleaned, frozen and thereafter slices of it are examined
under a microscope to determine the muscles biochemistry and nutrition
(Wilmore and Costill, 2004). The unit of measurement of glycogen in the
muscle tissue by this method is millimole of glycogen per kilogram wet
weight muscle tissue (mmol/kg ww). The rate at which muscle glycogen is
remade in the muscle is then measured as mmol/kg/h. The upper capacity
of muscle glycogen storage is about 100 mmol/kg (Coyle, 1991).

How the timing of carbohydrate intake affects muscle glycogen stores

The average rate at which glycogen is remade after exercise is about 5–8
mmol/kg/h (Coyle, 1991). The first 2 hours after exercise is the ideal time
to replenish glycogen stores through carbohydrate intake. This is because
of the enzyme (glycogen synthase) that is activated when glycogen stores
are depleted (Ivy et al, 1988; Wojtaszewski et al, 2001) and facilitates the
making of more glycogen. A further reason is that exercise causes an increased sensitivity to insulin (Richter et al, 1988), which allows more glucose to enter the muscle tissues. These increased rates of glycogen storage
do not last forever, but only during the critical 2 hours after exercise, after which time the remaking of glucose returns to a more normal rate of
around 4.3 mmol/kg (Ivy et al 1988) to 5 mmol/kg (Coyle, 1991). These
studies show that 20–24 hours are required for normalisation of glycogen stores, and in specific sports like running, up to 25 hours of high-
carbohydrate intake are needed before any further running is done to fully
recover glycogen stores.

Studies on football players have reported that muscle glycogen levels recover very slowly post-match when there is an inadequate carbohydrate
intake and continued training with short recovery periods. The muscles
may also be damaged (such as after eccentric exercise), which further limits the storage of glycogen.

How the amount of carbohydrate intake affects muscle glycogen stores and exercise performance

The benefits of carbohydrate intake for exercise performance have been
reviewed extensively (Coombes and Hamilton, 2000; Noakes, 2001; Rodriguez et al, 2009; Castell et al, 2010).

Every time an athlete exercises the muscle glycogen stores are used,
and the longer and harder they train the more they deplete their stores,

affecting their performance in training sessions or competition. Hence, stores must be continually refilled from carbohydrate in the diet. Costill and Miller (1980) looked at the effect of prolonged (3 days) daily exercise sessions (2 hourly bouts of running for 16.1 km) on recovery of muscle glycogen stores. They demonstrated that the recovery diet is vital for maintaining peak levels of carbohydrate stores that influence performance for training and competition. When following a low-carbohydrate diet (40–50% of total energy) as compared with a high-carbohydrate diet (70% of total energy), muscle glycogen stores decline as each day passes. A further disadvantage to the athlete is that as each day passes on such a low-carbohydrate diet, the muscle glycogen stores cannot be restored to its original state. At the time, the authors suggested 150–650 g CHO/day is required to normalise muscle glycogen stores. This would equate to about 0.7–1.0 g CHO/kg BW every 2 hours over the 24-hour recovery period is required, which will achieve a re-synthesis rate of around 5 mmol/kg muscle/h. Due to factors explained in the previous text, the first 2 hours after exercise is vital, and some suggest a higher rate of intake of 1.5 g CHO/kg BW within the first 30 minutes after exercise (Reilly and Ekblom, 2005). However, as the rate of glycogen re-synthesis is limited (Coyle, 1991), carbohydrate intake over and above 525–648 g (roughly 7–9 g CHO/kg BW) intake per day or 24 hours will not result in a further increase in glycogen stores. Therefore, a carbohydrate intake of 50–75 g (1–2 g CHO/kg BW) every 2 hours, or at comfortably frequent intervals after exercise, would be sufficient to recover glycogen stores.

Requirements for carbohydrate in sport and exercise

As energy is required mostly in the form of carbohydrates (expressed as a percentage of energy intake for the day), studies on muscle glycogen confirm that athletes need a higher amount of the energy they consume to come from carbohydrate-rich foods. Although dietary guidelines for the general population encourage a carbohydrate-rich diet (more than 50% of daily energy intake), for athletes the proportion of energy that is needed is about 60–65% of the total energy in the diet. The rest of the daily energy needs will come from protein (12–15%) and fat (20–35%).

Surveys have shown that the average western diet falls short of these recommendations, as it is low in carbohydrates (41% CHO of daily energy intake), moderately high in protein (17%) and high in fat (37%) (Brotherhood, 1984).

Similarly the National Diet and Nutrition Survey of Britons reveal that their diet is lower in carbohydrates and higher in protein, fat and alcohol than is recommended for athletes. Adults (19–64 years) have dietary proportions as follows:

- *Carbohydrate intake*: 47.7% of total energy intake for men and 48.5% for women
- *Protein intake*: 16.5% of total energy intake for males and 16.6% for females
- *Fat intake*: 35.8% of total energy intake for men and 34.9% for women
- *Alcohol intake*: 6.5% of total energy intake of the total sample of men and women consume 3.9% of total energy intake from alcohol (intakes are even higher when only the alcohol consumers are considered (>8% alcohol of total energy intake for men and >5% for women)

Henderson et al (2003)

This is the first significant sign that the diet of the athletes could be compromised and may not meet the energy and nutrient needs required for strenuous exercise of long duration or high intensity, or both. Therefore, consuming the average western diet may compromise athletes' increased needs for carbohydrate and protein.

For example, a 70 kg athlete who consumes 3000 kcal (12,600 kJ)/day and who consumes the average western diet of 41% CHO will achieve a carbohydrate intake of ~300 g CHO/day.

3000 kcal × 41%CHO ÷ 4 kcal = 300 g CHO/day

or

Expressed g CHO/kg BW/day:

300 g ÷ 70 kg = ˜4 g CHO/kg BW/day

This amount of carbohydrate may be enough to meet the needs of recreational athletes involved in less than 1 hour of physical activity a day.

Based on data of muscle glycogen stores, this amount of carbohydrate may not be enough to sustain energy needs for athletes involved in high-intensity or prolonged exercise. While athletes with a low training load or on a weight loss diet may require only 3–5 g CHO/kg BW/day (Castell et al, 2010) the carbohydrate needs of the majority of athletes will be met by an intake of 5–10 g/kg BW/day (Coyle, 1991; Rodriguez et al, 2009), although intensity and duration of training should be considered for more competitive athletes. Athletes with extremely high training loads may require more or less than ~12 g CHO/kg BW/day (Burke et al, 2004; Castell et al, 2010).

Castell et al (2010) summarises the carbohydrate requirements for *daily recovery* to be consumed throughout the day as follows:

- *3–5 g/kg BW/day*: athletes with light training

- *5–7 g/kg BW/day*: athletes on moderate exercise programme (1–1.5 h)
- *7–12 g/kg BW/day*: endurance athletes, 1–3 hours moderate to high-intensity exercise
- *≥10–12 g/kg BW/day*: extreme exercise load, >4–5 hours moderate to high-intensity exercise

How the type of carbohydrate intake affects muscle glycogen stores

Carbohydrates are found in different forms. Fructose is the carbohydrate in fruit. Starch or glucose polymer is the carbohydrate in bread. These different types of carbohydrates define the lengths of the carbohydrates in the food. These have to do with the chemical structure indicating how short or how long the chain of molecules is in the carbohydrate food. In the past, carbohydrates were classified according to their structure and were known as simple (sugars) and complex (starches) carbohydrates. Advice about carbohydrates was based on these two distinct groups. In 1981, Jenkins and colleagues provided a new classification system for carbohydrates. Although initially developed for diabetics, it proved very useful to athletes, and other groups of the population (i.e. obese subjects).

   The GI is a ranking of carbohydrate foods according to how quickly the food is converted to glucose and is absorbed into the bloodstream. The GI is indicated by a factor that represents a measurement of the effect of a carbohydrate food on blood glucose levels within a 2-hour period after ingesting the food. Only foods high in carbohydrate are measured, as they have the largest effect on blood glucose levels compared with proteins and fats that have a very small effect. When comparing GI values, all carbohydrate foods must contain the same amount of nutrient carbohydrate (usually 50 g) and are measured against the same reference food, usually glucose (Wolever et al, 1991). Jenkins et al (1981) original GI list used mean values of testing 5–10 individuals, and great variation was seen between values of the same food. Since then, the glucose response of many foods has been tested in several different countries. Foods are classified into three divisions by their effect on blood glucose. High-GI foods are quickly converted to glucose and absorbed into the blood. Moderate GI foods take longer to convert and low-GI foods are slow to convert to glucose and enter the bloodstream. In most tables, high GI is defined as a factor over 65 or 70, moderate GI as a factor between 50 and 70 and low-GI foods are below 50. Most healthy eating guidelines that use the GI factor recommend the use of low- to moderate-GI foods, to assist with weight loss and to manage blood glucose levels in diabetes. Low GI may also be useful to people with high blood lipids levels (hyperlipidaemia), as a low-GI diet is associated with lower triglycerides levels and/or favourable HDL cholesterol levels (Wong et al, 2009). For athletes, the whole range of GI can be applied in sport and exercise. The GI values for some common carbohydrate foods are as follows:

High-GI carbohydrate-rich foods:

- White bread
- Corn flakes
- Mashed potatoes
- Rice cakes
- Honey (regular, not raw)
- Energy bar
- Sports drinks
- Watermelon

Intermediate-GI carbohydrate-rich foods:

- Pita bread
- Oats porridge
- Canned sweet corn
- Fruit jam
- Rice
- Banana
- Raisins

Low-GI carbohydrate-rich foods:

- Swiss-type muesli
- Yoghurt
- Pasta
- Baked beans
- Corn on the cob
- Popcorn
- Apples
- Strawberries

The Glycaemic load (GL) takes into account the amount of available carbohydrate in the food and its blood glucose response. GL values range from low to high GL: <5, <10, <15 and <20. Typically, watermelon has a high GI value (72) (Miller, 1996). Overweight individuals and diabetics have been advised to avoid fruits like watermelon as it has a high GI value. However, a 25-mm slice of watermelon has a low GL (<5), that means it has very little available carbohydrate and can be part of a healthy eating plan for these groups and the general population. GL, therefore, complements the GI tables making sense of the latter for use in these client groups, and for athletes who want to lose weight or have diabetes or high blood lipid levels.

How to apply GI in sport and exercise

The GI is not only a practical guide to the benefits of carbohydrates for the general public but it is also a very useful tool for athletes.

Studies have been conducted on the effects of GI and its effect on the body's use of muscle glycogen, response of insulin, maintenance of blood glucose and free fatty acid concentrations and exercise performance. The research has looked specifically at:

- the pre-event meal;
- competition nutrition strategies; and
- recovery meals.

Early studies examined the effects of glucose (a high-GI food) as a pre-exercise snack and the findings inspired one of the earliest studies to apply the GI to sports nutrition. Thomas et al (1991) wanted to prove that low-GI foods eaten before exercise provide a slow-release source of glucose (that maintain blood glucose and free fatty acid concentration), without a rise in insulin. They demonstrated that eating a low-GI food (pre-soaked boiled lentils) 45 minutes before prolonged strenuous exercise, improves endurance capacity or time to exhaustion in cycling at 65–70% VO_2max by 20 minutes when compared with eating a high-GI food of baked potato.

The use of GI has similar effects on cyclists. Thirty minutes before cycling, trained cyclists ate 1.5 g CHO/kg BW in the form of fruit, cereal and dairy foods. Each meal had either a low GI or a high GI factor, had the same component of carbohydrates, although the low-GI meal of All-Bran cereal, apple and unsweetened yoghurt had more fibre, fat and protein. The cyclists then cycled for 2 hours at 70% VO_2max, and to exhaustion at 100% VO_2max. The study found that the low-GI meal maintained higher blood glucose at the end of the 2-hour trial, and produced a significant advantage in the performance trial where time to exhaustion in maximal cycling exercise was 59% longer than in the high-GI trial (DeMarco et al, 1999).

Similar performance benefits were found in runners. Wu and Williams (2006) compared the effect of ingesting a low-GI (with factor 37) or high-GI (with factor 77) meal on endurance capacity over two running trials. The subjects consumed either meal 3 hours before running to exhaustion at 70% VO_2max on a treadmill. The run time was 8 minutes longer on the low-GI trial as compared with the high-GI trial. These results were unlike an earlier study from this group (Wee et al, 1999) who found no difference in endurance capacity between high-GI and low-GI trials. The later 2006 study attributed the difference to the content of the low-GI meal and the glycaemic responses it elicited. In the 1999 study, subjects ate lentils and in 2006, common breakfast-type foods were eaten, like All-Bran, skim milk, apples, peaches and apple juice.

Improved glucose tolerance can also be achieved by a single low-GI meal the evening before a high-GI breakfast and a 60-minute run at 65% VO_2max. In this study, both high-GI and low-GI dinners had no effect on fuel use during exercise (Stevenson et al, 2005).

Low-GI foods taken before prolonged exercise improve endurance capacity or time to exhaustion/fatigue. Eating a low-GI meal like a cereal with yoghurt or milk and a glass of apple or orange juice will provide sustained energy levels and can be a good pre-training or pre-competition snack or meal.

High-GI foods can help to maintain blood glucose levels during exercise (Walton and Rhodes, 1997). From the beginning of exercise, muscle and liver glycogen stores are being depleted. During exercise lasting longer than 1 hour there is a heavier reliance on blood glucose, and the athlete can start to use high-GI foods that supply glucose rapidly into the bloodstream. This glucose provided during the exercise sustains the level of intensity or pace of the exercise, which may be a steady marathon pace or during intermittent high-intensity exercise such as a tennis match or a hockey game. At some point, usually late in aerobic exercise or during bouts of intense shorts bursts of anaerobic exercise, all the muscle and liver glycogen stores will be used up. Muscle glycogen stores are usually the first to deplete; thereafter, liver glycogen can supply glucose to the exercising muscles. Athletes will be able to keep going at the same pace or intensity as long as there is enough glucose available from the blood, and in late stages of prolonged exercise, blood glucose can be supplied by consuming high-GI foods and fluids. At this point, to continue exercising at the same intensity, it is critical to supply the blood with glucose. High-GI foods and fluids are rapidly absorbed and converted to energy. It is literally available in seconds, especially if the simplest molecule of carbohydrate (glucose) is given, which is immediately absorbed into the bloodstream without the process of breaking it down (digesting it) to make it simpler for the capillaries in the gut wall to absorb it into the bloodstream. It should be noted that if insufficient glucose is available, and there is a greater reliance on fat stores, exercise can be continued but at a much slower pace or lowered intensity (due to longer fat oxidation rates).

It appears GI is relevant to recovery of muscle glycogen stores. High-GI foods are more suitable after exercise, especially during the initial stages of recovery. Burke et al (1993) found a 30% increase in muscle glycogen storage of cyclists in the first 24 hours of post-exercise recovery, when consuming a high-GI carbohydrate-rich diet compared with low-GI diet with the same amount of CHO. Kiens and Richter (1996) investigated the effect of GI on recovery of muscle glycogen stores of moderately active men. The men consumed a low-GI and high-GI diet over 30 days and comparisons between the two trials showed lower muscle glycogen content and muscle triglyceride following the low-GI diet.

Using the GI list, the athlete can apply GI to specific parts of their train-ing programme, i.e. pre-event snack, competition and recovery. From the athlete's perspective, after carbohydrate have been digested and absorbed, glucose may subsequently be available as energy immediately (from high-GI foods), or over a longer period of time (from moderate- to low-GI foods), and excess amounts of carbohydrate that are not used are stored.

What to eat before exercise: preparing for a competition event

The aforementioned studies show the effects of different carbohydrate diets on glycogen stores, demonstrating that a high-carbohydrate diet pro-duced the greatest benefit in terms of glycogen storage and performance. Therefore, the main goal of pre-exercise nutrition is to maximise carbohy-drate stores to benefit performance. This is a key advantage that enables the athlete to begin exercise or participation in sport with their maximum amount of muscle and liver glycogen. They may be able to exercise longer or more intensely, or to their own maximal potential. Various strate-gies may be used in the days and hours before competition, including increasing or super-compensating the glycogen stores by following a carbohydrate-loading regime or using the GI tables, or both.

Preparing for competition

Origin of the carbohydrate-loading regimen (also known as glycogen loading)

A number of studies in the 1960s were led by Scandinavian researchers Bergstrom and Ahlborg (Bergstrom and Hultman, 1966; Ahlborg et al, 1967), whose investigations discovered that training and a diet high in carbohydrates affected glycogen synthesis and storage. Using this infor-mation, carbohydrate loading or glycogen loading was developed to en-hance the glycogen stores of athletes 1 week prior to an endurance event. Research in this area clearly demonstrated its effects on muscle glycogen stores (Astrand, 1967; Bergstrom et al, 1967). The goal of researchers was to increase subjects' glycogen stores above normal levels, by developing a test protocol using various dietary and exercise interventions. Hence came about the well-known classical super-compensation model of car-bohydrate (muscle glycogen) loading. The 7-day diet and exercise model suggested 1 day of exhaustive exercise, followed by a period (3 days) of carbohydrate deprivation to deplete glycogen stores. This diet consisted of a low-carbohydrate (25% CHO of total energy intake), high-protein and high-fat diet. A further exhaustive exercise bout was done on day 4, and following this, a very high-carbohydrate diet (70% CHO) was consumed in the last 3 days before the competition. The comparison of glycogen levels (80–100 mmol/kg ww) of inactive subjects on a mixed diet with the super-compensation protocol Astrand (1967) proved that it was possible to increase muscle glycogen stores to twice its normal level to above 200 mmol/kg ww (range, 80–212 mmol/kg ww).

However, there were drawbacks of this classical model of carbohydrate loading that was documented in the 1970s and 1980s. Athletes who follow this regimen may experience the following issues:

During the low-carbohydrate phase and exhaustive training sessions:
- Difficulty with preparing for, and carrying out such an unusually low-carbohydrate, high-protein and high-fat diet
- Discomfort with the training regime (exhaustive sessions during the low-carbohydrate phase and *no training* for most days)
- Fatigue, irritability, nervousness and tiredness
- Low blood glucose leading to muscle weakness and disorientation
- Gastrointestinal discomfort such as diarrhoea on the high-protein, high-fat diet
- Poor recovery from exercise and an increased risk of injury

During the high-carbohydrate phase:
- Gastrointestinal discomfort such as feeling bloated and weight gain (as every 1 g of glycogen is stored with 3 g of water) following a very high carbohydrate intake
- Implications for athletes with elevated blood fats, as a high-carbohydrate diet can increase triglyceride levels

An updated carbohydrate-loading plan

Since many athletes experience one or more of these difficulties when following the super-compensation model, studies have been conducted to test a more moderate regimen for optimum glycogen loading before an endurance event. Sherman et al (1981) tested three types of glycogen-loading protocols in runners. All trials involved 6 days of tapered training and various diet protocols. Subjects consumed either a mixed diet of 50% CHO or the classical super-compensation diet regimen or a mixed diet for 3 days followed by a 3-day high (70%) carbohydrate diet. The 6-day training regimen was the same for all protocols and involved reducing the time of a 90-minute run at 75% VO_2max at day 1, and then tapered to no exercise training on the last day. They did not include the exhaustive exercise sessions that were part of the original carbohydrate-loading regimen.

Muscle glycogen stores peaked at 211 mmol/kg ww in the classical super-compensation protocol. However, Sherman and colleagues proved that a modified regimen of a mixed diet followed by a high-carbohydrate diet was just as effective and produced glycogen stores of 204 mmol/kg ww.

Muscle glycogen stores of trained endurance athletes benefit the most from a moderate to high-carbohydrate diet that includes a rest day (no exercise training).

Performance benefits of carbohydrate loading

It appears that not all athletes or events will benefit from carbohydrate loading. Time plays a role, and the longer the endurance event, the greater the reliance on muscle and liver glycogen. Athletes participating in events lasting longer than 90–120 minutes will benefit most from carbohydrate loading, in terms of endurance capacity (exercising for longer before exhaustion, or time to exhaustion) and performance (achieving the best time for a set distance) (Figure 4.1). Higher than normal carbohydrate stores improve endurance capacity by 20% and endurance performance by 2–3% (Hawley et al, 1997). Even moderate carbohydrate loading (6 g CHO/kg BW/day) does not match higher glycogen storage that is achieved with a high carbohydrate-loading regimen (9 g CHO/kg BW/day). However, in this trial, researchers found no difference between the two regimens in cycling performance (measured as time to complete and peak power output) in a 100-km time trial distance during which a carbohydrate drink was consumed (Burke et al, 2000). They speculated that similar performance between the two regimens may be related to the placebo effect

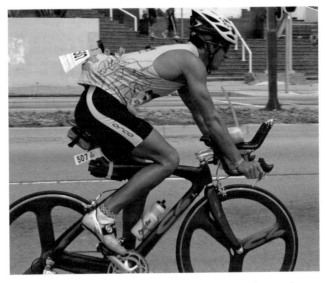

Figure 4.1 Carbohydrate loading can benefit long-distance cycling performance and ultra-distance events.

(by the moderate carbohydrate trial). A further study on cyclists made a comparison between a high-carbohydrate (loading) diet and a low-carbohydrate diet, using the previously established carbohydrate-loading diet and exercise tapering regimen of Sherman et al (1981). During 45 minutes of high-intensity (82% VO_2max) cycling, the study found no significant difference in cycling exercise between the two trials (Kavouras et al, 2004).

In addition to the benefits of carbohydrate loading to endurance athletes, athletes involved in intermittent exercise also achieve performance benefits from a high-carbohydrate diet. An early study on elite soccer players showed that a high-carbohydrate diet may be beneficial to players' glycogen stores and performance when playing two consecutive matches over 3 days. Players who consumed the high-carbohydrate diet maintained higher glycogen stores that corresponded with greater distances covered and better running performance in both halves of the matches, when compared with athletes who consumed a normal (control) diet (Saltin, 1973). More recently, a study found that performance in intermittent high-intensity running may also benefit from carbohydrate ingestion (Foskett et al, 2008). More research is needed in this area to confirm the benefits of carbohydrate loading on soccer and other team sports that involve intermittent high-intensity exercise.

Effect of high-protein diet on exercise performance

Recently, Macdemid and Stannard (2006) compared cycling performance between a group of cyclists on a 7-day high-protein, moderate-carbohydrate (4–6 g/kg BW) diet and a high-carbohydrate diet (7–10 g kg BW). Both diets had the same amount of energy and fat, just different proportion of protein and carbohydrate. The study found that self-paced endurance cycling performance was impaired on the high-protein diet when compared to the high-carbohydrate diet providing further evidence that favours the high carbohydrate-loading regimen.

Thus, research trials have used a modified carbohydrate-loading regimen and can be summaries as follows:

Day 1–3:
- Depletion phase
- Mixed diet (50% CHO or 6 g/kg BW/day, 35% fat, 15% protein)
- *Day 1*: 90 minutes training at 74–76% VO_2max
- *Day 2–3*: reduce volume of training, 60 minutes training at 74–76% VO_2max

Day 4–6:
- Loading phase
- High-carbohydrate diet (70% CHO or 8–9 g/kg BW/day, 13% fat, 17% protein)

- *Day 4 and 5*: reduce training volume: 20 minutes. Maintain intensity at 74–76% VO$_2$max
- *Day 6*: High-carbohydrate diet, no exercise.
  Day 7:
- Competition

Thus, in a modified carbohydrate-loading regimen, training is tapered by 50% from day 1 to 3, reducing duration of exercise but maintaining the intensity. On days 4 and 5, training is tapered by a further 50%, maintaining intensity. There is no exercise on day 6 as athletes continue the high-carbohydrate diet.

Putting theory into practice may not be so easy for athletes due to lack of knowledge of food composition, poor food preparation skills, inadequate meal planning or lack of time. A dietary survey of long distance runners found that in practice, runners' nutritional intake did not meet the requirements of the high-carbohydrate phase of the carbohydrate-loading regimen (Burke and Read, 1987).

1-day carbohydrate loading

In light of the fact that athletes may not have the time, knowledge or skills to adequately apply a rigorous carbohydrate-loading regimen, the evidence from a more recent study may prove much more useful to this group of athletes. Bussau et al (2002) found that it is possible to super-compensate muscle glycogen levels prior to an endurance event. This is achieved with 1 day of rest and consuming 7–10 g CHO/kg BW/day.

Example: How to calculate carbohydrate needs for training and carbohydrate loading

An endurance athlete weighing 70 kg trains 2 hours a day and requires 7 g CHO/kg BW/day: 70 × 7 = 490 g CHO. To convert nutrients into real food choices, athletes need to know the carbohydrate content of foods. Students can use standard food tables (i.e. McCance and Widdowson's The Composition of Foods Sixth Summary Edition (Food Standards Agency, 2002). In practice, packaged foods and nutritional supplements with wrappers and food labels provide useful nutritional information that can also be used. The carbohydrate-rich servings in Table 3.1 and Table 4.1 provide some examples for the diet. With regards to GI, moderate- to low-GI food should be eaten between exercise sessions, low-GI snacks and meals before exercise and high-GI snacks, fluids and meals are the ideal choice during and immediately after exercise.

Using the carbohydrate-rich food list, the exact amount of portions is determined to make a meal plan and a menu of food items.

Since the athlete in the aforementioned example requires 490 g CHO/day, converting these amounts to food portions are done in the following way:

490 g CHO ÷ 15 g CHO servings = 33 serves of carbohydrate-rich foods (32.666 rounded off to 33)

A typical training menu based on the aforementioned example is shown in Table 4.2.

To adjust the menu to 700 g CHO, during carbohydrate loading, 210 g CHO can be added by one of the following:

- 14 or more servings of carbohydrate-rich starchy foods (bread, cereal, rice, pasta)
- 8 servings of fruit, fresh or juiced, and include 4–6 larger servings of vegetables or vegetable juice or thick vegetable soup
- 8 high-energy gel sachets
- 4 servings of carbohydrate recovery drink (at 42 g CHO per serve)
- 2.5 L of concentrated (8% CHO) energy drink

Some athletes' energy and carbohydrate requirements may be very high, i.e. the ultra-endurance cyclist, ultra-marathon runner or an Ironman triathlete who trains and competes many hours a day. The athlete may need 10–12 g CHO/kg BW equivalent to about 700 g CHO/day (current guideline for a 70 kg athlete with a very strenuous daily endurance training programme). For practical reasons such as time constraints and volume of food required, many more energy-dense carbohydrate-rich foods, snacks and nutritional supplements may be used to make up the daily requirements.

Pre-competition meal: What to eat in the hours before competition

One important factor that should not be overlooked is the overnight period between the last meal on the evening prior to the event and the next morning. This is usually an overnight fast of about 8–10 hours, during which time the carbohydrate stores suffer some depletion. As most endurance events occur in the morning after this overnight fast, athletes have to take advantage of the pre-competition meal and start eating as soon as possible after they wake up. It is a good idea to be well prepared and plan ahead. Athletes may be distracted by other issues such as equipment, clothing or the journey to the venue, or competition anxiety may affect the appetite. For these reasons, it may be helpful to set out the food and utensils the night before. Rehearsing a routine with the ideal meal during special training sessions like time trials may help the novice, inexperienced competitor to be better prepared for competitive events.

Table 4.2 A typical training menu showing the carbohydrates servings and relative food items.

Meal	Menu	Servings Providing 490 g CHO
Breakfast	$1\frac{1}{2}$ cups high-fibre cereal or porridge	3 CHO
	1 glass of fruit juice	2 CHO
	1 apple	1 CHO
	$1\frac{1}{2}$ tablespoons of raisins	1 CHO
	2–3 raw nuts, crushed	
	1 glass of low-fat milk	$\frac{1}{2}$ CHO
	2 t honey	$\frac{1}{2}$ CHO
		Total = 8 CHO
		~24% of total CHO
Snack	4 wheat crackers	2 CHO
	2 T peanut spread or low-fat hummus	
	300 mL carbohydrate drink (4–6% CHO solution)	1 CHO
		Total = 3 CHO
Lunch	4 thin slices low-GI bread	4 CHO
	90 g tuna, drained	
	2 tablespoons low-fat mayonnaise	
	1 tablespoon low-fat spread	
	Tossed vegetable salad	1 CHO
	500 mL fruit juice	4 CHO
		Total = 9 CHO
Snack	50 g energy or cereal bar	1 CHO
	1 cup low-fat fruit yoghurt	1 CHO
		Total = 2 CHO
Dinner	2 cups cooked spaghetti	4 CHO
	100 g grilled chicken breast	
	1 can tomatoes	2 CHO
	Side salad of coleslaw (carrots and cabbage, fresh	2 CHO
	or with a dash of low-fat mayonnaise)	
	1 cup of strawberries	1 CHO
		Total = 9 CHO
Snack	1 hot or cold milky drink	$\frac{1}{2}$ CHO
	3 oat cookies	2 CHO
		Daily Total = ~33 CHO

Source: material from Hayley Daries Practice.
In this example 1 CHO serving contains 15 g CHO.
CHO, carbohydrate.

Muscle glycogen can be increased up until 3–4 hours before an event, i.e. less than 3 hours before the event; eating carbohydrate will increase liver glycogen and blood glucose levels. If the athlete has only 1–2 hours before an early event, it is important to prioritise carbohydrate intake during exercise that will assist the liver to maintain blood glucose levels during exercise.

Provided that there is enough carbohydrate available during exercise, 140–330 g carbohydrate before exercise will increase glycogen stores (Coyle et al, 1985), improve intermittent high-intensity running (Foskett et al, 2008) and 100 g CHO eaten 3 hours before prolonged cycling exercise at 70% VO$_2$max enhances endurance capacity (Schabort et al, 1999). It appears the benefits of eating carbohydrates are not only limited to the performance in the event or competition, Fallowfield et al (1995) found that it will also enhance *subsequent* exercise performance when the recovery period is short (around 4 hours).

Ideas for pre-competition meals, 2–3 hours before competition. Refer also to recipes for breakfast (Chapter 3), sandwiches and spreads (Chapter 6) and recipes rich in carbohydrates at the end of the chapter. *Most of the following foods are low GI*:

- Bran* cereal with milk, served with apple juice
- Maize or oat* porridge with milk, raisins and cinnamon
- Muesli, granola and yoghurt
- Banana or raisin bread with light spread
- Muffins or pancakes with maple syrup, jam or honey
- Beans on toast
- Toast with low fat hummus or banana and peanut butter mix
- Pasta and vegetables with tomato-based sauce, add a serving of lean chicken, fish or vegetarian option.
- Baby (new) potato salad with boiled egg and light dressing
- Seed bread filled with either cooked and skinless chicken breast and pineapple, or tuna and corn, or cottage cheese and salad.

*Caution: Some cereals have very high fibre content and may cause gastrointestinal symptoms. Always try a brand at training before using it in a pre-competition meal.

Pre-competition meal: what to eat 30–60 minutes before competition

Carbohydrate intake in the hour before competition serves to provide rapidly available form of carbohydrate (e.g. glucose or sugar). When consumed in liquid form in a carbohydrate-electrolyte beverage, it provides fluid for optimal hydration, delays fatigue and benefits performance in prolonged endurance exercise (Coombes and Hamilton, 2000).

Hargreaves et al (2004) have reported studies showing the negative metabolic effects of pre-exercise carbohydrate ingestion. It starts with a surge of blood glucose and insulin, this then leading to several metabolic effects that suggest unfavourable consequences during exercise. There is little or no reason to avoid carbohydrate before exercise, and as the researchers have concluded that carbohydrate ingestion in the hour before exercise does not weaken performance. Glucose, sucrose, fructose and the effect of GI have been studied extensively to determine what constitutes the ideal pre-exercise meal. There appears that solid or liquid feeds are equally appropriate, it is more important that the athlete consume known (preferred) foods high in carbohydrates. Foods high in fibre (e.g. high-fibre breakfast cereals, bread and beans) and high-fructose foods or drinks may cause gastrointestinal discomfort (cramping, diarrhoea or vomiting) for some athletes.

Overall, provided that sufficient carbohydrate is ingested during pro-longed exercise, the GI of the pre-exercise meal will not affect metabolism or performance. Burke et al (1998) found that when cyclists ate either potato (high GI) or pasta (low GI) in a pre-exercise meal, and con-sumed a glucose electrolyte during 2.5-hour cycling exercise, neither their metabolism not performance was affected.

A recent review of studies shows that in the 75-minute period before ex-ercise, differences in neither the timing of carbohydrate ingestion, amount of carbohydrates nor the GI affect exercise performance. However, some athletes do experience hypoglycaemic symptoms during exercise if they consume carbohydrates during this period. Hypoglycaemia may be pre-vented in susceptible athletes if they consume carbohydrates shortly be-fore exercise (within the 5 minutes before) or altogether avoid it in the last 90 minutes before exercise (Jeukendrup and Killer, 2010).

Suggested carbohydrates intake 1 hour or less before exercise should be around 50–100 g (1.0–1.5 g/kg BW), and tolerance of any foods and fluids should be determined during training not on competition day. Higher in-takes (1–4 g/kg BW eaten 1–4 hours before exercise) have been suggested for athletes partaking in prolonged exercise (Castell et al, 2010).

Pre-race snacks and fluids, consumed 30–60 minutes before competi-tion, should concentrate on convenient low-bulk snacks like cereal or en-ergy bars, fruit or yoghurt smoothies or fresh fruit or fruit juice (high fruc-tose may cause gastrointestinal symptoms in some athletes).

Carbohydrate intake during exercise

In practice, athletes often consume fruit, energy bars, energy (sports) drinks and high-energy gels during exercise training and competition. Dur-ing exercise, it is in the athlete's best interest to choose the most efficient fuel that will supply energy as rapidly as possible especially when fatigue sets in during intense exercise or late stages of endurance exercise.

The ideal type of carbohydrate to be consumed during exercise is dependant on how quickly the nutrient is absorbed and oxidised. Previously, oxidation rates of glucose, sucrose, maltose and glucose polymers (long chains of glucose) were reported to be quickest at 1.0 g/min and are readily available as a fuel source for the muscles during exercise. However, trials with carbohydrate mixtures have resulted in higher oxidation rates than was previously found. A combination of glucose with fructose and sucrose (2.4 g/min ingested) resulted in oxidation rates of 1.70 g/min, and when glucose was combined with fructose only (at 2.4 g/min ingested), the oxidation rates rose to 1.75 g/min (Jentjens et al, 2004; Jentjens and Jeukendrup, 2005). Later, Currell and Jeukendrup (2008) showed how cycling performance increased by 8% by consuming a glucose + fructose mixture as compared with glucose only feedings, subsequently used by Dutch cyclists in the Tour de France. High-fructose drinks could lead to stomach upsets for certain athletes.

Researchers have found that carbohydrate intake during exercise should be no less than 50 g/h, and up 70 g/h (i.e. about 0.5–1.0 g CHO/kg BW) (Coggan and Coyle, 1991; Jeukendrup and Jentjens, 2000; Castell et al, 2010).

The addition of protein to a drink may assist in fluid retention during exercise, up to 15% greater than when just a carbohydrate-electrolyte drink is consumed (Seifert et al, 2006). Further details of protein ingestion during and after exercise follow in Chapter 5.

The days are long gone when only water or hypertonic drinks (e.g. colas) were available during endurance competitions. Most endurance and ultra-endurance events are well organised and sponsors have taken advantage of scientific findings, using the platform to promote their sports drinks, bars and gels. Pre-race packs are provided with snacks and fluids and during the races there is a supply of water and fluids along the route. Sometimes sandwiches and fruits are provided in prolonged events. Chapter 8 will explore fluid replacement in sport and exercise in further detail.

Carbohydrates for recovery

Carbohydrate is vital during the recovery from prolonged exercise or intermittent high-intensity exercise. The aforementioned studies show that muscle glycogen stores decline after just 30 minutes, a series of single short sprints can heavily deplete stores and after 2–3 hours of exercise, very little if any muscle glycogen stores remain.

It has already been established that in order to be ready for the next training session or competition, and hence have saturated glycogen stores in the liver and muscle, the athletes needs to take full advantage of the 1–2 hour period after intense exercise or competition when the muscles are more likely to take up glycogen (greater glycogen uptake rate). There is only this window of opportunity for 2 hours, after that the glycogen uptake rate drops making it more timely to saturate the glycogen stores to their optimal level. Around 1.0–1.5 g high-GI carbohydrates (50–100 g) should be consumed in the first 30 minutes after completion of exercise, and a total of 7–10 g CHO/kg BW over 24 hours for athletes with a heavy training load. Quick ways to achieve a high-carbohydrate intake is provided in the following examples. Carbohydrate-strong beverages, smoothies or nutritional shakes may be good low-bulk options that deliver the most energy at more comfortable volumes. Bulky high-fibre foods may neither be convenient nor ideal as the fibre and bulk of the foods deter the athlete from eating enough to replenish glycogen stores. In any event, after exercise, quite a number of athletes hang around talking to friends or fellow competitors and may miss out on topping up stores.

Athletes in a glycogen-depleted state may benefit from the addition of protein to carbohydrate-based drinks or foods in the recovery phase after exercise (refer to Chapter 5).

Post-race recovery snacks and fluids should provide the first 50 g CHO in 30 minutes, repeated after 30-minutes and then every two hours, adding some protein, within the daily allowance per individual.

High-GI carbohydrate foods for first 1–2 hours post-exercise

- 2 energy gels
- 2 cereal or energy bars
- 1 high-energy sports bar (CHO–Protein mix)
- 2 English muffins with jam, honey or syrup
- 625 mL (8% CHO) sports drink (*Note*: fluid intake volume largely depends on post-exercise hydration levels, i.e. if dehydrated or intoxicated with fluid – refer to Chapter 8)
- 1 large bake potato with tuna and tomato sauce
- 1 large pancake with baked apple and sugar filling
- 1 long roll with baked banana, peanut butter and honey filling
- small 67 g packet of sweets, like fruit gums, pastilles or jelly beans

Creating 'plate space' for carbohydrate foods

Carbohydrates-rich foods should take up the most plate space as it is the preferred fuel of the muscle. Athletes are advised to fill two-thirds of their plate with vegetables, fruits, pasta, potatoes, rice, bread or other fibre-rich grains. In this way, they are guaranteed to get a good supply of carbohydrate in the diet. Plate space is important especially as carbohydrates compete with other nutrient-rich energy dense foods on the plate for space. For example, protein-rich foods and fat-rich foods can easily increase the energy of the meal and be eaten as a preference at the expense of a carbohydrate-rich diet.

This is especially evident when an athlete eats meals outside the home, at a restaurant or food canteen. Even if athletes choose high-carbohydrate base dishes like pasta or pizza, the accompaniments of rich sauces, meaty fillings and cheeses will inevitably make it a protein- and fat-rich dish, not a carbohydrate-rich dish as assumed (refer to Table 3.2 for ideas of carbohydrate-rich dishes and recipes).

Chapter summary

- Carbohydrate contains 4 kcal (17 kJ)/g and is the rapid source of fuel for the exercising muscles.
- Carbohydrate-rich foods include fruit, vegetables, grains, cereals and legumes, with a good amount from milk and milk products.
- Carbohydrate-value is defined as the amount of carbohydrate per serving of carbohydrate-rich food. Servings of food from the same group contain the same amount of nutrient (carbohydrate).
- Glycogen, the storage form of carbohydrate, is also found as glucose in the blood and the brain.
- The muscle biopsy technique measures the amount of glycogen in muscle tissue.
- The suggested carbohydrate intake for athletes is often expressed as g/kg BW/day and ranges from 3 to 12 g CHO/kg BW/day, depending on exercise load and dietary goals.
- The best time to replace depleted glycogen stores is the first 2 hours after exercise when glycogen synthase is activated and insulin sensitivity is increased.
- The Glycaemic Index (GI) is a ranking of carbohydrate-rich foods based on their effect on blood glucose values.
- A low-GI pre-event meal improves endurance performance and time to exhaustion.
- High-GI foods and fluids can help maintain blood glucose during exercise, and therefore, help athletes to maintain the intensity or 'pace' of exercise for longer.
- High-GI foods help restore muscle glycogen levels in initial recovery stages after exercise.
- The glycaemic load (GL) takes into account the available carbohydrate in the food and its blood glucose response.
- Super-compensation of muscle glycogen stores before competition can be achieved by following a carbohydrate-loading regime.

- A modified carbohydrate-loading regimen is a useful pre-competition strategy that will benefit endurance athletes who compete in events that last 90 minutes or longer. Athletes can double their glycogen stores and enhance endurance capacity and performance.
- The 7-day carbohydrate-loading regime involves a mixed diet for days 1–3 with a corresponding carbohydrate intake of 6 g/kg BW/day. Carbohydrate intake increases on days 4–6, to 8–9 g/kg BW/day, before competition takes place on day 7.
- A 1-day carbohydrate loading is achieved with rest and a carbohydrate intake of 7–10 g/kg BW/day.
- The amount of carbohydrate recommended for a pre-event meal is 140–330 g CHO, helps to increase glycogen levels and exercise performance and can be eaten 3 hours before the event.
- During exercise, athletes can consume a minimum of 50 g CHO and up to 70 g CHO per hour.
- 50–100 g of CHO ($\sim$1–1.5 g CHO/kg BW) can be consumed within the first $\frac{1}{2}$ hour after exercise is completed, the amount being dependent on the level of training and duration of exercise. This is repeated after 30 minutes and then every 2 hours (at $\sim$1–2 g CHO/kg BW), adding protein within the daily allowance for these nutrients.

Pasta, Potatoes and Soups

The following recipes are a selection of carbohydrate-rich meals to complement any level of sport and exercise training.

Classic Pea and Ham Soup

(Serves 4–6)

Ingredients

25 mL sunflower oil
2 onions, chopped
2 cloves garlic, crushed
1 bay leaf
300 g (11 oz) ham, cooked or smoked and cut into 2 cm cubes

400 g (14 oz) frozen or fresh peas
Salt and freshly ground pepper
1 L vegetable stock
Extra ham, chopped

Method

1 Sauté the vegetables, cloves and bay leaf in the oil for 5–7 minutes in a large pot.
2 Add the ham and peas and simmer for 20 minutes.
3 Blend the soup and season with salt and pepper.
4 Serve hot with toast and garnish with extra ham.

Nutrition analysis per portion

Energy	248 kcal (1040 kJ)
Protein	20 g
Carbohydrate	8 g
Fat	15 g
Cholesterol	36 mg
Fibre	10 g

Food note: Peas are rich in vitamin C, although it contains less protein than other pulses.

Jacket Potato with Tuna and Mayonnaise filling

(Serves 4)

Ingredients

4 medium potatoes

50 g onion, chopped

100 g canned tuna, drained

75 g mayonnaise

Pepper

Method

1 Pick the potatoes with a small sharp knife.
2 Cook in microwave for 10–14 minutes or until soft.
3 Combine chopped onions, tuna and mayonnaise.
4 Carefully cut open the top of the potatoes and fill with tuna mayo mixture.
5 Season with pepper.
6 Serve immediately.

Variation:

1 Replace the filling with cheddar cheese, goat's cheese or feta and garlic and parsley.

Nutrition analysis per portion

Energy	200 kcal (842 kJ)
Protein	11.2 g
Carbohydrate	30 g
Fat	2.5 g
Cholesterol	5 mg
Fibre	3 g

Food note: Canned tuna is a lean protein source and rich in B vitamins. Fresh tuna retains all its natural oils and is rich in omega-3 fatty acids.

Sundried Tomato Risotto

(Serves 4)

Ingredients

30 mL sunflower oil

1 onion, finely chopped

100 g (4 oz) sundried tomatoes, roughly chopped

1.25 L vegetable stock

10 mL fresh parsley, chopped

1 leek, finely chopped

2 garlic cloves, crushed

500 g (1 lb; 2 oz) Arborio rice

Salt and pepper

60 mL parmesan cheese, for garnishing

Method

1 Sauté the leeks, onions and garlic until translucent.
2 Add the tomatoes and rice and sauté for another minute.
3 Add 1 ladle of the stock. Simmer until most of the liquid has been absorbed, then add another ladle of stock. Follow this procedure until all the stock has been used.
4 Season the risotto. Remove from heat and serve.
5 Sprinkle the parsley and parmesan over the risotto.
6 Serve immediately.

Nutrition analysis per portion

Energy	198 kcal (833 kJ)
Protein	7.3 g
Carbohydrate	25 g
Fat	7 g
Cholesterol	6 mg
Fibre	2 g

Food note: Tomatoes and tomato products are known for their vitamin C content, although it is a major source of *lycopene,* a powerful antioxidant that protects against free radical damage. Lycopene concentration is higher in ripe, cooked tomatoes.

Tomato and Basil Pasta Sauce

(Serves 2)

Ingredients

15 mL olive oil

$\frac{1}{2}$ small red onion, chopped

2 garlic cloves, crushed

1 × 400 g tin whole or chopped tomatoes

15 mL (3 tsps) fresh basil or 5 mL dried basil

5 mL (1 tsp) honey (optional)

Salt and pepper

300 g cooked whole-wheat spaghetti

Method

1 Sauté the onions in the olive oil for 2 minutes. Add the garlic and sauté for another minute.

2 Add the tin of tomatoes and bring to the boil. Reduce the heat and allow the tomatoes to simmer for 15 minutes.

3 Add the basil, honey and seasoning. Remove from the heat and serve with any type of pasta.

Nutrition analysis per portion (with cooked spaghetti)

Energy	341 kcal (1432 kJ)
Protein	10 g
Carbohydrate	46.4 g
Fat	8.4 g
Cholesterol	0 mg
Fibre	9.2 g

Food note: Adding garlic in the diet provides a natural antibiotic for the body and has many healing properties.

Tuna and Anchovies with Basil Pesto

(Serves 4)

Ingredients

300 g (12 oz) tagliatelli pasta

30 mL sunflower oil

150 g (5 oz) fresh tuna steak

50 g (2 oz) anchovy fillets, copped

pecorino cheese, grated (optional)

basil pesto (see recipe)

Basil Pesto:

50 g (2 oz) basil leaves

20 g coriander leaves

30 g (1 oz) pine nuts, toasted

125 mL olive oil

Salt and pepper to taste

Method

1 Cook the pasta in salted boiling water until soft, but tender. Drain off the excess water.
2 Sear the tuna steak in the heated oil.
3 To prepare the Basil pesto, place all the ingredients into a blender. Add seasoning to taste.
4 Mix the pasta with the pesto and dish the pasta into four pasta bowls.
5 Top with the shredded tuna, chopped anchovies and pecorino cheese.
6 Serve immediately.

Nutrition analysis per portion
Light meal

Energy	329 kcal (1381 kJ)
Protein	12.6 g
Carbohydrate	10.6 g
Fat	24.7 g
Cholesterol	13 mg
Fibre	4.3 g

High-energy meal

Energy	641 kcal (2693 kJ
Protein	25 g
Carbohydrate	21 g
Fat	48 g
Cholesterol	25 mg
Fibre	8 g

Food note: Anchovies are oily fish (omega-3 fatty acids) that are an excellent source of calcium as both the bones and flesh can be eaten.

Warm Potato and Grilled Pepper Salad

(Serves 4)

Ingredients
2 large red peppers, seeded and cut into shapes
2 large yellow peppers, seeded and cut into shapes
10 mL olive oil
600 g new potatoes, halved
1 small red onion, thinly sliced
200 g cocktail tomatoes, halved
Dressing
75 mL orange juice
40 mL olive oil
10 mL honey
Salt and pepper

Method
1 Roast the peppers in the oil for 10 minutes at 200°C.
2 Boil the potatoes in lightly salted water, until tender.
3 For the dressing, mix all the ingredients together.
4 Mix the peppers, potatoes, onion and cocktail tomatoes. Drizzle the dressing over.
5 Serve warm.

Nutrition analysis per portion
Side Dish

Energy	92 kcal (387 kJ)
Protein	1.3 g
Carbohydrate	11 g
Fat	4 g
Cholesterol	0 mg
Fibre	1.7 g

Main Course

Energy	294 kcal (1235 kJ)
Protein	4 g
Carbohydrate	35 g
Fat	13 g
Cholesterol	0 mg
Fibre	5.4 g

Food note: Peppers (capsicums) become sweeter as they ripen. They are rich in vitamin C (especially green peppers), beta-carotene and minerals.

CHAPTER 5

Protein

Key terms

Protein	Anabolism
Amino acids	Catabolism
Essential amino acids (EAAs) (indispensable)	Nitrogen balance
	Protein synthesis
Non-essential amino acids (NEAAs) (dispensable)	Protein breakdown
	Muscle hypertrophy
Biologic value (BV)	Allergens
Whey	Glycoproteins
Casein	Food allergy
Protein turnover	

Here is a nutrient that has received unrivalled attention, from ancient Greek Olympians to present day world champions. Like carbohydrate, protein[1] is an energy-giving nutrient that yields 4 kcal (17 kJ) of energy per gram. Protein is one of the most abundant nutrients in many structures such as cells, organs and tissues. In lean body tissue (that includes muscle tissue), water and protein make up the major parts.

Popular terms used when referring to proteins are amino acids, whey protein and casein. Amino acids are the building blocks of protein, the simplest form of the nutrient. Amino acids contain and supply nitrogen to the body along with other elements such as sulphur, phosphorous and iron. There are 20 amino acids, of which 8 are essential for adults and 9 are essential for babies, children and stressed elderly persons. Essential amino acids (EAAs) cannot be made in the body and can only be obtained from food sources. Human growth and survival depends on dietary intake of EAAs, namely histidine, isoleucine, leucine, lycine, methionine, phenylalanine, threonine, tryptophan and valine. The 11 or so other amino acids

Nutrition for Sport and Exercise: A Practical Guide, First Edition. Hayley Daries.
© 2012 Blackwell Publishing Ltd. Published 2012 by Blackwell Publishing Ltd.

Table 5.1 Foods rich in protein energy.

Each serving contains ~10 g protein

(a) *Each following food item contains EAAs to support growth*:

      2 small eggs, or 80 g extra large egg

      300 mL semi-skimmed milk

      200 g low-fat yoghurt

      40 g medium cheddar cheese

      1 slice (35 g) cooked lean meat

      1 slice (40 g) lean chicken breast (cooked)

      45 g tuna canned in brine

      50 g sardines canned in tomato sauce

      3 grilled fish fingers

      1 cup (250 mL) soy milk

      100 g soy meat

(b) *Each following food item lacks one or more EAAs[a]*:

      100 g muesli

      90 g porridge oats

      100 g dry weight couscous

      360 g (4 $\frac{1}{2}$ heaped tablespoons) boiled rice

      275 g boiled spaghetti

      200 g baked beans

      50 g mixed nuts

      3 tablespoons sunflower seeds

Source: Material from Hayley Daries Practice.

[a]Vegetarians can eat a variety of foods in the (b) group to get a full complement of the essential amino acids.

EAA, essential amino acids.

are not essential (non-essential amino acids (NEAAs), dispensable), which means that they can be made by the body using other (essential, indispensable) amino acids.

Rich food sources of amino acids or proteins are predominantly in animal-derived products, such as meat, poultry, fish, eggs and milk products. Animals obtain their nitrogen-containing amino acids from dietary sources. Some protein is also found in plant sources, which make their own amino acids from nitrogen in the soil, e.g. vegetables, soy beans, legumes (pulses like lentils), nuts, seeds and grains (breads, cereals, rice). Table 5.1 provides a few examples of foods rich in protein energy. Each food has the equivalent amount of proteins (~10 g) per serving, and is grouped by the foods that contain all EAAs to support growth, and foods that contain some but not all EAAs.

In order for growth, tissue repair and maintenance to occur, a new protein must be created. For this to occur successfully in the body all nine EAAs must be ingested or protein synthesis would be impossible. Animal proteins are regarded as high-quality (complete) proteins because they

Table 5.2 Complementary proteins for vegetarian meals.

Food combination	Meal idea	Recipes available in this book
Grains[a] and milk	Bran cereal and milk	Muesli and granola breakfast (serve with yoghurt)
Bread and milk products	Sesame seed bagel with a glass of milk	Mozzarella, tomato and pesto on rye bread
Rice *or* pasta and cheese	Pasta with grated mozzarella cheese	Sundried tomato risotto with parmesan cheese
Grains and legumes	Lentil and rice curry (i.e. Biryani curry)	Brown rice and lentil salad Bean curry (serve with rice, quick-cook couscous, polenta or quinoa)
Bread, rice *or* corn and beans	Baked beans on toast	Beans and chickpeas on toast Bean and Lentil Burgers
Seeds/nuts and legumes	Spicy bean burger on a sesame seed roll.	Banana and peanut butter smoothie
Vegetables and grains/nuts/seeds/dairy products	Stir-fry vegetables with nuts, served with rice	Roasted sweet potato salad with (mint) yoghurt dressing

Source: Data of 'food combination' from Escott-Stump (1992) and material from Hayley Daries Practice.
[a]Grains refer to rice, cereals or bread.

contain all nine EAAs, whereas most individual plant proteins do not contain all nine EAAs and are regarded as low-quality (incomplete) proteins (except for soy). Quinoa, a grain-like staple from South America, is also a complete protein and hailed for its rich protein content. However, combining a variety of foods from plant sources together will ensure that all EAAs are present to be used by the body for tissue growth and repair. Table 5.2 gives a few examples of complementary protein meals, useful for vegetarians or vegans. Vegetables go with nuts, and grain/rice with beans. So, baked beans on toasted bread makes a complete protein, although the combination does not have to be consumed at one sitting by adults, as long as both are eaten over the course of the day.

An EAA from an animal source is no more superior than the same EAA from a plant source. This knowledge is useful for vegetarian athletes whose protein intake may be compromised, and who are uncertain of the protein quality of plant sources. All protein is measured against the amino acid profile of egg white, which is regarded as the gold standard of protein-rich food. It has one of the highest biologic values (BV) and is quality rated at 100 for comparison with other protein-rich foods. Factor 100 denotes the percentage of nitrogen absorbed that is retained by the body. Although

Table 5.3 Biologic value (BV) of food protein.

Food protein	Biologic value
Egg	100
Cow's milk	93
Meat, Fish, Casein	75
Soy	74
Corn	72
Wheat protein (gluten)	44

Source: Data from Robinson et al (1986).

studies cite that some proteins have a higher biological value than egg, i.e. whey protein (20% of milk protein is in the form of whey, 80% casein), which has a biological value of 100 or more (104 reported by Renner (1983)), it does not mean that 100% of the nitrogen in the food is incorporated into the body and not excreted. A protein with a BV of over 70 can support growth, provided that the total daily energy needs are met (Robinson et al, 1986). Values below 70 cannot support growth but may be able to maintain tissues. Table 5.3 provides the BVs of some food proteins. Interestingly enough, human milk has a higher BV (100) as compared with the BV of cow's milk (93).

Protein reserves

Protein is part of all cells and nearly all fluids in the body, including hair, skin, nails, bones, ligaments, teeth and blood. Examples of proteins are enzymes, genes and hormones, as well as immune proteins, blood proteins (haemoglobin) and contractile proteins for muscle contraction. The largest concentration of proteins is found in skeletal muscle, and regular resistance training can be a stimulus for further muscle hypertrophy. Unlike stores of fat (in adipose tissue), carbohydrate (as glycogen in liver and muscles) or certain fat-soluble vitamins, protein is not stored in one place, but is available from all body tissues in an emergency. Proteins are constantly being depleted and replenished, and the rate of turnover differs from tissue to tissue. A 70 kg man has a protein turnover rate of about 25 g protein/day (Noakes, 1992). Protein turnover is also increased in infection and fever, burns, surgery, bone fractures, severe trauma, sepsis, as well as in healthy people involved in intense physical exercise, and even in growing children and pregnant women who require synthesis of new protein tissue. Protein turnover assists the estimation of protein requirements for athletes, and is discussed later in the chapter.

Functions of proteins, at rest

Protein has structural and functional roles in the body. It is responsible for maintenance and growth of tissues, and plays a role in several metabolic and physiological regulation processes. The functional roles of proteins include enzymatic, transport, hormonal, immune and buffering actions (Thomas and Bishop, 2007). Thus, the digestion and absorption of food, vitamin and mineral transport, the immune response, fluid balance and maintenance of acid–base balance, are among the bodily processes that depend on proteins. Protein provides energy for the body, providing 4 kcal/g, and contributes 5–15% of total energy expenditure at rest.

Functions of proteins, during exercise

Increasing exercise duration and intensity, and heavy strength and power training increases the need for dietary protein. Studies have suggested specific roles of protein during exercise (for reviews see Tipton and Wolfe, 2004; Kumar et al, 2009).

In endurance athletes, protein is needed:
- to provide an added fuel source during exercise;
- to maintain, recondition and increase lean body mass;
- to facilitate protein synthesis of enzymes; and
- to replace protein breakdown and repair exercise-induced muscle damage.

In strength or power athletes, which includes high-intensity team sports, protein is needed:
- to maintain and increase lean body mass (due to hypertrophic stimulus of resistance exercise); and
- to maintain and increase muscular strength and power.

Another possible benefit of protein is that it aids fluid retention. Seifert et al (2006) found that when protein (1.5 g/100 mL) was added to a carbohydrate-electrolyte drink (6 g carbohydrate/100 mL), fluid retention was 40% greater than when water was ingested, and 15% greater than when just the carbohydrate-electrolyte drink was consumed. This could be explained by the fact that proteins enhance sodium and water absorption in the intestine. For this reason, experts suggested early on that amino acids should be added to an oral rehydration solution (Gisolfi et al, 1990).

Specific requirements for protein may be dependent on type of sport, intensity and duration of exercise and gender of the athlete. Recall that carbohydrates play a large part in the provision of fuel during exercise and that they are the preferred fuel for exercising muscles. Some protein catabolism occurs during exercise, and although protein's contribution during exercise is small compared with carbohydrate and fat, protein breakdown does increase further when energy intake is low or carbohydrate stores are depleted. Some body proteins are 'fixed' and not available for energy. However, under the aforementioned circumstances, protein from the liver and muscle supplies the liver with fuel that is converted to glucose (via the gluconeogenesis in the alanine–glucose cycle in exercise).

For example, during endurance exercise, the contribution of energy from protein (amino acid oxidation) ranges from 1% to 6% of the total energy cost of exercise. The branched chain amino acid, leucine, plays an important role during endurance exercise since its oxidation increases to ~25% (compared to ~4–7% at rest) (Tarnopolsky, 2004).

Glycogen availability or depletion will influence amino acid oxidation during exercise and protein requirement. In a study by Howarth et al (2010) glycogen-depleted cyclists consumed either a high-carbohydrate (~71%) or low-carbohydrate (~11%) diet for ~44 hours, followed by periods of by rest, exercise and recovery. The study showed that glycogen depletion affected protein metabolism during exercise. The availability of carbohydrate during exercise was lower in the low-carbohydrate diet whether at rest, after exercise or after recovery resulting in increased protein breakdown and reduced protein synthesis late in exercise, when compared with the high-carbohydrate diet. This finding supports recommendations for athletes to follow a high-carbohydrate diet that provides sufficient energy.

Not only is glycogen spared with carbohydrate ingestion during exercise (see Chapter 4), but glucose ingestion during exercise in fed cyclists without glycogen depletion can also spare endogenous protein (van Hamont et al, 2005). Hulston et al (2010) found that during endurance exercise, protein co-ingested with carbohydrate may not reduce muscle protein breakdown or increase muscle protein synthesis.

The role of protein after exercise

Protein has a role after exercise, to rebuild muscle tissue that has broken down during exercise. Although a small percentage of protein is broken down *during* exercise, which is accompanied by a reduction in protein synthesis, *after* exercise there is some protein breakdown but with a higher rate of protein replenishment. Resistance training is a stimulus for protein anabolism. Muscle protein synthesis increases by ~40–150% after a single bout of resistance training. Food consumption and exercise stimulates muscle protein synthesis, but even when no food is consumed the muscle protein synthesis is sustained for 48 hours (Burd et al, 2009). Provided enough energy is consumed, strength training results in increased muscle size and mass. Strength and power athletes aim to maintain a highly positive nitrogen balance, so as to achieve their highest level of muscle mass, strength and/or power, which involves the right combination of training, rest and recovery and diet.

Protein synthesis not only increases following resistance exercise, but also after endurance training that results in muscle tissue damage that is subsequently repaired. Review of studies suggests that protein synthesis increases by ~40–70% in the recovery phase after aerobic-type exercise (Kumar et al, 2009). High-level athletes participating in prolonged exercise of high intensities, such as ultra-marathon races, prolonged cycle tours or ultra-distance triathlons may be affected.

Thus, higher than normal (reference nutrient intakes (RNI)) protein, and energy intakes are required by resistance-trained and endurance athletes (Lemon, 1995; Tarnopolsky, 1999) and will be discussed in the following text.

Further advantages for protein intake appear apparent for athletes who are involved in glycogen-depleting exercise. Timing of ingestion is a factor that influences protein balance since muscle protein synthesis is enhanced when protein is consumed as soon as possible after intense exercise, rather than waiting for more than 2 hours or longer before consuming protein (Burd et al, 2009; Kumar et al, 2009). When protein is co-ingested with carbohydrate *in the recovery phase after exercise*, it may have the following effects:

- It increases mixed skeletal muscle fractional synthetic rate (Howarth et al, 2009).
- It improves net protein balance (Rasmussen et al, 2000; Howarth et al, 2009; Hulston et al, 2010).
- It enhances glycogen re-synthesis (Ivy et al, 2002).
- It attenuates muscle soreness (Luden et al, 2007).

Estimating protein requirements

Protein requirements are most frequently determined by measuring nitrogen balance. As protein contains nitrogen (1 g nitrogen is equivalent to 6.35 g protein), when the intake of nitrogen (protein) is equal to nitrogen (protein) excretion, a state of nitrogen balance or nitrogen equilibrium is achieved. Whether the body is in an anabolic state (building up tissue and muscle) or catabolic state (breaking down tissue and muscle), when protein is metabolised nitrogen is excreted by urine, faeces, sweat and other secretions (skin, hair, nails). The amount of nitrogen excreted in the urine, faeces and sweat can be measured as a reflection of protein breakdown in the body.

A nitrogen balance of >5 g/day (measured by urea content in urine) is considered to be positive (nitrogen balance) for healthy adults (Todorovic and Micklewright, 2000), although in exercise and sport, training adaptations may improve protein retention to a greater extent.

Nitrogen balance (g/day) = nitrogen intake − nitrogen output

However, although 90% of nitrogen excretion is through urea, this way of measurement would underestimate nitrogen losses for healthy individuals like athletes, as it does not take into account the increasing amount of nitrogen lost through sweat as a result of intense exercise training. In the aforementioned equation, nitrogen output *does* take into consideration obligatory nitrogen losses through hair, skin and faeces, although just 2–4 g nitrogen loss/day are considered. Consolazio (1983) reported a much higher increase in daily sweat nitrogen losses (up to 16–18 g protein/day), which accompany increasing physical activity and high environmental temperatures. Increased nitrogen losses in sweat during exercise is an important consideration for estimating protein requirements, especially in a low-carbohydrate diet (or a carbohydrate-depleted state) (Lemon and Nagle, 1981) when protein breakdown increases.

Positive nitrogen balance is when nitrogen (protein) intake exceeds nitrogen excretion. It occurs when new protein tissues are synthesised, and is favourable for tissue maintenance, and muscle growth and development. Negative nitrogen balance is when nitrogen excretion exceeds nitrogen intake. It occurs when energy intake is low and protein tissue is used for energy, or if protein intake is inadequate or as a result of catabolic disease states.

As protein is needed in growth and development and the maintenance of tissues, the RNI for each group of the population that has been estimated, and is based mainly on age, gender and the lifecycle.

Protein requirements for exercise and sport training and recovery

In the United Kingdom, the RNI for protein in adults is set at 0.75 g of protein/kg BW/day, equivalent to 55.5 g protein/day for men aged 19–50 years, and 45.0 g protein/day for same-aged women (DH, 1991). Inconsistencies in the literature exist with regards to establishment of protein requirements by athletes, most likely due to techniques used to study protein and amino acid metabolism, which range from simplistic measurements to invasive and expensive techniques. Nitrogen balance is the most common method used to determine protein requirements, and has frequently been used to establish the protein needs of endurance and resistance-trained athletes. Other methods that have provided more evidence for protein metabolism during exercise include measurement of urea in urine and sweat, arterial and venous blood differences and metabolic-tracer technologies.

For many years, experts argued that the RNI values (UK) or Recommended Dietary Allowances (RDA) of other countries were sufficient to meet the needs of exercise training, and that extra supplementation or increased dietary intake would not be necessary. No additional protein recommendations have been stipulated for active individuals in the RNI/RDA tables. Further evidence for the notion was provided by dietary intake studies of populations, which reveals that adults consume more protein than the RNI. For example, the average daily intake of protein in the United Kingdom is higher than the RNI. The National Diet and Nutrition Survey showed that men consume 88 g of protein, and women, 64 g, providing about 16% of total energy intake in the (average) British diet (Henderson et al, 2003).

Although protein is not the fundamental energy-giving nutrient contributing to exercise performance, participation in exercise and sport does increase the requirement for protein beyond normal levels, especially after exercise in the recovery phase, to repair muscle damage caused by endurance exercise and to stimulate protein anabolism following resistance exercise. Experts have established that trained athletes have higher protein requirements than the RDA of 0.8 g protein/kg BW/day (Lemon, 1995; Tarnopolsky, 1999). Since endurance training stimulates and increases the muscle's oxidative capacity and resistance training augments gains in muscle size and strength, the optimal protein intake may be different for these two groups of athletes. Intensity and duration of exercise and dietary intake also play a role in the level of protein requirement by individual athletes. Recommendations from the literature suggest that endurance athletes require between 1.2 and 1.4 g protein/kg BW/day, whereas resistance-trained and strength and power athletes require 1.7 g protein/kg BW/day (Lemon, 1995; Tipton and Wolfe, 2004; Rodriguez et al, 2009). Although, it has been suggested that 1.6 g protein/kg BW/day is the *maximal* requirement for top-level athletes (Tarnopolsky, 2004). As a proportion of total energy intake, protein should ideally provide 12–15% of total energy intake. Burke and Deakin (2006) provide recommendations for other groups of athletes, such as recreational endurance athletes, novice and experienced resistance athletes and women. They suggest that recreational endurance athletes who exercise for four to five times a week for 30 minutes at <55% VO_2max, require between 0.8 and 1.0 g protein/kg/day, not more than the requirements of sedentary men and women. Experienced, well-trained resistance athletes (in the steady state of training) require enough protein only to maintain protein balance, i.e. 1.0–1.2 g/kg/day. They suggest that when calculating protein needs of women, their requirements are set at approximately 15% lower than male athletes.

Dietary intake studies show that the habitual diets of many athletes already contain the aforementioned (increased) protein values (more than the RNI/RDA) and do not require additional protein. Groups with the highest consumption of protein are most commonly strength and power athletes, who consume a high proportion of total energy intake from protein-rich foods. Strength athletes not only consume high calorie intakes of around 6400 kcal (Alway et al, 1992), but elite male body builders have protein intakes of more than twice the RDA (2.1 g/kg BW/day) and females as much as three times the RDA (2.8 g/kg BW/day) (Kleiner et al, 1990), which may increase further as they prepare for competition.

Similar findings were reported by Van Erp-Baart et al (1989), regarding Tour de France cyclists who consume a 63% carbohydrate-rich diet. A close relation was found between energy intake and protein. Reported energy intakes were high (6500 kcal) and as energy intake increased, so did protein intake. Cyclists ingested an average of 2.5 g protein/kg BW/day, and in extreme cases, up to 3 g/kg BW/day. Energy balance seems to be equally or more important factor than nitrogen (protein) intake in determining nitrogen balance. When exercising men were given varying energy and protein intakes, nitrogen balance improved as energy intake increased, irrespective of the nitrogen intake (Todd et al, 1984).

Typically, other endurance athletes also consume more than the RNI/RDA for protein. Studies show their daily intake to be well within the recommendations for athletes, around 1.2–1.7 g protein/kg BW/day. On average, protein from the diet of elite endurance athletes provides 10–17% of total energy intake (Van Erp-Baart et al, 1989; Coetzer et al, 1993; Onywera et al, 2004).

Even recreational (non-elite) athletes are consuming protein in excess of the RNI/RDA values. Studies of athletes of various sports codes have found that athletes consume between 1.2 and 1.4 g protein/kg BW/day that is close to 17% protein energy (Hinton et al, 2004). One study found that male recreational triathletes consumed as much as 2.0 g protein/kg BW/day (16% protein energy), while females consumed 1.6 g protein/kg BW/day (15% protein energy) (Nogueira and Da Costa, 2004).

The habitual diets of British adults similarly reveal a diet high in protein and sufficient to cover the needs of a vast majority of athletes. For athletes with increased energy demands, it appears from the literature that as long as energy expenditure is matched by adequate energy intake, protein intake is sufficient and there is no need to supplement the diet with additional protein.

Mass building: increasing muscle size

Muscle hypertrophy refers to an increase in muscle size. Although hereditary factors and level of testosterone play a role in an individual's basic muscle size, with resistance training, muscles can grow an additional 30–60% in size (Guyton, 1984). Gains in muscle size are associated with gains in strength.

Protein, specifically amino acids, has been hailed as nutrients that enhance the size and strength of muscles. Misunderstanding about sports nutrition and inadequacies regarding the translation of theory into practice is still rife in resistance and strength-trained athletes. To add to the confusion, in an effort to lure athletes to buy their products, supplement companies use theories about proteins to make claims about its performance- and strength-enhancing abilities. They produce products containing individual amino acids or protein derivatives with little scientific evidence to back the claims. Many 'mass builder' products adorn the shelves of pharmacies and health shops and these products endorse the theory that excessive quantities of amino acids or protein alone causes weight gain. As a result, many athletes are convinced that they need extra protein or supplementation because a sufficient amount of, and/or good quality protein cannot be obtained from diet (food) alone.

Amino acids do stimulate muscle protein synthesis and as little as 6 g EAAs(indispensable) alone can achieve muscle protein synthesis after resistance exercise (Børsheim et al, 2002). Consumption of ∼20 g of a high-quality protein such as whole milk protein, supplies enough protein for the maximal synthetic response, demonstrating that there is no benefit of ingesting more protein (Kumar et al, 2009). Successful weight gain is dependant on a positive nitrogen balance, especially for an extended period of time, and will provide an opportunity for increase in muscle size and strength. However, as the aforementioned literature shows, energy intake is equally or more important than protein intake when it comes to nitrogen balance.

The use of branched chain amino acids, namely isoleucine, leucine and valine, has been widely promoted in resistance-trained athletes. Leucine is known to stimulate protein synthesis and anabolism. However, claims that leucine increases muscle mass during resistance training are unsupported in humans (Tipton, 2010), since *added* leucine ingestion does not enhance the anabolic response to resistance exercise above that of whey protein alone (Tipton et al, 2009). Hence, evidence-based supplement programmes no longer support the use of branched chain amino acids supplementation by athletes.

The requirements for protein based on body weight for athletes in the early stages of high-intensity (or load) resistance training, is higher than in the later maintenance stage/steady-state, or when there no further increase in load to the muscles. In the early stages of resistance training, increased protein breakdown is indicated by negative nitrogen balance, which heralds higher protein intakes to facilitate protein synthesis. However, negative nitrogen balance last only for about 12 days of training, and as protein retention improves, nitrogen equilibrium is reached (Gontzea et al, 1975).

Therefore, recommendations for protein intake in the early stages of resistance training would be higher (1.6–1.7 g protein/kg BW/day), due to increases in muscle load and to achieve a highly positive nitrogen balance, than in the steady state of training where maintenance is required (1.0–1.2 g/kg BW/day). Muscle hypertrophy can occur with much lower rate of protein intake (1.2 g/kg BW/day) (reported by Phillips (2009)).

However, far greater protein intakes have been reported, as in a nationwide survey of body builders, who had high recorded intakes of 2.5 g protein/kg BW/day (Van Erp-Baart et al, 1989). Even if athletes consume higher protein intakes than what is needed, the excess will simply be oxidised.

Muscle gains may be achieved more effectively by concentrating on the composition of ingested protein and amino acids, timing of ingestion, and the co-ingestion with other nutrients (Tipton and Wolfe, 2004). To promote muscle growth by stimulating protein synthesis, Børsheim et al (2004) showed that after resistance training, a mixture of 17.5 g whey protein, 4.9 g amino acids and 77.4 g carbohydrate stimulated muscle protein synthesis to a greater extent than a 100 g (isoenergetic) carbohydrate drink alone. By adding protein to the amino acid and carbohydrate mixture, the response also lasted longer, beyond the 1st hour after intake.

Similar findings were reported by Rasmussen et al (2000) whose participants ingested a 6 g EAAs and 35 g carbohydrate mixture. Although, when one study compared *timing* of intake using the same mixture, they found a greater net muscle protein balance when the mixture was ingested *before* exercise than when ingested immediately after exercise (Tipton et al, 2001).

As long as energy expenditure is matched by energy intake, extra protein *beyond* the recommended amount for strength athletes will not provide any further benefits. These athletes are better off focusing on the composition of their diets and timing of nutrient intake after training. Besides, excessive protein intake may not be advantageous, it may only be oxidised, and in extreme cases may pose some serious health risks.

Harmful effects of high dietary intakes of protein

Extra protein intake beyond the need of the body is in fact an expensive and wasteful way to gain weight, and is unlikely to cause gains in lean body tissue as much of the protein cannot be stored or added to body cells and tissues that are already in positive nitrogen balance. In effect, there is a limitation to how much protein tissue can be accumulated (Butterfield, 1987). Extra protein intake provided by excessive protein intake is either used as energy (converted to glucose in the liver), or stored as fat, which increases nitrogen excretion in the urine. Furthermore, a high protein intake above recommended levels (15% of total energy intake) can lead to ketosis, dehydration, calcium loss, gout and stress to the kidney (Mahan and Arlin, 1992) and liver.

- *Ketosis*:
  Ketosis is brought on by a low-calorie, low- or no-carbohydrate diet. Ketones are excreted in the urine, disturbing the acid-base balance in the body.
- *Dehydration*:
  As protein intake increases, so does nitrogen waste, which in turn increases water loss (through urine, sweat and other secretions). About 50 mL of water is lost with each gram of urea in urine (McArdle et al, 2006). Dehydration is also a symptom of ketosis, as water and electrolytes are lost with ketones in the urine.
- *Calcium losses*:
  High-protein diets increase calcium losses in the urine, compromising bone health and increasing the risk of bone demineralisation that lead to bone-related disease later in life.
- *Gout*:
  Gout, manifested by sudden and recurring attacks of painful arthritis, is triggered by intake of large amounts of protein-rich foods, among other factors (Escott-Stump, 2002).
- *Kidney damage*:
  High protein intake puts undue stress on the kidneys as they force them to excrete excess nitrogen as urea. People with reduced kidney function (in the case of having one kidney or kidney disease) or who want to maintain kidney function (diabetics) are at risk of kidney damage if they consume high-protein diets.
- *Increase in blood fats (lipoproteins)*:
  A high intake of protein-rich foods from animal sources leads to a high saturated fat and cholesterol intake, which are risk factors for heart disease and certain cancers. Individuals with a family history of heart disease or hyperlipidaemia should focus on healthier protein choices, including plant sources.

It seems that in some individuals, high-protein diets are not suitable and may lead to damaging effects on their health. However, most healthy athletes are unlikely to suffer the effects of high-protein diets and are advised to pay attention to the following dietary practices:

- Consume enough fluids.
- Be aware of dietary calcium RNIs and ensure that calcium needs are met.
- Choose leaner cuts of red meat and reduce consumption; rather choose poultry, fish, pulses, nuts and seeds to make up protein requirements.

Protein: role in weight management

Protein makes up a large part of muscle. A high proportion of muscle mass raises the metabolic rate and burns more energy, facilitating fat loss. Eating more protein improves satiation and thermogenesis (non-voluntary physical activity such as fidgeting) (Westererp-Plantenga et al, 1999), although evidence for the amount of protein optimising weight management is lacking. Protein also improves insulin sensitivity, discouraging the storage of fat, especially abdominal fat.

Proteins and allergic reactions

Many proteins are an integral part of the immune system, and therefore, have a role in immunity. As the immune system distinguishes self from non-self, sometimes a food substance is treated as non-self, thus bringing forth an allergic (immune) response. Allergens are usually proteins or glycoproteins that are able to invoke an immune response causing adverse health effects (allergy). The allergen may be food related, or other environmental allergen (e.g. airborne allergen). Although a wide variety of foods from all food groups can cause allergic reactions, many of the common food allergens are protein-rich foods. Table 5.4 lists the common food allergens. Allergy is not such a common occurrence in adults. Its prevalence is in 1% of adults, with adverse reactions to food (food intolerance) occurring in 1–2% of adults. Symptoms of food allergy include itching, redness and swelling of the mouth, throat and skin, vomiting, diarrhea, hives, eczema and respiratory symptoms including the life-threatening anaphylaxis. Adverse food reactions (food intolerance) can manifest in various body systems such as the skin, gut and the respiratory system. Symptoms can include (among others) abdominal pain, constipation, irritable bowel syndrome, asthma, migraine, attention deficit hyperactivity disorder

Table 5.4 Common foods provoking food allergy.

Food allergen
Cow's milk
Hen's eggs
Peanuts
Various tree nuts
Soy legumes
Fish
Shellfish
Wheat
Other foods
Fruits and vegetables

Source: Adapted from Buttriss (2002).

(ADHD, in children), vaginal discharge and rheumatoid arthritis (Buttriss, 2002).

Protein foods that are high in fat

In an attempt to improve protein quality of their diets, athletes could use the following guidelines to obtain better quality protein in their diets. It is useful for certain athletes, i.e. those who are on weight-reducing programmes or competitive athletes on a carbohydrate-loading regime to know that foods like cheese, sausage and other processed meats (e.g. bangers) have a high fat content and are more fat-rich than protein-rich. Eating these foods frequently could affect the proportion of protein and fat in the diet.

Further tips to improve the quality of protein foods are as follows:
- Remove the skin of poultry and the fat of meat before cooking.
- Choose white meat without the skin, like chicken breast, rather than dark meat (chicken drumstick or wing).
- Choose medium-fat or low-fat dairy products (cheese, milk, yoghurt).
- Reduce consumption of red meats, especially fatty meats like lamb.
- Use healthy cooking methods like grilling, steaming, oven baking, quick stir frying, microwaving or barbecuing food rather than frying or roasting food. Avoid burnt food.
- Use minimal oil when preparing meat, chicken or fish, and avoid lard, ghee or butter when preparing food.
- When purchasing tinned fish, choose fish in water, brine or tomato sauce, rather than fish tinned in oil or mayonnaise.

Chapter summary

- Amino acids are the building blocks of protein, the simplest form of the nutrient that contain and supply nitrogen to the body along with other elements such as sulphur, phosphorous and iron.

- Essential amino acids (EAAs) namely histidine, isoleucine, leucine, lycine, methionine, phenylalanine, threonine, tryptophan and valine, cannot be made in the body and can only be obtained from food sources.

- Foods containing proteins are from animal-derived products, such as meat, poultry, fish, eggs and milk products and plant sources such as vegetables, soy beans, legumes (pulses like lentils), nuts, seeds and grains (breads, cereals, rice).

- Combining a variety of foods from plant sources together will ensure that all EAAs are present to be used by the body for tissue growth and repair, e.g. baked beans on toasted bread.

- All proteins are measured against the amino acid profile of egg white, which is regarded as the gold standard of protein-rich food with a score or rating, known as biologic value (BV) of 100. Factor 100 denotes the percentage of nitrogen absorbed that is retained by the body.

- Protein are not stored in one place but is part of all cells and nearly all fluids in the body, including hair, skin, nails, bones, ligaments, teeth and blood. The largest concentration is found in skeletal muscle, and regular resistance training can be a stimulus for further muscle hypertrophy.

- Protein is responsible for maintenance and growth of tissues, and plays a role in several metabolic and physiological regulation processes. During exercise, it provides an added fuel source during exercise, maintains, reconditions and increases lean body mass, facilitates protein synthesis of enzymes, replaces protein breakdown, repairs exercise-induced muscle damage, maintains and increases lean body mass (due to hypertrophic stimulus of resistance exercise) and maintains and increases muscular strength and power.

- Protein synthesis increases in the recovery phase after aerobic exercise, especially in athletes who are involved in glycogen-depleting exercise.

- Proteins co-ingested with carbohydrate in the recovery phase after exercise may improve net protein balance, enhance glycogen re-synthesis and reduce muscle soreness.

- Protein contains nitrogen and a nitrogen balance of >5 g/day (measured by urea content in urine) is considered to be positive (nitrogen balance) for healthy adults, although training adaptations in exercise and sport may improve protein retention to a greater extent.

- Reference nutrient intake (RNI) for protein in adults is 0.75 g of protein/kg BW/day, equivalent to 55.5 g protein/day for men aged 19–50 years, and 45.0 g protein/day for same-aged women.

- Protein recommendations for endurance athletes are between 1.2 and 1.4 g protein/kg BW/day, whereas resistance-trained, strength and power athletes may require 1.7 g protein/kg BW/day.

- Muscle hypertrophy can occur at protein intake rates of 1.2 g/kg BW/day. However, current recommendations suggest an intake of 1.6–1.7 g/kg BW/day in the early stages of resistance training due to increases in muscle load and to achieve a highly positive nitrogen balance, and 1.0–1.2 g/kg BW/day in the steady state of training where maintenance is required.
- Extra protein intake beyond the needs of the body is unlikely to cause gains in lean body tissue as much of the protein cannot be stored or added to body cells and tissues that are already in positive nitrogen balance. Excessive protein intake is either used as energy (converted to glucose in the liver) or stored as fat, which increases nitrogen excretion in the urine.
- The risks associated with high protein intakes above recommended levels can lead to ketosis, dehydration, calcium loss, gout, stress to the kidney and liver and can raise blood fat levels.
- Protein has a role in weight management as it improves insulin sensitivity, discouraging the storage of fat, especially abdominal fat. A high proportion of muscle mass raises the metabolic rate and burns more energy.
- Many proteins are an integral part of the immune system and many of the common food allergens are protein-rich foods, including cow's milk, hen's eggs and shellfish.

Note

1 The word protein comes from the Greek word meaning 'to take first place', or 'of prime importance'.

Protein-Rich Dishes

Recall that protein reserves are found in all forms in the body and dietary protein is, therefore, an essential part of the diet. Whether you prefer plant proteins or a combination of plant and animal proteins, either can provide complete proteins for tissue growth and maintenance. A variety of foods in the diet will ensure that the EAAs are obtained.

Bean and Lentil Burgers

(Serves 4)

Ingredients

10 mL sunflower oil

1 large onion, chopped

2 garlic cloves, chopped

3 mL curry powder

1 × 400 g (14 oz) red kidney beans, drained

1 × 400 g (14 oz) lentils, drained

10 mL lime or lemon juice

5 mL coriander, chopped

5 mL parsley, chopped

Salt and freshly ground pepper

Breadcrumbs, for coating

8 slices wholegrain bread

4 tomatoes, sliced

100 g lettuce, shredded

Method

1 Sauté the onion and garlic in the oil. Add the curry powder and sauté for another minute.
2 Add the beans and lentils. Cook for 3 minutes and set aside to cool for 30 minutes.
3 Transfer the mixture to a food processor and add the rest of the ingredients (blend till a coarse puree).
4 If necessary, add a little breadcrumb for a firmer mixture.
5 Form 4–8 burgers and coat them with breadcrumbs.
6 Grill or fry the burgers for 2–3 minutes on each side.
7 Serve with wholegrain bread, lettuce and tomatoes.

Nutrition analysis per portion

Energy	457 kcal (1919 kJ)
Protein	22 g
Carbohydrate	63 g
Fat	5.2 g
Cholesterol	0 mg
Fibre	17 g

(Continued)

(*Continued*)

Food note: This recipe is a healthy vegetarian option providing a grain (bread) with legumes (kidney beans and lentils) to make a complete protein. The high carbohydrate content makes it ideal for loading and refuelling glycogen stores.

Bean Curry

(Serves 4–6)

Ingredients

20 mL sunflower oil

1 onion chopped

2 garlic cloves

1 bay leaf

10 mL mild curry powder

10 mL turmeric powder

300 g new potatoes, quartered

2 × 400 g tins soya beans, drained

1 × 400 g tin split red lentils, drained

Salt and pepper

Parsley

Method

1 Sauté the onions and garlic in the oil until translucent.
2 Add the bay leaf, curry and turmeric powders. Fry for 1 minute and add the potatoes. Cover with water and boil until tender, but not soft.
3 Add the beans and lentils and simmer for 15–20 minutes.
4 Season with salt and pepper.
5 Garnish with parsley.

Nutrition analysis per portion

Energy	528 kcal (2217 kJ)
Protein	36 g
Carbohydrate	35 g
Fat	20 g
Cholesterol	0 mg
Fibre	15.3 g

Food note: Turmeric contains *curcumin*, which has anti-inflammatory properties.

Lemon and Honey Chicken

(Serves 4)

Ingredients

8 chicken thighs and drumsticks, skinned   Thyme
4 cloves garlic, crushed   Salt and freshly ground pepper
3 lemons, zest and juice   20 mL olive oil
90 mL honey, melted

Method

1 Preheat the oven to 190°C.
2 Marinate the chicken in the garlic, lemon zest and juice, honey and
   thyme for 1 hour.
3 Season the chicken and place them in an oiled baking dish.
4 Bake for 30–40 minutes, or until golden brown (Be sure to turn the
   chicken once during the cooking process and baste it with the gravy
   accumulating in the baking dish. This will ensure that the chicken stays
   moist).
5 Serve with mashed butter beans.

Tip: for quicker preparation use a roasting bag and cook the dish in the
microwave. It may save half the cooking time.

Nutrition analysis per portion

Energy	355 kcal (1489 kJ)
Protein	34 g
Carbohydrate	25 g
Fat	10.3 g
Cholesterol	86 mg
Fibre	5 g

Food note: Lemons bring out the natural flavour of chicken, together
they are a good combination as the vitamin C in lemons are good for
immunity and protection of blood vessels.

Peppered Beef Fillet with Haricot Bean Mash

(Serves 4)

Ingredients

Beef Fillet:

400 g beef fillet

30 mL olive oil

10 mL freshly ground pepper

Salt to taste

5 mL sunflower oil

Mash:

250 g potatoes, boiled

1 × 400 g haricot beans, drained

180 mL low-fat milk, heated

1 garlic clove, crushed

Salt and pepper

Method

1 Preheat the oven to 200°C.

2 Rub the olive oil onto the fillet, followed by the salt and ground pepper

3 Heat a large pan and add the sunflower oil. Heat until smoking point.

4 Sear the beef fillet for 1 minute and rotate until all the sides have been seared.

5 Remove the fillet from the pan and bake for 20 minutes in the oven.

6 Mash the beans and potatoes together and add the heated milk, garlic, salt and pepper.

7 Serve the fillet and mash while warm with vegetables.

Nutrition analysis per portion

Energy	450 kcal (1892 kJ)
Protein	40 g
Carbohydrate	27 g
Fat	17.5 g
Cholesterol	96 mg
Fibre	6 g

Food note: A high-protein dish. Beef is rich in iron and zinc. The combination of the haricot beans with mashed potato lowers the GI of the dish.

Roasted Spicy Chicken

(Serves 3–6)

Ingredients

5 g chilli, red, chopped

2 mL ground mustard seeds

5 mL lemon juice

6 different chicken cuts, skinned

5 mL ground turmeric

2 mL freshly ground black pepper

40 mL olive oil

Method

1 Preheat the oven to 190°C.

2 Mix the spices, lemon juice and oil together to form a paste.

3 Rub the paste into the chicken.

4 Bake the chicken for 30–40 minutes or until done.

5 Serve with peas or couscous.

Nutrition analysis per portion

Energy	186 kcal (780 kJ)
Protein	33 g
Carbohydrate	0.7 g
Fat	5.4 g
Cholesterol	86 mg
Fibre	0.3 g

Food note: A lean protein-rich dish. Chicken is also rich in niacin, zinc and iron. The dark meat is higher in fat than white chicken but it has a higher mineral content.

Seafood Curry

(Serves 4)

Ingredients

20 mL sunflower oil
4 shallots, chopped
2 garlic cloves, crushed
3 g fresh ginger, chopped
10 mL/5 g mild curry powder
10 mL/3 g turmeric powder
1 × 400 g can reduced-fat coconut milk
1 kg (2.25 lb) seafood mix (500 g black shell mussels (scrubbed and beards removed); 250 g monkfish fillets (cubed); 250 g prawns) *or* marinara mix
20 mL/5 g coriander leaves, roughly chopped

Method

1 Sauté the shallots, ginger and garlic in the oil until translucent.
2 Add the curry and turmeric powders and sauté for another minute.
3 Pour in the coconut milk and simmer for 15–20 minutes.
4 Add the seafood mix and simmer for 10–20 minutes (*Hint*: if the sauce has a very runny consistency, grate in a medium-sized potato and simmer).
5 Stir in the coriander and serve with rice.

Nutrition analysis per portion

Energy	406 kcal (1704 kJ)
Protein	58 g
Carbohydrate	14 g
Fat	13 g
Cholesterol	235 mg
Fibre	1.5 g

Food note: Very high protein dish that can easily provide ~60–70% of the daily protein needs for most athletes. Shellfish is rich in minerals and while it is a source of cholesterol, it does not tend to raise blood fat levels.

Smoked Cod Risotto

(Serves 4)

Ingredients

20 mL sunflower oil	1.5 L fish stock/vegetable stock/water
2 onions, chopped	50 g frozen peas
3 garlic cloves, crushed	400 g smoked cod fillets, cubed
100 g button mushrooms, sliced	Salt and freshly ground pepper
350 g Arborio rice	

Method

1 Sauté the onions and the garlic in the oil until translucent.
2 Add the mushrooms and rice, sauté for another 2 minutes.
3 Add the stock and add little at a time until the stock has been absorbed by the rice. Use all the stock.
4 Add the peas and fish. Simmer for another 5 minutes. Season to taste.

Nutrition analysis per portion

Energy	292 kcal (1227 kJ)
Protein	29 g
Carbohydrate	27 g
Fat	6.4 g
Cholesterol	79 mg
Fibre	2 g

Food note: Arborio rice is a short-grained plump and chewy rice that is rich in carbohydrates. It is highly absorbent but does not cook as soft as other rice.

Sweet and Sour Pork with Noodles

(Serves 4)

Ingredients

400 g pork fillet, cut into strips

60 mL low-sodium soya sauce

5 g ginger, chopped

1 clove garlic, chopped

20 mL honey

1 red chilli, seeded and chopped

10 mL peanut oil

2 zucchinis, sliced

Pepper

250 g egg noodles

Method

1 Marinate the fillet in the soya sauce, ginger, garlic, honey and chilli for 1 hour.

2 Stir-fry the pork in the peanut oil for 5 minutes.

3 Add the zucchini and stir-fry for another 4 minutes. Season with pepper.

4 Soak the egg noodles in boiling water until tender.

5 Serve warm and spoon the pork onto the noodles.

Nutrition analysis per portion

Energy	333 kcal (1401 kJ)
Protein	34.5 g
Carbohydrate	20 g
Fat	12 g
Cholesterol	106.5 mg
Fibre	2 g

Food note: A good eat-in menu as it is lower in fat and salt than the take-away version.

CHAPTER 6

Fats

Key terms

Dietary fats
Free fatty acids (FFAs)
Triglyceride
Essential fatty acids (EFA)
Lipoproteins
Saturated fat (SFA)
Unsaturated fat
Monounsaturated fat (MUFA)
Polyunsaturated fat (PUFA)
Intramuscular triacylglycerol (IMTG)
Phospholipids
Cholesterol
Linolenic acid
Linoleic acid

'Fat loading'
Long chain triglycerides (LCT)
Medium chain triglycerides (MCT)
Hyperlipidaemia
Obesity
Android fat distribution
Gynoid fat distribution
'Apple shape'
'Pear shape'
Waist circumference
Weight management
Very low calorie diets (VLCD)
Excess post-exercise oxygen consumption
   (EPOC)

Fats and oils are just some of the many lipids, a group of organic compounds, that do not dissolve in water. Other fat-like substances, like cholesterol, add to the diversity of lipid forms that also include the following:
- Free fatty acids (FFAs)
- Plasma triacylglycerol/triglycerides (triglyceride is regarded as a trivial name for triacylglycerol)
- Intramuscular triglyceride (IMTG)
- Essential fatty acids (EFA), i.e. linoleic acid and linolenic acid
- Sterols (plasma triglyceride), including cholesterol, steroid hormones, vitamin D and bile salts

Nutrition for Sport and Exercise: A Practical Guide, First Edition. Hayley Daries.
© 2012 Blackwell Publishing Ltd. Published 2012 by Blackwell Publishing Ltd.

- Phospholipids, including lecithins, cephalins and sphingomyelins
- Glycolipids (cerebrosides and gangliosides)
- Sulpholipids
- Lipoproteins (LDL, HDL and VLDL)
- Fat-soluble vitamins A, E and K

The most important dietary simple lipids are triglycerides. It consists of 1 unit of glycerol and 3 units of fatty acids. Although the simplest fat or building block is a fatty acid, which occurs in food and is part of every cell in the body, most fats are in the form of triglycerides that is constantly being broken down, transported and rebuilt. Fatty acids are either saturated or unsaturated. Most fat-rich foods and liquids contain a measure of saturated fat (SFA) or unsaturated fat. SFA is derived mostly from animals, which are solid (beef, lamb fat and butter fat) or semi-solid (chicken or pork fat) at room temperature, and regarded as hard fats. Some plant sources contain SFAs that are liquid at room temperature, such as palm oil and coconut oil. Of all the commonly eaten dietary fats, coconut oil has the highest proportion of SFA (92%). In comparison, butter fat is 66% saturated and sunflower oil is 11% saturated. Fat is dense in energy, providing 9 kcal (37 kJ) per gram of energy. A small amount of fat contains many calories. Desiccated coconut, the type used on coconut marshmallows, in sweets and cakes, contains 661 kcal per 100 g (or 66 kcal per tablespoon). A diet high in SFA has adverse health effects and can lead to certain types of cancer, increased blood fats and heart disease. The SFA in coconut does not have the same detrimental health effects as hard animal fats. It may actually be good for health.

Unsaturated fatty acids include monounsaturated fatty acids (MUFAs) and polyunsaturated fatty acids (PUFAs), and are derived mostly from plant sources and some animal sources. Classification of fatty acids is based on the highest concentration of either SFA, MUFA or PUFA. For example, olive oil is considered as a MUFA, as 77% of it consists of MUFAs, with 14% saturated and 9% polyunsaturated. Canola oil is also a MUFA, and in contrast with other oils, it has the lowest proportion of SFA (6%).

A group of PUFAs cannot be synthesised by the body and has to come from dietary sources. These are called essential fatty acids (EFA). Alpha-linolenic acid, an EFA, is synthesised from omega-3 fats in the diet, i.e. from oily fish, walnuts and flaxseeds. Linoleic acid, the other EFA, is synthesised from omega-6 fats like sunflower, cottonseed and soybean oil. Non-essential fatty acids are synthesised in the body by either alpha-linolenic acid or linoleic acid. Docosahexaenoic acid (DHA) and Eicosapentaenoic acid (EPA) are synthesised from alpha-linolenic acid. Dihomo gamma-linolenic acid and Arachidonic acid is synthesised in the body by linoleic acid. Table 6.1 provides a list of plant and animal sources of fatty acids.

Table 6.1 Food sources of fats.

Fatty acid	Major food sources (with highest concentration of the fatty acid)	
	Plant	Animal
Polyunsaturated	Cornflower oil, safflower oil, sunflower oil, flaxseed oil, cottonseed oil, soybean oil, sunflower spread, rapeseed oil, walnuts, brazil nuts, sunflower seeds, pumpkin seeds	Fish oil, oily fish such as canned and fresh sardines, pilchards, mackerel, herring, kippers, salmon, anchovies, trout and fresh roe, fresh tuna (bluefin)
Omega-3	Flaxseed oil, pumpkin seeds, hemp oil	(as above)
Omega-6	Safflower oil, corn oil, sunflower oil, soybean oil, walnut oil	None
Monounsaturated Omega-9	Hazelnuts, avocado pears, olive oil, almonds, rapeseed oil/canola oil, peanut oil, groundnut oil, sesame oil, olive spread, canola spread, cashew nuts, pecan nuts	None
Saturated fat	Palm kernel oil, coconut oil, desiccated coconut, hard margarine, vegetable fats, coffee creamers	Butter, lard, ghee, cream, butter, full cream milk, eggs and cheese, sausage, processed meats, fat of bacon, meat, pork, skin and fat of chicken and turkey, desserts, biscuits, pies, pastries
Other dietary fats Cholesterol[a]		Organ meats, egg yolk, some shellfish, caviar, red meat (beef, lamb, mutton) and pork, tongue, duck, chicken, turkey, dairy products like butter, cream, full cream milk and cheese
Trans fat	Partially hydrogenated vegetable oils, fried foods, hard margarines, cooking fats, some soft margarines, manufactured baked products, e.g. pies, pastries, biscuits, cakes	

Source: Material from Hayley Daries Practice.
[a]Many other animal foods contain cholesterol, although just some of the highest sources are listed.

Functions of fat

Primary function: energy source

Fat is the most concentrated source of energy and is twice as calorie dense as carbohydrates and proteins. Although fats are easily stored, circulating glucose and amino acids not used are manufactured into fats and stored. Fat in the body is comprised of storage fat (under the skin, in muscle tissue and in the abdomen between the organs) and essential fat (i.e. bone marrow lipids and central nervous system lipids). A tiny amount of fat circulates in the plasma as FFAs. Fat is stored as triglyceride (triacylglycerol or TG) in small amounts in the circulation. TG is bound to albumin in plasma or integrated into lipoproteins. Such examples are, among others, low-density lipoproteins (LDL or 'bad cholesterol') or high-density lipoprotein (HDL or 'good cholesterol'). There are also abundant stores of TG in adipose tissue. In muscle, a small amount of fat (intramuscular triacylglycerol or IMTG) can be found between muscle fibres, and as fat droplets within muscle cells. Fat from adipose tissue and IMTG act as a near limitless fuel for exercise.

Fat stores in healthy, non-obese adults range between 8% and 25% of the body in men and between 21% and 36% in women, more so in obese individuals. While levels of 10% body fat is considered low by most standards, lower fat levels are reported in elite athletes. Dangerously low fat levels can lead to deterioration in exercise performance and other serious health consequences. For a female weighing 55 kg, 20% body fat equates to 11 kg, and for a male of 75 kg, 16% body fat equates to 12 kg. Most of these fat stores are in the subcutaneous layer (under the skin) that contains 50% of all adipose tissue. In a ~75 kg person with 16% body fat (12 kg), the endogenous fat stores comprise of the following:

- 0.4 g (3.6 kcal) plasma FFAs
- 4 g (36 kcal) plasma TG
- 300 g (2700 kcal) IMTG
- 12,000 g (108,000 kcal) adipose tissue

McArdle et al (2010)

Since a healthy, non-obese male has between 9 and 15 kg of body fat (body weight around 70–80 kg), with just 9 kg of adipose tissue, he has enough fat stores to run continuously at a slow pace (low intensity) for roughly 4320 minutes or 3 days.

Fat weight, not total body weight determines health risk. Various methods are used to measure body composition (fatness and lean mass), and some include determination of fat tissue mass (refer also to Chapter 2, Table 2.1):

- *Dual Energy X-ray Absorptiometry (DEXA)*: It passes small doses of radiation through the body to measure bone mineral content and density, fat tissue mass and lean tissue mass.

- *Hydrostatic (underwater) Weighing (HW)*: It estimates total body fat by using the difference between weight measurements on a standard scale, and then submerged in water.
- *Bioelectrical Impedance Analysis (BIA)*: It is based on the conduction of a low-level electrical current in the body and the differences in the ability to conduct electricity between the fat and water components of the body. The more the resistance (or *impedance*) against the current, the higher the body fat reading.
- *Skinfold measurements*: It measures Skinfold Thickness (SF) of the fat layer directly under the skin (subcutaneous fat) using a calliper. Some sites of measurement include triceps, subscapular, suprailiac and thigh skinfolds.
- *Body mass index (BMI)*: It is a height–weight index and has a close relation with estimates of body fatness. A BMI of 20–25 is considered healthy.

Since DEXA is the most accurate way to determine body fat, other methods of estimating body fat percentage have been compared with it. BIA has been found to underestimate body fat percentage compared with DEXA (Eisenkölbl et al, 2001), while other researchers suggested that *DEXA* overestimates body fat percentage compared with BIA (Bolanowski and Nilsson, 2001). Skinfold equation(s) (using skinfold measurements) more accurately estimated body fat percentage compared with BIA (Eckerson et al, 1996). Although all of the aforementioned methods to estimate body fat percentage are used in research and practice, factors such as accessibility to the equipment and technician skill are some considerations to take into account before deciding which method may be most appropriate or useful in a given situation.

Phospholipids are fats that are a primary part of all cell membranes. It is found abundantly in the brain, liver and nervous tissue. Even cholesterol (a sterol) is an essential structural component of cell membranes, and of lipoproteins that carry fat in the blood.

Fat provides insulation and organ padding. The subcutaneous fat layer insulates against cold and prevents heat loss. Critical organs such as the kidneys and the heart are padded by fat for protection.

Fat carries fat-soluble vitamins A, D, E and K, and EFA, linolenic and linoleic acid.

Fat for exercise

Fat is an important source of energy and its contribution to energy supply during exercise is dependent on exercise intensity and duration. Increased FFA oxidation occurs as exercise duration increases, and fat is the major fuel at low exercise intensities. The 'crossover' concept and substrate partitioning of carbohydrate and fat oxidation during exercise are discussed in

Chapter 2. Due to the ample supply of stored fats (triglyceride) in adipose tissue and within muscle fibres, an increase in FFA oxidation may be beneficial to endurance or ultra-endurance athletes. Increasing the reliance on fat can spare muscle and liver glycogen and delay nutrient-related fatigue during prolonged exercise.

Endurance training increases fat oxidation, which decreases the reliance on liver and muscle glycogen stores. Further training adaptations of endurance exercise includes increased fat breakdown, reduced glycogen breakdown, increased number of capillaries and increased fatty acid transport.

IMTG has received interest as a fuel relied on during endurance exercise, with concerns raised about its replenishment after exercise. Spriet and Gibala (2004) highlighted IMTG use during endurance exercise and re-examination of post-exercise recommendations for fat intake. Such new nutritional practices may influence adaptations to training, particularly metabolic changes in fat mobilisation, and oxidation that occur in skeletal muscle.

Dietary fats

All fat-rich foods contain a mixture of different types of fatty acids. Some fat is synthesised in the body and some can only be obtained from dietary sources as the body does not manufacture it. Fats and oils are classified according to the concentration of fatty acid present in the food. Table 6.1 provides some examples of fat-rich foods, classified by fatty acid concentration. Plant sources of fats contain PUFAs including omega-3 and omega-6 fatty acids, MUFAs including omega-9 fatty acids and SFAs. Animal sources of fats contain PUFAs and SFAs.

Dietary Intake of fat

Fats are a very concentrated source of energy and should comprise about one-third of total energy intake, ideally less than 35% of total energy intake. In Britain, the average fat intake in men is 87 g fat (36% of food energy) and in women, 62 g (35% of food energy) (Henderson et al, 2003). The same national survey found that SFA intake is higher (13% of food energy) than recommended (11% of food energy).

The dietary intakes of athletes are discussed in Chapter 2. Most recreational and elite athletes appear to achieve a prudent fat intake within the recommended values. However, certain groups of athletes have higher fat intakes, notably in runners and aquatic athletes. Van Erp-Baart et al

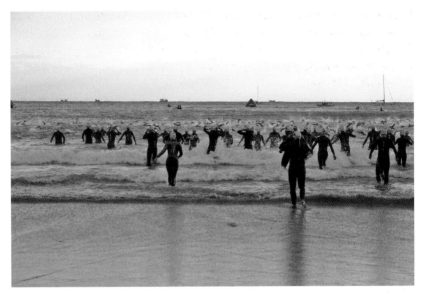

Figure 6.1 Aquatic athletes often consume higher fat intakes, although some groups of elite athletes are prudent consumers of dietary fat.

(1989) and Coetzer et al (1993) found that runners have a high average fat intake per kg body weight, in excess of 1.7 g/kg BW/day (including elite black South African runners studied by Coetzer). In contrast, some groups of African runners (of Kenyan Kalenjin ethnicity) consume very low-fat diets (46 g fat/day or 13.4% of food energy) during training (Onywera et al, 2004). Aquatic athletes have been shown to have higher fat intakes. Greek male swimming and water-polo athletes consume around 40% of food energy in the form of fat, and female aquatic athletes eat 33.9% of food energy as fat (Farajian et al, 2004). Not all female aquatic athletes consume high-fat diets, as Felder et al (1998) found that elite female surfers consume a prudent 27% of energy as fat (Figure 6.1).

Recreational athletes representing various sports consume a moderate amount of fats, as both male and females consume 1.0 g/kg BW/day (Hinton et al, 2004) and recreational triathletes consume on average ~1.2 g/kg BW/day (Worme et al, 1990).

'Fat-loading' diets

Any dietary manipulation that allows the body to use more fat during exercise will be of benefit to endurance athletes, which may explain why some groups of athletes (i.e. endurance-trained athletes) may opt for higher fat consumption levels during training or pre-competition phases. Studies show that athletes achieve enhanced fatty acid oxidation and glycogen sparing after fat-loading diets of 5–7 days, followed by 1–3 days of carbohydrate loading (Burke et al, 2000, 2002; Carey et al, 2001). No performance benefit of high-fat diets (>65% of energy or ≥4 g fat/kg BW/day) could be established in any of the aforementioned trials. Kavouras et al (2004) observed no major effect of a high-fat diet (66% of energy) on 45-minute strenuous cycling performance, compared with that observed following an isocaloric high-carbohydrate diet (75% of energy). High rates of fat oxidation are observed for endurance-trained athletes involved in high-intensity interval training (±86% VO_2 max) who followed a 3-day fat-loading diet (4.6 g fat/kg BW/day), compared with a high-carbohydrate diet. However, although similar performance was observed for both trials, athletes had higher ratings of perceived exertion on day 4 of the high-fat diet (Stepto et al, 2002). Therefore, individual tolerance of high fat intakes should be considered before attempting to start a fat-loading diet.

As fat is oxidised slowly, there are limitations to its consumption *during* exercise. Due to the impracticality of consuming fatty acids during exercise, most dietary fat is consumed as long chain triglycerides (LCTs). LCTs remain in the stomach for over 3 hours and require the enzyme lipase to convert it to FFAs. Medium chain triglycerides (MCTs) are soluble in water and are oxidised almost as quickly as glucose. It is often combined with glucose for quicker gastric emptying and absorption. However, large amounts of MCTs will cause gastrointestinal upset, therefore, intake is restricted. Additionally, a review of evidence shows that MCTs do not benefit exercise performance in most instances (Coyle, 2004).

For health reasons, athletes who want to consume high-fat diets could focus on heart-healthy fats, i.e. essential fats and fats mostly from plants sources, rather than high intakes of hard animal fats. The use of MUFA (olive oil, rapeseed oil) and PUFAs (sunflower oil; fish oils; oily fish) and less SFAs from animal sources, baked goods, cakes and desserts is recommended.

High-fat diets and detrimental health effects

High fat intakes lead to over-consumption of calories, leading to overweight and obesity. A high-fat diet can also raise blood fats, leading to hyperlipidaemia and associated heart disease. Athletes are advised not to follow high-fat diets if they have a family history of raised lipids, heart disease or stroke. For the rest, caution is advised when using high-fat diets for a long term. PUFAs such as omega-3 fats reduce bad cholesterol (LDL) and triglyceride levels; MUFA reduce LDL and can improve good cholesterol

(HDL) levels. SFAs and trans fats increase total cholesterol and LDL, and reduce good cholesterol levels.

It is useful to know which dietary fats increase (↑) or reduce (↓) blood fat levels, and make the necessary changes to consumption levels. Recommended fat intake as a percentage of energy is 35%, of which the average contribution of fatty acids should be as follows:

- Not more than 11% from SFA
- Not more than 2% trans fats
- 6.5% from PUFAs
- At least 0.2% omega-3 fats
- At least 1% omega-6 fats
- ~13% from MUFAs

(Department of Health, 1994)

Overweight and obesity

Obesity (an excess fatness) can negatively affect exercise performance. The factors that affect performance include:

- strength,
- agility,
- mobility,
- muscular appearance,
- speed,
- power, and
- endurance.

Excess fat mass can reduce some or all of these performance indices. For example, excess fat or 'dead' weight will reduce the endurance and speed required by a marathon runner. In weight-category sports such as boxing, leanness is favoured for optimal strength and power, the aim is to have a higher muscle mass to fat ratio.

With regard to the general population, the prevalence of overweight and obesity is rising, especially in developed countries where it has become a major health problem. Globally, there are more than 1 billion overweight people, of whom more than 300 million are obese (WHO, 2003). In Europe, there has been a dramatic rise in obesity, between 10% and 50%, in the last 10 years. More alarmingly, UK surveys report that obesity has risen three-fold or more since 1980. Between 1980 and 1991, obesity (defined by BMI $\geq$25 kg/m^2) in men aged 16–64 years increased from 6% to 13% of men. Over the same period, obesity in women increased from 8% to 16% (Knight, 1984; White et al, 1991). White and colleagues showed that BMI is significantly associated with age, social class and educational qualifications of the UK population.

The Health Survey for England (Department of Health, 1999) revealed that the prevalence of obesity is continuing to rise. The 1999 survey found that in the United Kingdom, 46% of men were overweight and 17% were clinically obese. They found that 32% of women were overweight and 21% were clinically obese. By this time, already, almost half of adults were overweight and at this rate, experts had suggested that 25% of the population would be obese by the year 2010. In fact, the 2009 Health Survey of England showed the increase in obesity prevalence in both men (13–22%) and women (16–24%) since 1994. Overall, 61.3% of adults (aged 16 years and older) were overweight or obese. Sixty-six percent of men were overweight and 22% obese. The percentage of overweight women was 57% and nearly a quarter of women were obese (24%).

Obesity is strongly age related. By 2003, three times as many adult men in age groups of between 35 and 75 years of age were obese (25–28% obese) as those between 16 and 24 years (8% obese). Obesity in woman also increases with age. By 2003, 14% of 16–24 year olds were obese, which rose to 18% in 25–34 year olds, and 30% in 65–74 year olds (Department of Health, 2004).

By 2009, the prevalence of overweight and obesity was still lowest in the 16–24 year olds and continued to rise with age up to 75 years (Craig and Hirani, 2009).

Treatment of obesity comes at a great cost to the National Health Service (NHS), and was estimated to be more than £0.5 billion a year (NAO, 2001). In 2007, direct costs were estimated at £4.2 billion. The Foresight project further reported that without action, obesity-related diseases would cost the wider economy an extra £49.9 billion per year by 2050.

The scale of the problem is even greater in the United States. There, estimates show that 55–60% of the population are overweight (defined by BMI ≥ 25 kg/m^2) and 20–25% are obese (BMI ≥ 30 kg/m^2).

There remain health implications and psychological consequences to obesity. Obesity increases the risks of osteoarthritis, gallstones, gout, fertility problems and sleep apnoea. The metabolic complications of obesity include type 2 diabetes, heart disease, cancer, hyperlipidaemia and hyperinsulinaemia (WHO, 2003).

These metabolic abnormalities are closely linked to intra-abdominal fat in the abdominal wall (Ashwell, 1992). Body fat distribution that is central is known as android fat distribution and also referred to as 'apple shape'. Peripheral fat distribution is known as gynoid fat distribution and referred to as 'pear shape'. The 'apples' appear to have greater health risks. Thus, a simple and practical method for assessing health risk is to measure the waist circumference. The circumference of the waist indicates fat deposition in the abdominal area and is an adequate estimation of intra-abdominal fatness when compared with computer techniques

(Seidell et al, 1987). A raised waist measurement or upper body obesity is associated with a greater risk of developing degenerative diseases that are coupled with obesity (mentioned previously), and include hypertension and some bone and joint disorders. Healthy waist circumference is ≤ 80 cm ($31\frac{1}{2}$ inches) for women and ≤ 94 cm (37 inches) for men. A waist circumference of >88 cm ($34\frac{1}{2}$ inches) in women and >102 cm (40 inches) in men substantially increases health risk.

Apple shape is the typical pattern of fat storage in men. Women are usually pear shape, as most of their fat tends to be stored around the hips and thighs (peripherally), as opposed to around the abdomen. This latter fat distribution carries least risk, and is not associated with many metabolic consequences, although 'pear shapes' will still be prone to bone and weight-bearing joint disorders.

Obesity is multi-factorial. However, the following three factors govern energy balance and affect appetite and metabolism:

1 Diet
2 Physical activity
3 Genetics, and family eating habits

Diet

Obesity is defined as an excess or abnormal fat accumulation in adipose tissue caused by consuming more energy than is expended. In effect, an energy imbalance must exist in the following equation for weight gain to occur.

Energy input = energy out + energy stored

Either energy intake is increased or energy output in decreased, leading to overweight and obesity, which has its associated health problems. It is probable that increased intake of food away from the home (i.e. fast food) is a contributory factor to the rise in obesity in western countries (Binkley et al, 2000). No persuasive evidence exists that explains differences in eating behaviours between lean and obese people, although in dietary studies, it is not uncommon for overweight subjects (or unsuccessful dieters) to underreport food intake or overestimate their level of physical activity. The cause of obesity can also be traced to a change in the nutrient density of the diet, with most industrialised countries consuming a higher proportion of fat in the diet. Globally, the increased intake of caloric-dense foods that are high in SFAs and sugars are listed as major contributing causes of obesity (World Health Organization, 2003). However, in adults and children, absolute fat intakes are decreasing in the United Kingdom (DEFRA, 2000) and Europe (Ahmun et al, 2002), although fat consumption (proportion of total energy) is still higher than recommended. Trends in energy expenditure suggest that a reduction in physical activity is a greater contribution to obesity than, perhaps, energy intake.

Physical activity

Physical activity is a global term that refers to any bodily movement produced by skeletal muscles that result in energy expenditure (Caspersen et al, 1985).

Physical inactivity doubles the risk of heart disease and is a major risk factor for stroke. In the Women's Health Study involving 37,878, the risk of diabetes was reduced as the amount of physical activity increased (Weinstein, 2004). Being inactive is estimated to cause 1.9 million deaths globally, and also causes certain cancers and diabetes (WHO, 2003). The Health Survey for England (Department of Health, 1999) showed that only 37% of men and 25% of women were involved in activity to benefit their health (30 minutes moderate physical activity on 5 or more days a week). The percentage of adults who are participating in enough activity declines with age. The study showed that in the 16–24 years age group, 58% of men are active and 32% of women, compared with the 65–74 years age group when only 17% of men and 12% of women are active. Recently, a survey of 363,724 adults showed that 33% of people aged 16–24 years regularly exercise/participate in sport. Activity levels continue to decline with age as only 20% of adults in the age group 45–54 years are active, and even less active (12%) are those of retirement age (65–74 years). In this survey, only 21% of adults were classified as regular exercisers, participating in 30 minutes of sport and active recreation of moderate exercise intensity (excluding DIY and gardening) at least 3 times per week (Sport England, 2006).

Genetics

Genetics play as role in determining where fat is distributed in the body. Over 40,000 US citizens were part of a national survey regarding the origins of obesity. Children of two lean parents were thinnest and of two obese parents were fattest. The study did not exclude the influence of environmental factors on obesity (Garn and Clark, 1976).

Successful weight management

Reducing energy intake or increasing energy output (exercise), or both, will create a negative energy balance that favours weight loss. Body fat stores are used to meet energy demands. Fat loss includes adipose tissue and supporting lean tissue, and represents approximately 7.2 kcal/g or 7200 kcal/kg. Although exercise alone often does not achieve the same scale of weight loss as that of reducing energy intake, there is evidence to support that it can work. Studies show that keeping the diet 'normocaloric' or constant, and reducing calorie intake by exercise alone, results in substantial weight loss (>5 kg per week) in both women (Hadjiolova et al, 1982) and men (Ross et al, 2000). However, an earlier review by Wilmore (1996) showed that formal exercise training done without significant changes in the diet does not result in substantial changes in body weight and composition. Over a period of 1 year, individuals involved in exercise training would lose 3.2 kg body mass, 5.2 kg fat mass and gain 2.0 kg fat-free mass. Reasons why weight loss through exercise does not match weight loss by dieting may be because of greater control of energy balance with diet, and/or because individuals increase their energy intake as exercise increases. This results in a failure to produce a negative energy balance (through exercise).

There is evidence that physical activity may increase food consumption, although large variations exist within individuals. Stubbs et al (2002, 2004) showed that over a period of 1 or 2 weeks of increased energy expenditure, daily energy intake did not remain constant. Over the 2-week period, they found that large individual variation existed in energy compensation. *On average* individuals compensated for about 30% of the energy deficit induced by exercise, although some compensated for as much as 100% of the energy deficit.

Thus, to lose weight, a negative energy balance must be created. An energy deficit of 500–1000 kcal/day will result in a weight loss of 0.5–0.9 kg (1–2 pounds) per week. At a weight loss rate of up to 1 kg per week, lean tissue may be spared (Garrow, 1988).

Studies of weight loss and maintenance suggest that unless weight loss of ≥10% of initial body weight is sustained, long-term health benefits are not maximised. Kramer et al (1987) found that maintaining 100% of weight loss over a 4-year period was nearly impossible for men (0.9% successful maintained weight loss), but less so for women. A larger percentage of women (5.3%) maintained all of the weight loss.

Successful weight maintenance has most notably been highlighted by the National Weight Control Registry (NWCR) (Klem et al, 1997; Kennedy et al, 2001) that involved a retrospective study to investigate weight maintenance strategies of successful weight losers. In this instance, successful was defined as maintaining a weight loss of 30 pounds (roughly 13.6 kg) for at least 1 year. Some of the findings that have been reported so far include the following key strategies used by most successful weight losers who maintained this weight loss for an average of 5.5 years:

Diet:
- Consume a low-calorie diet, an average of 1381 kcal/day (consider that 80% of registrants are female).

- Composition of the diet was low in fat (24% of total energy intake), high in carbohydrates (56% of energy intake) and 19% protein energy.
- Eat breakfast almost everyday.
- Very few people consume a low-carbohydrate diet (<1%), and those who do maintained their weight loss for less time and were less physically active.
- Consume roughly 5 meals a day.
- Eat at restaurants only once to twice a week.

Monitoring:
- Frequent self-monitoring, either of the dietary intake and/or body weight.
- Most monitor their dietary intake by keeping a food journal (diary) especially if they noticed a couple of pounds of weight gain.
- Three in four weigh themselves either daily or weekly.

Physical activity:
- Participate in more scheduled exercise (about 1 hour a day) and more lifestyle activity.
- Many have a high level of physical activity and walk as their main form of exercise, about 28 miles/week.
- Women expend on average 2545 kcal per week on exercise.
- Men expend on average 3293 kcal/week on exercise.
- One in five participates in weight training.

Individuals who regain weight report an increased fat intake, decreased physical activity by an average of 800 kcal/week and engage in less self-monitoring activities.

Three key strategies

Three key strategies to lose and maintain weight involve working on three cores areas, namely (1) energy intake, (2) physical activity and (3) behaviour modification (Figure 6.2).

Reduce energy intake

To reduce weight, cut calorie intake by 500–1000 kcal/day. Dietary reference values (DRV) for energy is 2200 kcal and 2900 kcal for women and men, respectively (Department of Health, 1991). Overweight or obese female athletes exercising more than 1 hour a day can consume 1500–1700 kcal/day (or ~25 kcal/kg ideal BW/day), while male athletes with similar exercise patterns could consume 2000–2400 kcal/day (or ~30 kcal/kg ideal BW/day) to lose excess weight. These recommendations for athletes are not set in stone and must take into account individual dietary needs

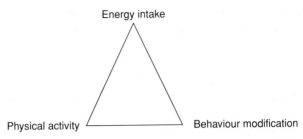

Figure 6.2 Three key areas to address in weight management. (Material from the Hayley Daries practice.)

and the athlete's current dietary intake before creating a calorie deficit of at least 500 kcal/day. Diets high in carbohydrate, low in fat and protein in moderation are recommended to athletes as they have a greater impact on weight loss (as shown previously) and associated with better long-term health outcomes.

Very low calorie diets (VLCDs) refer to diets that provide less 600 kcal – 800 kcal/day (3347 kJ/ day) for a period of 8 weeks or more. Most VLCDs became popular in the 1970s and are based on meal replacements, used as either total or partial substitution of meals. Following a number of sudden deaths due to cardiac arrhythmias (heartbeat irregularity), VLCDs were reviewed and their composition altered (National Task Force on the Prevention and Treatment of Obesity (NTFPTO), 1993). Current VLCDs are required to provide sufficient protein and meet the daily requirements for vitamins, minerals, electrolytes and EFA, and is advised not to be followed for periods longer than 12–16 weeks. Due to the severe calorie restriction and the potential side effects, medical and dietetic supervision is required when following VLCDs.

Studies that investigated long-term weight maintenance of such diets used <800 kcal/day diets. (For a review refer to Anderson et al, 2001). Athletes who may have only a small amount of weight to lose, VLCDs may not be the best route as lean tissue may be compromised. This is because average weight loss of 2 kg per week can be achieved with VLCDs, compared with 0.5 kg loss on low-energy diet (NTFPTO, 1993). Furthermore, as a case against it, VLCDs may cause a reduction in resting energy expenditure (REE) by 20% (Escott-Stump, 2002). This lowered metabolism could compromise long-term weight maintenance when calorie intake increases after the VLCD intervention.

The effect of glycaemic index (GI) and glycaemic load on weight loss has been studied extensively, and shows conflicting evidence. Although it appears that it is possible that reducing diet GI may reduce body weight (Wolever, 2006), the usefulness of each study should be approached with caution as the magnitude of weight loss is influenced by interpretation of GI, measurement and control of energy intake and weight regain in long-term studies. A review of studies show that low glycaemic index or load (LGI) diet interventions and short-term follow-up cause greater weight loss and improved lipid profiles (greater reduction in total cholesterol and LDL cholesterol), than when compared with high glycaemic index or load (HGI) diets (Thomas et al, 2007). Other studies have not supported the benefits of low-fat LGI diets for improved weight loss above that of low-fat HGI diets, although they also found greater reductions in total cholesterol and LDL cholesterol levels with low-fat LGI diets (Sloth et al, 2004). Raatz et al (2005) also found that lowered glycaemic load and GI of weight reduction diets did not provide any added benefit to calorie restriction in promoting weight loss in obese subjects. Similarly, Sichieri et al (2007) also found that long-term weight changes were not significantly different between the LGI and HGI diet groups, but that LGI diets caused favourable changes in lipid profiles (notably TG and Very Low Density Lipoprotein (VLDL) cholesterol).

Others have found that LGI diets have a beneficial effect on HDL cholesterol and triglyceride concentrations, but not LDL cholesterol levels, compared with a low-fat diet. LDL cholesterol improved more on a low-fat diet (Ebbeling et al, 2007). In the short-term, low-fat LGI diets may cause greater weight loss and improvements in blood lipids than low-fat HGI diets or other hypocaloric diets. However, in the longer term there is no added benefit of LGI diets on weight loss, but as long as fat intake is prudent, lipid profiles will improve. Therefore, at this stage, information that will help athletes to reduce fat intake may be more useful and practical to apply in pursuit of better health and weight loss. Table 6.2 provides guidelines for healthy, reduced-fat cooking methods and Table 6.3 provides a guide to reduced-fat meal options when dining out (refer also to Table 3.2. for low-fat carbohydrate dishes that are popular with athletes, as well as the many recipes provided in this book).

Increase physical activity

The caloric cost of activities of humans has been established from classic experiments measuring human oxygen consumption, referred to as indirect calorimetry. Since 1 L of oxygen consumed is equivalent to about 5 kcal of heat energy, charts and tables of energy expenditure at rest and during exercise have been established by using this reference. Activities from household chores to high-intensity sport activities have been measured (in kcal and kJ) and these figures provide a handy and practical reference for the average person or athlete, since the alternative involves using a spirometer or computer technology for the actual measurement

Table 6.2 Lower fat, alternative cooking methods.

Healthy cooking method	Examples of suitable food for the method
Grill	Meat, chicken, fish (excess fat trimmed) and certain vegetables (i.e. shitake mushrooms, tomatoes)
Poach	Eggs, fish
Barbecue	Lean cuts of meat, chicken, fish, lean sausage, variety of root and cruciferous vegetables or potato (wrap in foil and pack between hot coals) or corn on the cob. Sandwiches or rolls with onion, tomato and olives.
Pot roast	Meat, chicken or fish (fat removed), legumes and vegetables for stews and curries
Oven bake	Meat, chicken, fish, jacket potatoes and sweet potatoes, vegetables like whole onions, aubergine
Microwave	Jacket potato or sweet potato and vegetables
Steam	Vegetables, fish
Dry fry	Most cuts of meat and sausage

Source: Material from Hayley Daries Practice.

of oxygen consumed (McArdle et al, 1991). These methods are expensive and require trained staff, so it is not accessible to most people.

The following recommendations for participation in physical activity for adults (19–64 years) are based on current public health evidence of the impact of physical activity on health (Department of Health, 2011):

- at least five or more times per week, preferably all days;
- at least moderate-intensity physical activity;
- 150 minutes ($2\frac{1}{2}$ hours) over a week; or
- 30 minutes per day on at least 5 days; or
- 75 minutes vigorous-intensity exercise over a week; and
- do physical activity to improve muscle strength, at least 2 days per week

Several studies and reviews provide evidence supporting physical activity as a key component of fitness that promotes health and weight management, especially for long-term benefits (Gwinup, 1987; Zelasko, 1995; Fogelholm and Kukkonen-Harjula, 2000; ACSM, 2001; Blair and Church, 2004). Recommendations for participation in physical activity for adults who want to lose weight are as follows:

- Participate in endurance or aerobic-type exercise (e.g. cycling, walking, running, lap swimming, etc.)
- At least 30–60 minutes/day or 200–300 minutes per week
- Moderate-intensity exercise (55–69% of HRmax)
- At least five or more days of the week
- Expend ≥2000 kcal per week

Table 6.3 Reducing fat: better choices when dining out[a].

Fast Food/Take-away food

It is best to avoid fast food if you are trying to lose weight, have hypertension, raised lipids (i.e. cholesterol) or diabetes until your condition is well managed. Then, if you do eat out, have it as a main meal not snack. Have smaller portions and choose the vegetables, salads, fruit, whole grain/seed bread and 'light' sugar-free drinks. ALWAYS have the smallest burger, light drink and salad.

AVOID (>20 g fat)	BETTER choices (<20 g fat)
Meat pies and pastries; sausage	Sushi (*low fat, high omega-3*)
Potato salad (with usual mayo)	Bean salad (*high in fibre*), coleslaw (fresh or with reduced-oil salad dressing or light mayonnaise on side)
Potato fries, thin-cut	Mashed potato or baked potato
Double burger, with or without cheese; egg and/or bacon; white rolls	Smallest plain lean burger or vegetarian (bean) burger; choose whole-grain rolls or seed rolls
Fish and chips; deep-fried or fried fish burger	Grilled fish
Crumbed, deep-fried chicken; chicken and fried noodles	Grilled chicken breast or turkey sub sandwich or similar; grilled chicken tortilla wrap; steamed noodles or pasta
Pizza with cheesy topping or processed fatty meat toppings (salami/pepperoni); thick base or filled base.	Pizza with lean toppings like ricotta or mozzarella cheese and tomato, or vegetable, fruit or chicken and lean meat topping; Thin base.

Restaurant choices

When planning to eat a main dish at a restaurant, daily energy intake can be controlled by reducing food consumption for the rest of the day (i.e. if a substantial meal is eaten at lunch time, having fruit for breakfast and a light meal/sandwich or salad at dinner time will aid energy balance).
Refer also to Table 3.2. for healthy alternatives for favourite carbohydrate-based dishes.

Avoid high-fat choices	Best low-fat choices
Italian	
Antipasto, like salami	Minestrone/vegetable soup, no cream
Pesto/carbonara sauce	Tomato-based sauces
Fried dishes	Plain pasta + parmesan cheese and a salad
Buttery garlic breads, cheese breads	Plain, crusty Italian bread
Creamy pasta dishes	Ravioli + spinach + ricotta
Creamy desserts	Sorbets and low-fat desserts
Chinese	
Deep-fried dishes	Clear soups with noodles or vegetables
Crispy chicken	Steamed prawns and fish
Pork or duck dishes	Meat/chicken/fish + chilli/soy/oyster sauce
Fried rice or egg fried rice	Steamed rice or noodles
Indian	
Fried samosa, pakora, fried breads, some naan breads	Steamed basmati rice and Indian breads – chapatti
Fried pilau rice	
Butter, creamy nut sauces and deep-fried meat/vegetables	Meat dishes in yoghurt/tomato
Creamy soups and meaty curries (e.g. tikka masala)	Lentil (dahl) soups, Pickles, raita, onion salad; starter chicken/tandoori

---

Source: Material from Hayley Daries Practice.
[a]Alternatively, athletes can eat in using the recipes provided in this book.

- Supplement the endurance (aerobic component) with resistance exercise

Exercise is an effective strategy for weight loss, with or without dietary restriction. The effectiveness of aerobic exercise *without* dietary restriction was investigated in a group of obese women. Greater weight loss benefits were found through cycling (12% loss of body weight), compared with walking (10% loss) and swimming (no loss) (Gwinup, 1987). When combining exercise *with* diet, a review of studies showed that a 20% greater weight loss is achieved (than with diet alone) that is partially sustained after 1 year (Curioni and Lourenço, 2006). Increasing exercise intensity further results in greater weight loss (Shaw et al, 2006).

A further benefit of exercise is the increased metabolism even after exercise has been completed. During exercise, the level of oxygen needed and the level of supplied differs, as the body is slow to provide sufficient oxygen for exercise. An oxygen deficit occurs, which was previously referred to as the *oxygen debt*. The result is a temporary rise in the metabolic rate following exercise that can last from a few minutes to several hours. Today, this occurrence is referred to as excess post-exercise oxygen consumption (EPOC) (Wilmore and Costill, 2004). EPOC rises linearly as exercise intensity increases, but only up to 80% VO_2max; thereafter, as exercise intensity increases, the rate of EPOC is greater (Zelasko, 1995). The greater the intensity and duration of exercise, the greater the energy cost of EPOC, hence greater benefits for weight management are seen in athletes who take part in strenuous exhaustive exercise. Even after exercise, the level of oxygen consumption remains excessive.

Change behaviour around food and exercise

Behaviour modification is based on the concept that (food- and exercise-related) behaviours are learned and can be changed by influencing the environment or the reactions to the environment or events. Identifying barriers (i.e. problem behaviours) to compliance with diet and exercise programmes are an important aspect of any weight management programme. Behaviour change theories provide tools to overcoming such barriers and are as important as the diet or exercise component. There is evidence that behaviour therapy (BT) alone does result in some modest weight loss of around 2.3–6.8 kg (5–15 pounds) (Brownell, 1984), or more in some controlled trials (for review see Shaw et al, 2005). A combined intervention of BT, dietary modification and physical activity causes greater weight reduction. Increasing the intensity of the behavioural intervention increases the weight reduction, significantly. Cognitive-behaviour therapy (CBT), when combined with a diet and exercise intervention, was found to increase weight loss compared with diet and exercise alone (~4.9 kg). Therefore, both BT and CBT improve weight loss in people who are overweight or obese (Shaw et al, 2005).

Principal behavioural strategies

Principal behavioural strategies include the following:
- *Assessing readiness to change* that involves awareness of what a weight management programme is and determination of willingness to participate in such a programme.
- *Goal setting* ensures that goals are SMART, i.e.
  - *Specific*, identify the goals.
  - *Measurable*, every goal has an outcome measure.
  - Make goals *attainable* and *realistic*, and base them on rational expectations. An initial weight loss goal of about 5% of body weight is realistic.
  - Has a clear *time frame*, a goal has a date or a deadline.
- *Self-monitoring* focuses on observation of behaviour by using a food diary/record that can keep a record of time of eating, food type intake, cooking methods and may identify behaviour or emotions associated with eating. Self-monitoring activity may also be helpful with the use of an activity diary or calendar. This is effective at creating awareness about problems, behaviours, environmental barriers or emotional triggers that affect food intake and choice.
- *Stimulus control* involves identifying positive and negative stimuli, and limiting exposure to tempting situations (i.e. parties), or people, that encourage overeating or inactivity, or both. Managing stress through non-food-related coping mechanisms and problem-solving skills training are helpful tools.
- *Thought restructuring* and awareness of the mind–body connection can help to cultivate a healthier self-concept through positive thoughts and actions, and examining old beliefs about food and weight.
- *Social support* from family, friends, colleagues or groups and professional support are helpful to achieve and maintain weight loss.

Another behavioural approach is the anti-dieting programmes that use a non-diet approach, replace dieting with eating habits. These have shown to improve weight stability, eating behaviour and psychological well-being (Higgens and Gray, 1999).

Chapter summary

- Fats and oils are a group of organic compounds called lipids that do not dissolve in water. The diversity of lipid forms includes free fatty acids (FFAs), plasma triglycerides, intramuscular triglyceride (IMTG), essential fatty acids (EFA), sterols (like cholesterol), phospholipids, glycolipids, sulpholipids, lipoproteins and fat-soluble vitamins A, E and K.
- Most fat-rich foods and liquids contain a measure of saturated or unsaturated fat (i.e. MUFAs and PUFAs).

- Alpha-linolenic acid is an Essential Fatty Acid (EFA) synthesised from omega-3 fats in the diet, i.e. from oily fish, walnuts and flaxseeds; and linoleic acid, the other EPA, is synthesised from omega-6 fats like safflower, cottonseed and soybean oil.

- Fat is the most concentrated source of energy providing 9 kcal (37 kJ) per gram of energy, twice as calorie dense as carbohydrates and proteins.

- Fat is stored under the skin, in muscle tissue, in the abdomen between the organs, as essential fat in bone marrow lipids and central nervous system lipids, and a tiny amount of fat circulates in the plasma as FFAs.

- Fat from adipose tissue and intramuscular triacylglycerol (IMTG) (between muscle fibres and as fat droplets within muscle cells) act as the near limitless fuels for exercise.

- Fat stores in healthy, non-obese adults range between 8% and 25% of the body in men, and between 21% and 36% in women, although lower fat levels are reported in elite athletes.

- Methods to measure body composition (fatness and lean mass) include Dual Energy X-ray Absorptiometry (DEXA), Bioelectrical Impedance Analysis (BIA), Skinfold Thickness (SF) and Hydrostatic Weighing (HW).

- Fat is an important source of energy during exercise and is a major fuel during low exercise intensities and prolonged exercise.

- Training adaptations of endurance-trained athletes include increased fat oxidation, which decreases the reliance on liver and muscle glycogen stores, increased fat breakdown, reduced glycogen breakdown, increased number of capillaries and increased fatty acid transport.

- Fats are a very concentrated source of energy and should comprise about one-third of total energy intake, ideally less than 35% of total energy intake. The recommendation for athletes is a diet of <30% fat, or <73 g for female athletes and <97 g for male athletes.

- Athletes may achieve enhanced fatty acid oxidation and glycogen sparing after fat-loading diets but it may have no performance benefit, rather it has been shown that high-fat diet can cause higher ratings of perceived exertion.

- High fat intakes lead to over-consumption of calories, leading to obesity, risk of raised blood fats (hyperlipidaemia) and associated heart disease.

- Excess fat mass can reduce some or all of the following performance indices including strength, agility, mobility, muscular appearance, speed, power and endurance.

- Body fat distribution that is central is known as android fat distribution and also referred to as 'apple shape'. The circumference of the waist indicates fat deposition in the abdominal area and a healthy waist circumference for women is 80 cm ($31\frac{1}{2}$ inches) and 94 cm (37 inches) for men.

- The cause of obesity can also be traced to a change in the nutrient density of the diet, and globally there is an increased intake of caloric-dense foods that are high in SFAs and sugars.

- To lose weight a negative energy balance must be created and by an energy deficit of 500–1000 kcal/day a weight loss of 0.5–0.9 kg (1–2 pounds) per week will be achieved. At a weight loss rate of up to 1 kg per week, lean tissue may be spared.
- Key strategies used by most successful weight losers include consuming a healthy diet, frequent self-monitoring and increased physical activity.
- Reducing energy intake, increasing physical activity and changing behaviour are key strategies athletes can use to lose excess body fat. Principal behavioural strategies include assessing readiness to change, goal setting, self-monitoring, stimulus control, thought restructuring and social support.

Sandwiches and Spreads

Fats are a rich energy source. The recipes that follow contain a sample of easy-to-prepare dishes that are rich in all the healthy fats, i.e. MUFA and PUFAs, including the essential fatty acids. These meals are perfect for the packed lunch or a quick supper for the athlete *on the go*.

Gypsy Ham and Cheese Sandwich

(Serves 1)

Ingredients
1 whole-wheat roll, halved and toasted

10 mL olive oil

100 g (3 oz) gypsy ham

$\frac{1}{4}$ apple, cored and roughly chopped

75 g Swiss cheese

Method
1 Drizzle the olive oil onto the lower half of the whole-wheat roll.
2 Add the gypsy ham on top, followed by the chopped apple and cheese.
3 Place the roll under a preheated grill until the cheese is slightly melted.
4 Close the sandwich with the top half of the roll and enjoy while still warm.

Nutrition analysis per portion
Light meal

Energy	247 kcal (1037 kJ)
Protein	15.8 g
Carbohydrate	11 g
Fat	15 g
Cholesterol	44 mg
Fibre	1.6 g

High-energy meal

Energy	659 kcal (2769 kJ)
Protein	42 g
Carbohydrate	29 g
Fat	40 g
Cholesterol	117 mg
Fibre	4.2 g

Food note: Apples provide a good amount of soluble fibre that help lower blood fat levels.

Mozzarella, Tomato and Pesto on Rye

(Serves 2)

Ingredients

4 slices rye bread

90 mL parsley and coriander pesto (use *Tuna Pasta's* basil pesto recipe on page 88)

150 g (5 oz) mozzarella, cut into rounds

2 tomatoes, sliced

30 mL olive oil

Pepper

Method

1 Blend the pesto ingredients together and spread on each slice of bread, on one side only. Preserve some pesto to add at a later stage.

2 Arrange a layer of mozzarella over the spread, followed by a layer of tomato.

3 Season with pepper and drizzle with olive oil.

4 Add the leftover pesto over the sandwich.

5 Slice the sandwiches in half and serve.

Nutrition analysis per portion
High-energy meal

Energy	909 kcal (3818 kJ)
Protein	29 g
Carbohydrate	56 g
Fat	56 g
Cholesterol	594 mg
Fibre	17 g

Food note: Mozzarella cheese is lower in fat than hard cheeses like cheddar and Stilton. Cheese is a good source of calcium.

Salmon and Cottage Cheese Spread

(Makes 480 g of spread)

Ingredients

150 g (5 oz) smoked salmon, chopped $\frac{1}{2}$ lemon, zest and juice

250 g (9 oz) low-fat smooth cottage cheese 10 g (1 Tbsp) chives, chopped

---

Method

1 Mix all the ingredients together and refrigerate until needed in an airtight container.

2 Use as spread on sandwiches.

Nutrition analysis per portion

Energy	60 kcal (251 kJ)
Protein	6 g
Carbohydrate	1.1 g
Fat	4 g
Cholesterol	9 mg
Fibre	0.4 g

Food note: Salmon provides protein and essential fatty acids (omega-3s) in the diet. Of all cheeses, cottage cheese is lowest in fat. Choose low-fat or fat-free, smooth or chunky, plain or flavoured cottage cheese.

Smoked Mackerel Pitta

(Serves 2)

Ingredients

200 g (7 oz) smoked mackerel, roughly shredded

60 g ($\frac{1}{2}$ cup) dried apricots, chopped

$\frac{1}{2}$ red onion, chopped

30 g (1 oz) raisins

1 orange, juiced

$\frac{1}{2}$ lemon, juiced

75 g cooked mixed vegetables (corn, peas and carrots)

20 g mayonnaise

2 whole-wheat pitta breads

Method

1 Mix all the ingredients together and spoon into the pitta pockets.

2 Serve immediately.

Nutrition analysis per portion

Energy	650 kcal (2730 kJ)
Protein	26 g
Carbohydrate	74 g
Fat	24 g
Cholesterol	63 mg
Fibre	8 g

Food note: Mackerel is the highest source of omega-3 fats in the diet. Apricots are a rich source of beta-carotene, fibre and iron.

Spicy Chicken Wraps

(Serves 4)

Ingredients

4 chicken breasts, boned and skinned

20 mL sunflower oil

20 mL green masala spice

$\frac{1}{2}$ pineapple, peeled and cubed

1 small red onion, peeled and finely chopped

1 small red chilli, seeded

10 mL coriander leaves, finely chopped

150 g lettuce, shredded

whole-wheat tortillas/pitta breads

40 mL sweet and sour sauce

Method

1 Preheat the oven to 180°C.
2 Rub the oil and masala onto the chicken. Bake for 20 minutes or until done.
3 *For the pineapple salsa*: In a small bowl, add the pineapple cubes, onion, coriander and finely chopped chilli together. Mix well and refrigerate until needed.
4 To make the wraps, roughly shred the chicken (1 breast per tortilla) and place the chicken on the wrap, followed by the salsa, lettuce and sweet and sour sauce.
5 Roll the wraps up and serve.

Nutrition analysis per portion
Light meal

Energy	166 kcal (697 kJ)
Protein	15.4 g
Carbohydrate	8.4 g
Fat	7.3 g
Cholesterol	45 mg
Fibre	1.3 g

High-energy meal

Energy	602 kcal (2530 kJ)
Protein	56 g
Carbohydrate	30 g
Fat	26 g
Cholesterol	163 mg
Fibre	5 g

Food note: A high-protein dish. The pineapple adds vitamin C to the meal.

Turkey Burger

(Serves 3)

Ingredients

300 g (10 oz) turkey mince

2 egg yolks

1 celery stick, finely chopped

1 small red onion, chopped

$\frac{1}{4}$ cup breadcrumbs

5 mL parsley, chopped

Salt and freshly ground pepper

6 seed loaf slices

Method

1 Combine the mince, eggs, celery, onion, parsley and breadcrumbs together.
2 Season to taste and rest the mixture.
3 Shape the mixture into three equal balls and flatten them with the palm of your hand.
4 Place the burgers in a baking tray and grill for 5–7 minutes on each side.
5 Serve on the seed loaf slices with a tomato or pepper relish.

Nutrition analysis per portion

Energy	434 kcal (1824 kJ)
Protein	39 g
Carbohydrate	39 g
Fat	11 g
Cholesterol	241 mg
Fibre	5.4 g

Food note: Turkey is a low-fat protein-rich food source, high in B vitamins. Celery may help lower blood pressure.

Veal Steak Rolls

(Serves 2)

Ingredients

2 × 150 g veal escalope cuts (thinly sliced prime cut of veal; or thinly sliced beef steaks)

15 mL olive oil

20 g yellow mustard (regular)

2 granary rolls, sliced horizontally

10 g watercress or rocket

1 tomato, thinly sliced

Salt and freshly ground pepper to taste

Method

1 Set the oven on grill.
2 Season the escalope cuts or steaks with the salt and pepper.
3 Massage the meat with some of the olive oil.
4 Grill the meat for 5–7 minutes on each side. Set aside to rest for 2 minutes.
5 Spoon the mustard onto the roll, followed by the grilled meat.
6 Add the watercress/rocket and tomato slices.
7 Serve immediately.

Nutrition analysis per portion
Light meal

Energy	213 kcal (895 kJ)
Protein	13.8 g
Carbohydrate	13.8 g
Fat	10.5 g
Cholesterol	53 mg
Fibre	2.1 g

High-energy meal

Energy	688 kcal (2891 kJ)
Protein	44.5 g
Carbohydrate	44.5 g
Fat	34 g
Cholesterol	171 mg
Fibre	7 g

Food note: Veal is a good source of protein and vitamin B_{12}.

CHAPTER 7

Vitamins and Minerals

Key terms	
Micronutrients	Iron status
Dietary reference values (DRVs)	Iron deficiency
Reference nutrient intakes (RNIs)	Iron deficiency anaemia
Lower reference nutrient intakes (LRNIs)	Hepcidin
Megadoses	Sports anaemia
Toxic potential	Training-induced hypervolemia
Vitamin	'Dilutional pseudo-anaemia'
Primary vitamin deficiency	Haeme iron
Secondary vitamin deficiency	Non-haeme iron
Symptoms of deficiency	Food fortification
Water-soluble vitamin	Iron supplementation
Fat-soluble vitamin	Calcium
Mineral	Bone mineral density (BMD)
Mineral deficiency	Osteopaenia
Macrominerals	Osteoporosis
Microminerals	Sports amenorrhoea
Trace elements	Stress fractures
Electrolytes	Peak bone mass (PBM)
Supplementation	Bone mineral content (BMC)
Antioxidants	Calcium supplementation
Oxidative stress	Vitamin D
Oxygen radicals	Phosphorous
Reactive oxygen species (ROS)	Zinc
Delayed onset muscle soreness (DOMS)	Magnesium
Endogenous antioxidant defence system	Hypomagnesaemia
Iron	Supplement practices

Vitamins and minerals are termed micronutrients and although they are required in small quantities in the diet, their highly specific physiologic functions in the body are essential to life. Unlike the energy-giving

Nutrition for Sport and Exercise: A Practical Guide, First Edition. Hayley Daries.
© 2012 Blackwell Publishing Ltd. Published 2012 by Blackwell Publishing Ltd.

macronutrients, carbohydrates, proteins and fat, vitamins and minerals do not provide energy. Their requirements range from as little as a few micrograms (μg) (that is 1/1000th of a milligram (mg) or 1/1000000th of a gram) to 1 g or more per day. Dietary reference values (DRVs) estimates the amount of energy and nutrients needed by healthy people in the United Kingdom, and are age and gender related. DRVs also take into account stages of the lifecycle and other factors, for example during pregnancy, lactation, exercise and sport participation, illness and disease, energy and some nutrient requirements change. Reference nutrient intakes (RNIs), are estimates of protein, vitamins and minerals that are needed by most groups of healthy people. Lower reference nutrient intakes (LRNIs) are estimates for a small number of people with lower requirements. Vitamins and minerals are obtained from food sources and are also available in dietary supplement forms as individual nutrients or a variety of combinations. Safe intakes for vitamins and minerals have been established where not enough evidence is available to set an RNI. Since supplementation use is rising, safe micronutrient intakes can help to curb excessive intakes or 'megadoses' that may lead to toxic levels in the body. Certain vitamins have a greater toxic potential than others, i.e. vitamin A and D are ranked as the highest toxic potential (Combes, 1998).

RNI and specific recommendations for athletes are important for optimum health and to prevent deficiencies. However, the energy and nutrient demands in certain athletes may be higher than the RNI.

Vitamins are organic substances that are essential for growth, maintenance, development and reproduction. Adequate amounts of vitamins needed for physiologic functions, chemical processes and metabolic reactions cannot be synthesised by the body and must be obtained from food sources. When vitamin requirements are not met, it leads to deficiencies and related health problems. A variety of factors affect vitamin deficiencies. Reduced dietary intake of vitamins result in primary deficiencies, which are caused by poor food habits, ignorance and food taboos among other factors. Secondary deficiencies result when vitamins are not absorbed or used after ingestion. In this case, malabsorption, increased needs and increased losses of vitamins are among the causative factors (Combes, 1998). A specific set of symptoms characterise each vitamin deficiency, which can facilitate diagnosis and appropriate treatment.

Thirteen essential vitamins are classified as either fat-soluble or water-soluble. Fat-soluble vitamins, A, D, E and K, dissolve in fats from the diet and are easily stored in the body. Water-soluble vitamins, B-complex and C, dissolve in water and are not easily stored. Excessive intake of both fat- and water-soluble vitamins can cause toxicity. Table 7.1 lists summary of vitamins, their functions and signs of deficiency and excess.

Table 7.1 Summary of vitamins.

Vitamin	Main functions	Signs of deficiency	Signs of excess
Fat-soluble vitamins			
Vitamin A (retinol and carotenoids)	Vision, growth, immunity, anticarcinogenic properties, it protects against oxidative damage to cells	Night blindness, poor growth, risk of infections, dry skin and eyes	Headache, hair loss, joint pain, dry mucous membranes, liver damage
Vitamin D	Absorption and use of calcium and phosphorous, normal bone and tooth formation and maintenance	Rickets in children, osteomalacia in adults	Nausea, vomiting, calcium deposits, fragile bones
Vitamin E	Antioxidant properties, disarms free radicals, cell membrane stability, protective role in Alzheimer's disease and cardiovascular disease, anticoagulant properties	Rupture of red blood cells, nerve damage	Impaired vitamin K metabolism
Vitamin K	Blood clotting, bone mineralisation	Excessive bleeding, hip fractures	Jaundice in infants
Water-soluble vitamins			
Thiamin (B_1)	Releases energy to cells, carbohydrate metabolism, growth, protects against imbalances caused by alcohol intake	Beriberi, muscle weakness and wasting, Wernicke-Korsakoff syndrome	Respiratory failure
Riboflavin (B_2)	Releases energy to cells, carbohydrate and fat metabolism, growth	Cracks in corners of the mouth and lips, skins rashes	None known

Vitamin	Function	Deficiency	Toxicity
Niacin (B$_3$)	Releases energy to cells, carbohydrate, protein and fat metabolism	Pellagra (3 Ds – dermatitis, diarrhoea and dementia/death)	Skin flushing
Pantothenic acid (vitamin B$_5$)	Energy metabolism, synthesis of antibodies, healthy red blood cells	Fatigue, vomiting, leg cramps, burning feet syndrome	Diarrhoea
Vitamin B$_6$ (Pyridoxine)	Carbohydrate, protein and fat metabolism, healthy red blood cells, immunity, homocysteine metabolism	Convulsions in infants, anaemia, nervous disorders, skin disorders	Sensory nerve destruction
Vitamin B$_{12}$ (Cobalamin)	Protein metabolism, formation of blood cells and nerve cells, growth, homocysteine metabolism	Pernicious anaemia, megaloblastic anaemia, poor vision	None known
Folate (folic acid, folacin)	Protein metabolism, growth, haemoglobin formation, homocysteine metabolism, DNA synthesis, new cell and red blood cell formation	Extreme fatigue, megaloblastic anaemia, birth defects in newborn babies (spina bifida)	Neurological disorders
Biotin	Carbohydrate and fat metabolism	Skin inflammation (eczema), scaling skin, fatigue	None known
Vitamin C (ascorbic acid)	Antioxidant, collagen formation, wound healing and anti-inflammatory, blood vessel functioning, helps with absorption of iron	Fatigue, bleeding gums and loose teeth, easy bruising, scurvy (poor wound healing)	Bleeding (e.g. gums), prolonged wound healing, diarrhoea and gastrointestinal symptoms, kidney stones or gout in susceptible persons

Source: Data from Escott-Stump (2002).

Minerals are inorganic substances vital to health and well-being. Mineral matter makes up about 4% of body weight and is incorporated into structural components of the body tissues and is present in body fluids. Between 15 and 22 essential minerals need to be obtained from the diet and are classified by their proportion of (mineral) matter in the body. However, even minerals required in small daily quantities in the body (e.g. 140 µg iodine/day for adults) (Department of Health, 1991) have functions just as critical to health as those required in larger quantities (e.g. UK RNI for calcium is 700 mg/day for males and females, 19–50 years) (Department of Health, 1991). Major minerals (also known as macrominerals) are required in quantities greater than 100 mg/day (i.e. RNI for phosphorous is 550 mg, and for magnesium it is 300 mg for males and 270 mg for females aged 19–50 years) (Department of Health, 1991). Trace elements (or microminerals) are required in smaller quantities, i.e. RNI for the same age group for iron is 8.7 mg for males and 14.8 mg for females. Females with high menstrual losses may need supplementation in addition to the RNI. RNI for zinc is 9.5 mg for males and 7 mg for females (Department of Health, 1991). Electrolytes, namely sodium, potassium and chloride, are electrically charged ions that function as minerals essential for body water balance and chemical reactions. Table 7.2 provides a summary of minerals, their functions and signs of deficiency and excess.

Exercise and micronutrient requirements

Exercise increases micronutrient requirements because of the following effects:
- Increased stress to metabolic pathways
- Increased free-radical production
- DNA damage to cells
- Decreased absorption from the gut
- Greater micronutrient losses in sweat, urine and faeces
- Increased micronutrient turnover
- Increased maintenance and repair of lean tissue
- Increased retention of micronutrients in skeletal muscle
- Gastrointestinal blood loss in susceptible athletes during prolonged exhaustive exercise

(Jeukendrup and Gleeson, 2004; Wilmore and Costill, 2004; Rodriguez et al, 2009).

Table 7.3 summarises some common micronutrient deficiencies seen in athletes. Groups most at risk of low intake and compromised micronutrient status are athletes who consume low-energy diets.

Table 7.2 Summary of minerals.

Mineral	Main functions	Signs of deficiency	Signs of excess
Major minerals (macrominerals)			
Calcium	Bone and tooth formation, muscle contraction, nerve impulse transmission, blood clotting, heart rhythm/beat regulation, cell permeability	Weak bones and teeth, rickets in children, osteoporosis, muscle cramps, pre-menstrual syndrome (PMS)	Hypercalcaemia, kidney stones
Phosphorous	Bone and tooth formation, energy metabolism, acid–base balance	Weakness, rickets, osteomalacia	Poor bone mineralisation
Magnesium	Muscle contraction, energy metabolism, protein synthesis, activates enzymes, nerve transmission	Muscle weakness and pain, convulsions, behavioural disturbances (hyperactivity, hyperirritability), abnormal heart rhythms	Diarrhoea, palipitations, kidney failure
Macrominerals (electrolytes)			
Sodium	Fluid balance, nerve function, muscle contraction, acid–base balance, blood pressure regulation	Nausea, confusion	High blood pressure, increased calcium loss and excretion, heart failure
Potassium	Fluid balance, nerve impulse transmission, muscle contraction, protein synthesis, forms glycogen, acid–base balance	Muscle weakness and paralysis, irregular heartbeat	Heart disturbances, muscle weakness
Chloride	Acid–base balance, fluid balance	Disturbed acid–base balance	Disturbed acid–base balance
Trace Elements (microminerals)			
Copper	Iron metabolism, red blood cell formation, antioxidant	Anaemia, reduced immunity	Vomiting, liver disorders
Iodine	Part of thyroid hormones, energy metabolism	Goitre, poor foetal growth and brain development (in iodine-deficient pregnant women)	Interference with thyroid activity
Iron	Component of haemoglobin and myoglobin that transports oxygen, skeletal muscle function, cognitive function, immunity	Iron-deficiency anaemia, fatigue, reduced immunity, reduced learning ability	Liver cirrhosis, gastrointestinal upset
Selenium	Antioxidant, associated with sparing vitamin E	Muscle weakness and pain	Gastrointestinal upset
Zinc	Component of enzymes, energy metabolism, antioxidant, wound healing, cell membrane structure and function	Skin lesions, poor growth, reduced appetite, slow wound healing	Nausea, vomiting, diarrhoea, reduced copper absorption

Source: Data from Escott-Stump (2002).

Table 7.3 Common micronutrient deficiencies in athletes.

Micronutrient compromised	Consequences of low intake	Athletes at risk
All/any micronutrients	Micronutrient depletion	• Low energy intake or unbalanced diet • Severe weight loss regimes • Avoiding one or more food groups or dietary extremism • Consumption of large amounts of low-nutrient foods, at the expense of eating nutrient-dense foods
Calcium	Fractures; Stress fractures	• Female athletes with low energy intakes or unbalanced diet • Athletes who eliminate calcium-rich food groups, e.g. milk and milk products group • Those with menstrual dysfunction
Antioxidants (vitamin A, C, E, beta-carotene, selenium	Muscle soreness; Lipid peroxidation of cell membranes	• Athletes who follow a low-fat diet • Those who have restricted energy intakes • Those with limited intake of fruits and vegetables
Iron	Iron depletion; Iron deficiency anaemia leading to reduced exercise performance	• High requirements through increased red blood cell mass, especially during muscle growth phases • Increased iron losses in urine and sweat • Female athletes with heavy menstrual periods and blood loss • Athletes taking part in prolonged strenuous exercise, who are susceptible to gastrointestinal bleeding • Athletes with a poor energy intake (<1200 kcal) or an unbalanced diet • Avoidance of iron-rich food groups, e.g. meat, fish, poultry (a source of haeme iron) • Avoidance of iron-fortified foods, e.g. breakfast cereals, malted drinks, food products with white/brown flour • Excessive intake of tea, coffee, bran, eggs and legumes. • Athletes with copper deficiency • Vegan or new vegetarian athletes, with unbalanced diets • Specific groups of athletes, i.e. female long-distance runners • Taking calcium citrate or calcium phosphate supplements reduces the absorption of iron

Source: Material from Hayley Daries Practice.

A healthy, balanced diet including plenty of fruits and vegetables meets the micronutrient needs of most people, including athletes. There are some exceptions, as mentioned earlier, of groups of the population who may require vitamin and/or mineral supplementation, and will be discussed throughout the chapter. Women wishing to conceive, those already pregnant or lactating, people who do not get enough sunlight, the elderly and younger women will benefit in various ways from dietary supplementation. Other environmental factors such as smoking, alcohol consumption, low-calorie or low-nutrient diets and specialised or restricted diets, i.e. vegan or vegetarianism, affects micronutrient status and may lead to sub-optimal levels of vitamins and minerals. Athletes who are 'at risk' due to diet, environment or other factors or are being treated for a known deficiency require micronutrient supplementation (see Table 7.3). Furthermore, some vitamins and minerals have specific roles in exercise metabolism and performance and are an important aspect of the athlete's diet and potential supplement practice.

Vitamins with specific roles in exercise metabolism

Not all vitamins have been extensively investigated to determine their roles in exercise metabolism or athletic performance. For many micronutrients, their roles in exercise are unclear or unsubstantiated. Vitamins known to play a key role during exercise are the B-complex vitamins and vitamins with antioxidant properties, i.e. vitamin A, C, E and beta-carotene (pro-vitamin A). These will be discussed briefly.

B-complex vitamins

As energy needs increase in relation to the demands of exercise, so nutrient needs increase. Exercising muscles rely on energy produced from ingested food and fluids, and stored nutrients. Assimilating and metabolising carbohydrates, proteins and fats to produce energy are a function largely of the B-group vitamins that serve as co-enzymes in energy metabolism pathways. Exercising muscles also rely on oxygen that certain B vitamins (vitamin B_6, B_{12} and folic acid) function to transport.

Thiamin, riboflavin, niacin, pantothenic acid (vitamin B_5), vitamin B_6 and biotin have essential functions in releasing energy to cells. Carbohydrate metabolism is dependent on thiamin, niacin, riboflavin, as well as biotin and vitamin B_6. Protein (amino acid) metabolism is dependent on riboflavin, vitamin B_6, vitamin B_{12} and folic acid. Fat metabolism requires riboflavin, niacin, pantothenic acid and biotin (Escott-Stump, 2002).

Some of these vitamins also serve other vital functions including the formation of haemoglobin (Hb) (thiamin, folic acid and vitamin B_6) and blood cells (red blood cells (RBCs) by vitamins B_5 and B_6, and white blood cells and RBCs by vitamin B_{12}). Vitamin B_6 and biotin synthesise glycogen and glucose, respectively (via gluconeogenesis), and vitamin B_6 breaks down glycogen during exercise (Noakes, 1992). Growth involving protein synthesis and the maintenance and repair of lean tissue is function of vitamins B_1, B_2, B_6, B_{12} and folic acid (also of vitamin A). Niacin (B_3) and pantothenic acid have a role in fat synthesis. Vitamin B_6 can boost immunity. Thiamin (vitamin B_1) may help to treat anaemia. It can also protect against imbalances caused by alcohol consumption, since alcohol decreases thiamin absorption and increases its excretion (Wardlaw et al, 2004). Prevention of fatigue during exercise is a function of vitamin B_5 and riboflavin.

Vitamins with antioxidant properties

The aerobic energy pathway uses oxygen to form ATP, and during prolonged strenuous exercise muscle oxygen uptake may increase 100-fold (Gleeson, 2005). The result is that more free radicals are produced in skeletal muscle increasing oxidative stress that can weaken cell function and cause oxidative damage to DNA and lipid peroxidation of cell membranes. Muscle cells and other critical cells may be affected, such as erythrocytes (RBCs). Oxidative stress has health consequences, such as premature skin aging, and could result in more debilitating diseases like cancer and cardiovascular disease. Antioxidant vitamins A, C, E and beta-carotene intercept oxygen radicals and can repair, and work against, the damage it has caused. However, intense physical activity can disturb the balance between oxidative reactions and antioxidant capacity (Clarkson and Thompson, 2000).

Muscle fibre injury symptomised by muscle soreness or stiffness, among others, is often associated with unaccustomed eccentric exercise or vigorous training (Friden and Lieber, 2001). Eccentric exercise refers to exercise that involves lengthening of the muscle during activation resulting in damage to the muscle fibres (Jeukendrup and Gleeson, 2004). Downhill running and components of resistance exercise are considered largely to be eccentric exercise. The muscles may become damaged when they are over-exerted or over-trained, and micro-tears occur in the muscle fibres. This activates resident immune cells that trigger the inflammatory response, which stimulates nerve endings in the damaged muscle tissue. Although these immune cells act to heal the muscle, it involves the production of reactive oxygen species (ROS), which refers to oxygen-centred radicals and reactive derivatives of oxygen. ROS is associated with muscle damage markers, such as delayed onset muscle soreness (DOMS). Muscle

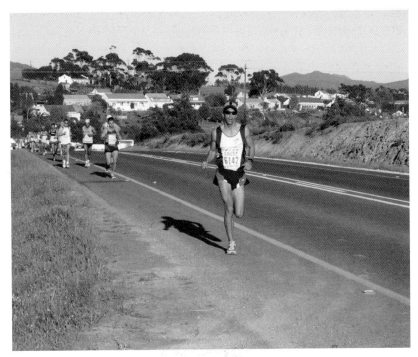

Figure 7.1 Severe exercise can damage muscle tissue of trained athletes, affecting glycogen stores and subsequent exercise performance.

soreness usually occurs within 24–48 hours of severe exercise in trained athletes, or within 4–6 days of unaccustomed exercise in untrained individuals. It is likely that there are several possible causes of muscle soreness (apart from free radical damage) such as muscle enzyme leakage, breakdown of protein and muscle cells and accumulation of phosphate (Noakes et al, 1991). Furthermore, damaged muscle is less able to re-synthesise and store glycogen, which may reduce exercise performance (Figure 7.1).

Compared to untrained individuals, trained athletes become adapted to higher oxidative stress by producing more antioxidant enzymes that enhances the enzymatic antioxidant system. Endurance training enhances the endogenous antioxidant defence system (Kanter, 1998). Thus, for majority of trained athletes, there appears no need to supplement with antioxidants in addition to RNIs provided they consume recommended intakes of micronutrients from dietary sources and have a replete antioxidant vitamin and mineral status. Table 7.4 lists of dietary sources of vitamin C, with reference values for this nutrient.

Supplementation intervention trials using high doses of antioxidant vitamins and/or minerals have attempted to reduce the increasing effects of (eccentric) exercise-induced muscle damage. Antioxidants, vitamin C, with its anti-inflammatory properties, and vitamin E, which ensures cell

Table 7.4 Food sources of vitamin C.

Food and portion size	Vitamin C
1 average guava (fruit)	165 mg
2 kiwi fruits	114 mg
1 medium orange	98 mg
1 cup fresh grapefruit juice	80 mg
6 brussels sprouts	78 mg
$\frac{1}{4}$ cup (2 tablespoons) sweet pepper, red	71 mg
1 slice ($\frac{1}{4}$ fruit) paw-paw/papaya	47 mg
1 cup tomato juice	45 mg
$\frac{1}{2}$ cup cooked broccoli	33 mg
$\frac{1}{2}$ cup raw cauliflower	23 mg
1 sweet potato	17 mg

Source: Material from Hayley Daries Practice.
**Reference values for adult males and females 19[+] years
(Department of Health, 1991)**.
UK RNI for vitamin C = 40 mg (Department of Health, 1991)
Supplemental doses = 60–3000 mg[1]

membrane stability, have been most frequently used in interventions. Muscle soreness is one of the muscle damage markers used in such trials, although other practical indicators are also used. For example, higher levels of muscle proteins such as creatine kinase (CK) are released from the muscle into the blood during vigorous exercise.

Mastaloudis et al (2006) studied 22 runners during a 50-km ultramarathon. The sample included both male and female ultra-marathon runners who were randomly allocated to one of two groups. Each group either received a placebo, or antioxidants in the form of 1000 mg vitamin C and 300 mg alpha-tocopheryl acetate (vitamin E). The intervention with supplementation lasted for 6 weeks. They found that antioxidant supplementation had no effect on muscle power, and although there were differences between men and women in the study (men had higher values of CK than women, indicating more muscle damage), 6-week antioxidant supplementation had no effect on exercise-induced increase in muscle damage or recovery. Similarly, some studies have shown no effect of antioxidant therapy to muscle damage and/or recovery in response to eccentric-type exercise (Warren et al, 1992; Beaton et al 2002), while other have shown a benefit (Bryer and Goldfarb, 2001; Bloomer et al, 2004).

However, an enhanced antioxidant defence system may not provide adequate protection for athletes who train extensively (Clarkson, 1995). Furthermore, dietary intake of antioxidants may be compromised in some athletes, i.e. those who follow a low-fat diet, who have restricted energy intakes and who have limited intakes of fruits and vegetable may be at risk due to poor antioxidant intakes (see Table 7.3). These athletes will clearly benefit from antioxidant supplementation to achieve daily requirements. However, if ideal supplemental doses differ to those of the general healthy population, then it requires further investigation since animal studies have found that *excessive* antioxidant supplementation can reduce exercise-induced adaptations and exercise performance.

Minerals and exercise metabolism

The interest in mineral intake of athletes lies in the fact that low mineral status (of a specific few minerals) is common in certain groups of athletes. Notably, athletes' intake of one or more select nutrients, i.e. iron, zinc, calcium and magnesium, are often compromised and their roles during exercise are discussed in the following text. Of these minerals, iron and zinc play a role in immune function, as does copper and selenium.

Iron

Iron is found in all body cells. Total iron in the body is a total of 3.8 g (about 50 mg per kg BW) in men, and a total of 2.3 g (about 35 mg per kg BW) in women. Body iron compartments consist of 2500 mg in erythrocytes, 1000 mg in stores and 115 mg in marrow (Zilva et al, 1988). Functional forms of iron are a crucial component of erythrocyte Hb (70% of all iron), a protein found in RBCs, myoglobin (5% of iron), a protein found in muscle, enzyme systems containing iron (cytochromes) and other cellular constituents (5% of iron). Hb transports oxygen from the lungs to the body tissues and myoglobin supplies oxygen to the mitochondria of muscle cells. Cytochrome enzymes help produce ATP (Mahan and Arlin, 1992). Storage forms of iron (20% of all iron) are known as ferritin and haemosiderin, and are found in the liver, spleen and bone marrow (Robinson et al, 1986; Zilva et al, 1988).

Iron status of athletes is assessed using serum iron, serum ferritin, Hb, haematocrit (Hct), RBC count and total iron binding capacity (TIBC).

Exercise, especially endurance exercise may contribute to low iron status. Iron is lost through sweat (0.3–0.4 mg/day), faeces (0.86 mg/day) and urine (0.1–0.15 mg/day) (Green et al, 1968; Jeukendrup and Gleeson, 2004). Blood is lost through gastrointestinal bleeding and/or urine (due to destruction of RBCs, i.e. erythrocytes), and in women, menstrual blood loss (0.3–0.4 mg/day or 16 mg per month) can be considerable (up to 1–1.4 mg/day) (Robinson et al, 1986; Zilva et al, 1988). In total, men lose about 1.0 mg iron/day, and premenstrual women lose 1.3 mg (up to 2 mg/day in women with heavy menstrual blood loss).

Furthermore, prolonged exercise or hard training may cause a drop in the concentration of circulating free iron. It could be induced by the acute-phase immune response to stress or inflammation (Sherman, 1992). The response elevates cytokine levels that causes the liver to produce more Hepcidin, a hormone that reduces iron transport and absorption (Peeling et al, 2008). It has also been suggested that exercise and muscular damage causes redistribution of blood and biochemical variables related to iron status (Córdova et al, 2002). An increase in plasma volume in the blood that is associated with endurance exercise and/or intense training could also 'dilute' free iron concentration, causing low levels of Hb, referred to as 'sports anaemia'. In sports anaemia, Hb levels approach those seen in clinical anaemia, i.e. 13 g Hb per 100 mL blood (dL) in women or 12 g Hb/dL blood in men. Training-induced hypervolemia, shown by a 20% expansion of blood plasma volume, occurs after just 4 days of sub-maximal exercise training, without a change in RBC volume (Green et al, 1987), or the amount of Hb functioning in the RBCs. This 'dilutional pseudo-anaemia' is likely to have no negative effect on the athlete (Shaskey and Green, 2000), since in this case the athlete may not be iron deficient because of the dilution of blood measures of iron status (i.e. serum iron, serum ferritin, Hct and Hb, serum transferrin receptor (sTfR) concentration).

Since pre-menopausal females generally are inclined to develop anaemia, female athletes, especially runners or vegan/vegetarian athletes, are at risk of iron-deficiency due to iron losses in sweat, urine and blood, and low iron intake (athletes' iron intake is discussed later in this chapter). Refer also to Table 7.3 for athletes at risk of iron depletion and iron deficiency anaemia.

Previous studies speculating that iron deficiency without anaemia may negatively affect sports performance (Clement and Sawchuck, 1984) has since been reviewed (Haas and Brownlie, 2001), confirming that iron deficiency leads to reduced physical work capacity. Six weeks of high-intensity interval cycle training can reduce iron stores (Wilkinson et al, 2002) and it appears that training volume affects rate of ion depletion. Magazanik et al, 1988 showed that more intensive physical training programmes (up to 8 h/day), resulted in fast iron depletion (as much as 65% drop in iron stores within 2 weeks). Such intensive physical training programmes can result in anaemia within 4 weeks in some female athletes. Similarly, some forms of exercise (running and strength training) may result in greater alterations in red cell function and more pronounced reductions in serum ferritin (Schobersberger et al, 1990; Schumacher et al, 2002).

Not all studies have reported changes in iron status following exercise training. Bourque et al, 1997 measured the effect of endurance training (weight-bearing and non-weight-bearing type exercises) on iron status of previously untrained women with normal iron stores (serum ferritin

>20 µg/L). They found that 12 weeks of moderate-intensity walking/running or cycling exercise, performed 3–4 days per week at 80% VO_2max, did not negatively affect iron status.

Athletes are recommended to regularly monitor iron stores and maintain normal serum ferritin and Hb levels. Consumption of adequate amounts of haeme iron and the nutrients that influence iron metabolism can prevent exercise-induced losses of iron, especially in young female athletes (Malczewska et al, 2000). Iron-deficiency anaemia responds well to iron supplementation, resulting in an increase in serum ferritin, unlike in sports anaemia, which does not respond to iron supplementation.

In the case of athletes who are iron-deficient without anaemia, iron supplementation may improve exercise capacity and physical performance (Hinton et al, 2000; Freidman et al, 2001; Brownlie et al, 2002, 2004) and can reverse mild anaemia (LaManca and Haymes, 1993). Other studies have not found improvement in aerobic capacity following iron supplementation (Newhouse et al, 1989; Klingshirn et al, 1992).

The maximum total safe daily intake is up to 1000 mg iron/day (Department of Health, 1991). However, iron supplements may cause constipation, and excessive iron intake can accumulate to toxic levels. Furthermore, overdosing on iron supplements (≥200 mg iron/day) will not increase the rate of Hb synthesis of 5–10 mg/day (Escott-Stump, 2002).

Iron in the diet

If iron intakes of athletes are already below the RNI, and they have increased losses of iron, an iron-depleted state may easily be reached. Furthermore, of ingested dietary iron, 10–30% of haeme iron is absorbed and only 2–10% of non-haeme iron is absorbed. Although absorption of haeme iron is not affected by food components, non-haeme iron is affected by the following factors:

Factors increasing iron absorption:
- Vitamin C
- Vitamin A
- Beta-carotene
- Riboflavin (vitamin B_2)
- Presence of haeme iron from meat, fish and poultry
- An iron-depleted state

Factors reducing iron absorption:
- Phytates/phytic acid in cereals, bran, pulses (legumes), spinach and soya products
- Tannins in tea
- Polyphenols in coffee and red wine
- Fibre in whole grains

- High amounts of calcium or calcium salts, i.e. calcium phosphate or calcium citrate
- Zinc supplements

Calcium citrate and calcium phosphate supplements (*but not calcium carbonate supplements*) reduce iron absorption (Cook et al, 1991). Calcium-containing foods also reduce absorption of non-haeme iron.

It is estimated that 40% of the world population is iron deficient (Escott-Stump, 2002), making it the single most common nutrient deficiency in the world. A fraction of this number, some ~15%, have iron-deficiency anaemia. Ways to increase iron status of individuals and vulnerable groups are imperative. Food fortification has become common practice especially in developing countries. Developed countries each have their own food legislation based on the needs of the population. Certain groups are more vulnerable to low micronutrient status, such as growing children and the elderly. White and brown flour (not wholemeal flour) is fortified with iron on a mandatory basis in the United Kingdom and must contain at least 1.65 mg iron per 100 g flour. Other foods like cereals are also fortified, albeit this is done voluntarily. Food sources of iron are provided in Table 7.5.

Some ways to increase iron absorption
- Increase intake of vitamin C-rich foods like guavas, kiwi fruits, oranges, grapefruit/tomato juice, sweet peppers, broccoli, etc. with meals (see Table 7.4).
- Eat enough meat, chicken and fish, and combine them with non-haeme foods.
- Avoid drinking tea and coffee with meals or non-haeme foods.
- Do not combine soya, bran or fibre with non-haeme foods.
- Take calcium supplements between meals, not with meals.

Calcium
Calcium is the most abundant mineral in the body, accounting for 40% of the total mineral content and amounting to 1200 g. It is needed for building and repair of bone tissue, maintenance of blood calcium levels, making acetylcholine for transmission of nerve impulses, activating enzymes including ATP, making cell membranes more permeable, helping vitamin B_{12} absorption from the intestine and for normal muscle contraction and relaxation, including cardiac (heart) muscle.

The balance between intake of calcium (absorbed from the diet), and loss of calcium (faeces and urine), in addition to adequate vitamin D, determines the total body calcium (Zilva et al, 1988). Since nearly all of the body's calcium is found in bone, bone mineral density (BMD) or assessment of calcium in the bone provides a standard measure for bone health. If dietary calcium intake is not adequate, the risk of low BMD

Table 7.5 Food sources of iron.

Food and portion sizes	Iron
haeme iron food, high bioavailability (cooked values)	
125 g sirloin steak	3.8 mg
50 g oysters	3.35 mg
50 g beef liver	3.15 mg
100 g tinned tuna in oil	1.6 mg
2 slices lean roast beef	1 mg
125 g roast chicken	1 mg
1 sandwich portion (45 g) of tinned tuna in oil	0.72 mg
100 g grilled salmon	0.5 mg
non-haeme iron foods, high bioavailability	
1 average portion (95 g) steamed broccoli	0.95 mg
non-haeme iron foods, low bioavailability	
1 cup Oat bran cereal	15 mg
1 average bowl of iron-fortified breakfast cereal (30–60 g)	3.6–7 mg (check individual brands)
1 cup kidney beans	5.3 mg
80 g cooked soya	4.1 mg
Medium portion (90 g) cooked spinach	3.2 mg
50 g dried apricots	2.4 mg
1 medium portion (135 g) baked beans	1.89 mg
1 slice wholemeal bread	1 mg
1 boiled egg	0.95 mg

Source: Material from Hayley Daries Practice.
Reference values for adult males and females 19[+] years.
UK RNI for iron = 8.7 mg (M), 14.8 mg (F) (Department of Health, 1991)
Supplemental doses = 2–60 mg/unit[2]

increases. Reduced bone mass (osteopaenia) can lead to osteoporosis (loss of bone mineral and reduced BMD). Athletes at risk of these bone disorders are female athletes, especially those who have low body weight and consume low-energy diets, i.e. endurance runners, dancers, gymnasts, those who avoid calcium-rich foods/food groups (dairy and soya group) and those with menstrual dysfunction (American College of Sports Medicine, 2009). Athletes with sports amenorrhoea (menstrual dysfunction among female athletes) (Burke and Deakin, 2000) are oestrogen deficient, and therefore, do not have oestrogen's protective effect on bone. This hormonal imbalance allows bone resorption and turnover, leading to reduced bone mineral content (BMC). Lack of calcium also increases tooth decay and the risk of lifestyle diseases (cancer, hypertension, diabetes). Table 7.6 provides food sources of calcium and relevant reference values for adults.

Table 7.6 Food sources of calcium.

Food and portion sizes	Calcium
100 g canned sardines in tomato sauce, with bones	460 mg
220 g serving of macaroni cheese	374 mg
30 g reduced fat cheddar-type cheese	252 mg
200 mL (small glass) of semi-skimmed milk	248 mg
150 g pot of low-fat fruit yoghurt	225 mg
100 g slice of pizza	180 mg
120 g serving of custard made with whole or full-fat milk	166 mg
90 g cooked spinach	144 mg
100 g tinned salmon, without bones	93 mg
150 g small can of baked beans	80 mg
1 tablespoon (12 g) of sesame seeds	8 mg
1 medium (160 g) orange	75 mg
56 g serving of dried apricots	52 mg

Source: The Dairy Council.
Reference values for adult males and females 19$^+$ years (Department of Health, 1991).
UK RNI for calcium = 700 mg
UK Maximum safe daily intake limit = 2 g/day

Inadequate calcium also increases the risk of stress fractures in athletes (Myburgh et al, 1990). Myburgh and colleagues studied elite female athletes suffering from lower leg stress fractures and matched them with controls who did not have stress fractures, but were of the same age, weight and height and had the same performance level. The stress fractures group showed signs of lower BMD than the control group, and also had lower calcium intakes and had fewer dairy products in their diet. Although biochemical factors are also implicated in injury rates in this study, diet is considered the primary causative role in stress fractures.

It is estimated that peak bone mass (PBM) is attained during adolescence and young adulthood (16–28 years of age), thereafter, bone loss occurs with aging. PBM is a primary determinant of osteoporosis risk later in life. PBM in these early years determines adults' BMD, and is positively related to calcium intake and weight-bearing activity. Some sports are less effective with regard to PBM. Female athletes involved in impact sports such as basketball, volleyball and gymnastics, have higher BMD than inactive people (Robinson et al, 1995b). Dancers also have higher BMD (on average 9% higher) than age- and weight-matched reference controls (Yannakoulia et al, 2004). Cross-sectional athlete studies of young adults show that the highest BMC and BMD values is found in strength and power-trained athletes, while endurance activities (i.e. long distance running and swimming) seem less affected with regard to PBM (Suominen, 1993).

However, since running is a weight-bearing exercise, it is associated with greater site-specific BMD than swimming or cycling (Duncan et al, 2002). However, spine BMD of female runners with amenorrhoea is 5–15% lower than those of non-runners (Cann et al, 1984; Drinkwater et al, 1990), and may be associated with intensive endurance training. Calcium supplementation boosts dietary intake of female athletes (Mehlenbeck et al, 2004; Winters-Stone and Snow, 2004) and in addition to dietary calcium intake equal to, or more than, adequate intake may offset cortical bone loss on young female runners (Winters-Stone and Snow, 2004). Consuming up to 120% of RDA appears to help BMD and bone development in athletes with amenorrhoea (Jeukendrup and Gleeson, 2004). Male cyclists involved in high-intensity cycle training risk adverse effects on BMD (Barry and Kohrt, 2008). Furthermore, having a long history of exclusive cycle training leads to low BMD in male master cyclists, compared to age-matched non-athletes, increasing cyclists' risk of osteoporosis as they get older (Nichols et al, 2003).

Optimal absorption of calcium with vitamin D

Vitamin D is required for absorption and use of calcium and phosphorous, normal bone and tooth formation, maintenance and neuromuscular function. In the presence of sunlight, skin cells can reliably make most of the vitamin D required, and the rest, a small amount, can be obtained from the diet (Wardlaw et al, 2004). Athletes who have compromised vitamin D status may risk their overall health and ability to train by affecting bone health, natural immunity and exercise-related immunity and inflammation (Willis et al, 2008).

Recommendations for adequate vitamin D include:

- regular safe sun exposure, 2–3 times a week;
- between 10 am and 3 pm;
- on the arms and legs for 5–30 minutes;
- amount of sun exposure depends on time of day, season, latitude, age and skin pigmentation; or
- dietary supplementation with 1000–2000 IU vitamin D per day.

(Wardlaw et al, 2004; Willis et al, 2008).

Other minerals

Phosphorous partners with calcium, and in bone the proportion of calcium to phosphorous is 2 to 1. It has a key role in bone and tooth formation, acid–base balance and as an essential component of ATP, it has a role in energy metabolism.

Zinc, as a component of enzymes, is an antioxidant, and has a role in energy metabolism, wound healing and cell membrane structure and function. Vegetarian athletes and those who avoid meat and seafood are at risk of zinc deficiency as well as athletes who consume low-energy diets, although megadoses of zinc supplements are not recommended (Gleeson, 2005).

Magnesium plays an important role on the formation of glycogen (Bock and Lambert, 1990). Other functions include muscle contraction, energy metabolism, protein synthesis, enzyme activation and nerve transmission. There is evidence to suggest that magnesium supplementation has no effect on performance (strength, anaerobic and aerobic systems) (Newhouse and Finstad, 2000), although more research with vulnerable groups (female athletes) should be considered. Increased losses of magnesium in the urine are seen in individuals with elevated blood glucose levels, leading to low blood levels of magnesium (hypomagnesaemia). Diabetics who are poorly managed are at risk of hypomagnesaemia (Escott-Stump, 2002).

Vitamin and mineral requirements

Most countries have their own reference values for nutrient intakes. Some of the leading developing countries have their own terms, and values also differ with respect to gender, age group and stage of the lifecycle, e.g.
- UK Recommended Nutrient Intakes (RNI)
- Australian Recommended Dietary Intakes (RDI)
- North American Recommended Daily Allowances (RDA)

Athletes at risk

Certain age groups and genders of the healthy population appear to have compromised micronutrient intakes. The UK Nutritional Survey (Henderson et al, 2003) reveals the following findings of micronutrient status and related dietary practices of healthy adults aged 19–54 years:
- In general, vitamin A, riboflavin (vitamin B_2), magnesium and potassium are compromised in men and women, especially the younger age groups (19–24 years and/or 25–34 years), and in women iodine is also compromised, especially the youngest age groups.
  Mean daily intakes from food sources, by gender:
- Women have low iron, magnesium, potassium and copper intake, below the RNI.
- Men have low potassium intake, below RNI.

Mean daily intakes from food sources, by age group:
- *Women, 19–24 years*: low vitamin A, iron, calcium, magnesium, potassium, zinc, iodine and copper, below RNI.
- *Women, most age groups*: low iron, magnesium, potassium, zinc and copper, below RNI.
- *Women, 19–24 years and 25–34 years*: over 40% have low iron intake.
- *Men, 19–24 years*: low vitamin A, magnesium, potassium, zinc and copper, below RNI.

  Mean daily intakes of supplements:
- 40% of women and 29% of men take 'extra vitamins, minerals or other dietary supplements'.

  Furthermore, only 13% of men and 15% of women meet the 5-a-day recommendation (for fruits and vegetables).

Athletes' micronutrient intake and supplementation practices

Dietary intake surveys of athlete's food practices and choices have been conducted extensively (Van Erp-Baart et al, 1989; Worme et al, 1990; Felder et al, 1998; Farajian et al, 2004; Hinton et al, 2004; Onywera et al, 2004) and are discussed in some detail in Chapter 2. Where athletes' diets are concerned, increased demands of exercise training should be matched with an energy-rich, well-balanced diet to meet all macronutrient and micronutrient requirements. Energy from protein, carbohydrate and fat may be easily met by increased food and drink consumption. However, it is possible that the nature of some athletes' diets may cater too much for meeting energy needs (with low-nutrient, energy-dense foods, drinks and supplements) and not fully regard the increasing vitamin and mineral needs associated with more intense exercise training and competition.

Low micronutrient intakes have only been reported in some groups of athletes, and in a select few studies. Iron deficiency is one of the single nutrient deficiencies that is commonly reported among athletes involved in regular exhaustive exercise. Low dietary iron intakes have been reported in both elite and recreational athletes. Many studies report mean iron intake among female athletes to be lower than RDA, compared with other (population-specific) reference values (Felder et al, 1998; Farajian et al, 2004; Gábor et al, 2010), more often reporting marginal intakes (below 70% of the RDA) or lower consumption. Most likely causes of low iron status are low intake of iron-rich foods, and/or replacing micronutrient-rich foods with low-micronutrient, energy-dense food.

Other studies have not found similar results and report adequate iron intakes among female (Hinton et al, 2004). Male athletes have been frequently reported to have iron intakes in excess of RDA or reference values (Worme et al, 1990; Farajian et al, 2004). Some studies have reported iron depletion, anaemia and iron deficiency anaemia in both male and female athletes, as Dubnov and Constantini (2004) observed in basketball players.

Besides compromised iron status, low intakes of one or more other micronutrients are also reported in dietary surveys of athletes, although more often in females than in males. Of these, athletes' intakes of calcium, magnesium, zinc, folate and B-vitamins often fall below RDA or reference values. Singh et al (1993) found that ultra-marathon cross-country runners had low levels of zinc in their diets, consuming a mean of only 65% of RDA for zinc.

However, some studies report adequate or excessive intakes of micronutrients either by food intake and/or vitamin and mineral supplementation. A recent study by Petroczi and Naughton (2008) examining the supplement practices of high-performing athletes in the United Kingdom, found the following results:

- 58.8% of athletes use of at least one nutritional supplement.
- 82.6% of users used more than one supplement.
- 11.5% reported use of more than five nutritional supplements.
- 72.6% of athletes used multivitamins.
- 70.7% used vitamin C.
- 36.1% used creatine, typically by males.
- 31.7% used whey protein.
- 30.9% used echinacea.
- 29.9% used iron, typically by females.
- 23.7% used caffeine.
- <11% said they used magnesium or ginseng.
- A 'typical' supplement user: male, 24–29 years of age, involved in professional sport and using a combination of supplements.
- Other users: male professional players (30–34 years), and female non-professional athletes (24–29 years).
- Non-users: most athletes over 40 years.

In contrast to studies that found increase supplement use by high-performance athletes, a follow-up study (between 2002 and 2009) found a downward trend in supplement use by Olympic athletes (Heikkinen et al, 2011). Further observations are needed to confirm if this trend applies to other athletes, or across all sport codes.

These surveys provide valuable information about nutrient intakes and supplement use by adults and athletes that can be used to indicate vulnerabilities in the diets of athletes and the nutritional issues that need to be addressed.

Chapter summary

- Vitamins and minerals are non-energy giving nutrients that are essential to life and have highly specific physiologic functions in the body.
- Vitamins are organic substances needed for physiologic functions, chemical processes and metabolic reactions and cannot be synthesised by the body but must be obtained from food sources.
- Primary and secondary vitamin deficiencies are defined by specific causes and a specific set of symptoms.
- There are 13 essential vitamins that are classified as either fat-soluble or water-soluble vitamins.
- Minerals are inorganic substances that make up about 4% of body weight and are incorporated into structural components of the body tissues and present in body fluids.
- Between 15 and 22 essential minerals need to be obtained from the diet including major minerals, trace elements and electrically charged ions that function as minerals namely, electrolytes.
- Exercise increases micronutrient requirements as well as other environmental factors.
- B-complex vitamins serve as co-enzymes in energy metabolism pathways assimilating and metabolising carbohydrates, proteins and fats to produce energy and transporting oxygen to the exercising muscles.
- Muscle oxygen uptake may increase 100-fold during prolonged strenuous exercise, resulting in more free radicals being produced in skeletal muscle.
- Antioxidant vitamins A, C, E and beta-carotene intercept oxygen radicals and can repair, and work against, the damage it has caused.
- Reactive oxygen species (ROS) is associated with muscle damage markers, such as delayed onset muscle soreness (DOMS).
- Trained athletes become adapted to higher oxidative stress by producing more antioxidant enzymes that enhances the enzymatic antioxidant system.
- Iron is found in all body cells, in erythrocytes, liver, spleen and bone marrow, as functional iron in haemoglobin (Hb), myoglobin, enzyme systems and other cellular constituents.
- Athletes lose iron through sweat, faeces, urine and blood.
- An increase in plasma volume in the blood that is associated with endurance exercise and/or intense training 'dilutes' free iron concentration, causing low levels of Hb, referred to as 'sports anaemia', not to be confused with 'dilutional pseudo-anaemia'.
- Iron deficiency leads to reduced physical work capacity. Intensive physical training programmes that involve high training volumes can cause fast iron depletion, and in some female athletes it can lead to anaemia.

- Iron-deficiency anaemia responds well to iron supplementation, resulting in an increase in serum ferritin, unlike sports anaemia, which does not respond to iron supplementation.
- Consumption of adequate amounts of haeme iron and the nutrients that influence iron metabolism can prevent exercise-induced losses of iron, especially in young female athletes.
- Absorption of non-haeme iron is affected by a number of food-related components, including vitamin C, A, beta-carotene, riboflavin, phytates, tannins, polyphenols, fibre, calcium and zinc supplements.
- Calcium is the most abundant mineral in the body. Assessment of calcium in the bone by measure of bone mineral density (BMD) provides a standard measure for bone health.
- Athletes at risk of these bone disorders (low BMD, osteopaenia or osteoporosis) are female athletes, especially those with low body weight who may consume low energy diets, those who avoid calcium-rich foods/food groups and those with menstrual dysfunction.
- Inadequate calcium also increases the risk of stress fractures in athletes, diet being considered the primary causative role in stress fractures.
- Vitamin D is required for absorption and use of calcium and phosphorous, normal bone and tooth formation, maintenance and neuromuscular function. In the presence of sunlight, skin cells make most of the vitamin D, and a small amount is obtained from the diet.
- Phosphorous, zinc and magnesium have a role in energy metabolism and other functions related to exercise.
- Dietary surveys of nutrient intakes from food sources and supplements such as the national *UK Nutritional Survey*, and surveys of athletes provide valuable information about current vitamin and mineral intakes of the general population and athletes, and their supplement practices.

Notes

1 Risk of diarrhoea at high vitamin C intakes (Department of Health, 1991)

2 Maximum total safe daily intake is up to 1000 mg iron/day (Department of Health, 1991), although overdosing on iron supplements ($\geq$200 mg iron/day) will not increase the rate of haemoglobin synthesis of 5–10 mg/day (Escott-Stump, 2002). Furthermore, iron supplements may cause constipation, and excessive iron intake can accumulate to toxic levels.

Avocado and Prawn Salad

(Serves 4)

Ingredients

2 large ripe avocado pears, halved
500 g (1 lb) pre-cooked, frozen prawns
200 g (7 oz) low-fat mayonnaise or low-oil dressing

1–2 small red chillies, seeded and chopped
40 mL lemon juice
Watercress leaves

Method

1 Boil the prawns for 10–15 minutes in water. Drain the water and set the prawns aside to cool.
2 Thinly slice the avocado pear halves and arrange decoratively on four serving plates. Sprinkle lemon juice over the sliced avocado pears.
3 In a bowl, mix the mayonnaise, prawns and red chillies.
4 Spoon the prawns over the avocado slices.
5 Serve immediately with watercress.

Nutrition analysis per portion
Side salad

Energy	185 kcal (755 kJ)
Protein	10.6 g
Carbohydrate	1.8 g
Fat	14.5 g
Cholesterol	105 mg
Fibre	1.5 g

Main dish

Energy	495 kcal (2077 kJ)
Protein	28 g
Carbohydrate	5 g
Fat	39 g
Cholesterol	281 mg
Fibre	4 g

Food note: Avocado is rich in the heart-healthy monounsaturated fats.

Brown Rice and Lentil Salad

(Serves 4–6)

Ingredients

500 g (16 oz) brown rice, cooked and cooled	50 mL parsley, chopped
100 g frozen mixed vegetables, steamed	1 lemon's juice
1 × 400 g tin lentils, drained	Salt and pepper
50 g sundried tomatoes, chopped	50 mL olive oil

Method

1 Lightly fluff the rice and combine all the ingredients.
2 Season to taste.
3 Refrigerate and serve cold.

Nutrition analysis per portion
Side salad

Energy	246 kcal (1031 kJ)
Protein	6.4 g
Carbohydrate	28 g
Fat	10 g
Cholesterol	0 mg
Fibre	5 g

Main dish

Energy	369 kcal (1550 kJ)
Protein	10 g
Carbohydrate	42 g
Fat	14.3 g
Cholesterol	0 mg
Fibre	8 g

Food note: A healthy vegetarian choice, the rice and lentils make a complete protein.

Salads and Fruit Recipes

Although required in small quantities in the diet, vitamins and minerals have a very important role in health and well-being and cannot be neglected at the expense of the energy-giving nutrients. To make sure your plate is colourful, add the dishes from the following recipes with your carb- and protein-rich meals.

Chicken Caesar Salad

(Serves 4)

Ingredients

4 slices whole-grain bread, cubed (for croutons)

2 chicken breasts

50 mL low-oil salad dressing

50 mL low-fat yoghurt

15 mL lemon juice

2 anchovy fillets, chopped

1 garlic clove, chopped

250 g (9 oz) cos lettuce, shredded

50 g (2 oz) parmesan cheese, shaved with a potato peeler

Method

1 Lightly toast the bread cubes in the oven at 200°C.
2 Grill the chicken breast for 5–6 minutes on each side. Cool and cut the chicken into pieces.
3 Combine the salad dressing, yoghurt, lemon juice, anchovies and garlic.
4 In a large serving bowl, mix the croutons, chicken and lettuce together.
5 Dish into four individual plates.
6 Drizzle the sauce over and sprinkle with the parmesan cheese.

Nutrition analysis per portion
Side salad or light meal

Energy	376 (1579 kJ)
Protein	36 g
Carbohydrate	19 g
Fat	16 g
Cholesterol	92 mg
Fibre	3 g

Food note: Lemons are rich in vitamin C (immune-boosting) and bring out the natural flavours of chicken and fish.

Greek Salad with Lemon Vinaigrette

(Serves 4)

Ingredients	**Lemon Vinaigrette:**
1 bag of mixed lettuce	2 lemons, juiced and zest
300 g (11 oz) cocktail tomatoes	3 mL fresh parsley, finely chopped
1 (250 g) English cucumber, thinly sliced	Salt and freshly ground pepper
2 small red onions/shallots, cubed	20 mL honey, heated
120 g (4 oz) pimento olives	125 mL olive oil
175 g low-fat Greek feta cheese, cubed	

Method

1 Toss all the vegetables and cheese in a deep serving dish.
2 For the vinaigrette, combine all the ingredients into a jug and beat with a fork.
3 Pour the vinaigrette over the salad.
4 Serve.

Nutrition analysis per portion
Small salad

Energy	75 kcal (315 kJ)
Protein	3.8 g
Carbohydrate	4.1 g
Fat	4.0 g
Cholesterol	5 mg
Fibre	1.9 g

Nutrition analysis per portion
Side salad

Energy	150 kcal (630 kJ)
Protein	8 g
Carbohydrate	8.2 g
Fat	8 g
Cholesterol	10 mg
Fibre	4 g

Large salad

Energy	279 kcal (1172 kJ)
Protein	14 g
Carbohydrate	15.2 g
Fat	15 g
Cholesterol	19 mg
Fibre	7 g

Food note: Red onions contain more *quercetin* than other onion varieties.

Mango and Chilli Juice

(Makes 2 glasses)

Ingredients

2 large ripe mangoes, peeled and cubed

2 large oranges, seeded and chopped

$\frac{1}{2}$ small red chilli, seeded and chopped

10 mL lime juice

250 g ice cubes

Mint leaves

Method

1 Blend all the ingredients together, except the mint leaves.

2 Garnish with mint leaves.

Nutrition analysis per portion (excluding mint leaves)

Energy	237 kcal (996 kJ)
Protein	2.5 g
Carbohydrate	47 g
Fat	0.7 g
Cholesterol	0 mg
Fibre	7.5 g

Food note: Mangoes are rich in antioxidants namely beta-carotene and vitamin C.

Melon Wrapped in Parma Ham

(Serves 4)

Ingredients

$\frac{1}{2}$ cantaloupe (sweet melon), seeded and sliced
$\frac{1}{2}$ honeydew melon (winter melon), seeded and sliced
16 (200 g) Parma ham slices
30 mL pomegranate juice

Method

1 Peel the melons and cut into thick slices.
2 Wrap a slice of Parma ham around each slice of melon.
3 Drizzle the pomegranate juice over and serve.

Nutrition analysis per portion

Energy	142 kcal (596 kJ)
Protein	11 g
Carbohydrate	16 g
Fat	3 g
Cholesterol	24.2 mg
Fibre	2 g

Food note: Melons are low in calories and have high water content.
They contain vitamin C (some varieties more than others).

Roasted Sweet Potato Salad with Mint Yoghurt Dressing

(Serves 4)

Ingredients

500 g (1 lb) sweet potatoes, washed and cubed
8 baby onions, peeled and halved
150 g (6 oz) baby carrots
4 garlic cloves, sliced in halves
Piece of fresh ginger root, cut into chunks
6 sprigs of thyme or rosemary
20 mL olive oil
Parsley
Salt and freshly ground pepper

Yoghurt Dressing (Optional):
200 mL low-fat Bulgarian yoghurt
50 mL fresh mint, finely chopped
20 mL honey

Method

1 Preheat the oven to 190°C.
2 Combine all the ingredients and bake for 25–30 minutes.
3 For the dressing, mix the yoghurt, mint and honey.
4 Serve the vegetable in four bowls and drizzle the dressing over.
5 Serve the vegetables hot or cold.

Nutrition analysis per portion (excluding mint leaves)

Energy	220 kcal (925 kJ)
Protein	5 g
Carbohydrate	32 g
Fat	6.3 g
Cholesterol	5 mg
Fibre	4.5 g

Food note: Sweet potatoes are rich in beta-carotene and have a lower glycaemic index (GI) than potatoes. Bulgarian yoghurt is a good source of calcium and live cultures containing *probiotics.*

Sardine Pasta Salad

(Serves 4)

Ingredients

300 g (11 oz) screw pasta
400 g (14 oz) smoked sardines, shredded
50 g (2 oz) raisins
1 apple, chopped
50 mL orange juice

50 mL lemon juice
1 spring onion, chopped
100 mL sweet and sour sauce
70 mL olive oil
Coriander, chopped

Method

1 Boil the pasta in salted water until 'al dente'. Drain and set aside to cool.
2 In a large serving dish, combine all the ingredients.
3 Serve chilled.

Nutrition analysis per portion

Energy	566 kcal (2379 kJ)
Protein	21 g
Carbohydrate	39 g
Fat	31 g
Cholesterol	47 mg
Fibre	3 g

Food note: Sardines are an excellent source of calcium and omega-3 fatty acids, therefore, the fat content of this meal is mostly polyunsaturated. Olive oil provides heart-healthy monounsaturated fat, the amount added can be adjusted to suit individual tastes.

Tofu and Vegetable Stir-fry

(Serves 4)

Ingredients

30 mL canola oil

2 leeks, sliced

4 garlic cloves, crushed

400 g (14 oz) tofu, drained and cubed

150 g (6 oz) carrots, julienned or thinly sliced

1 red pepper, seeded and sliced

250 g (9 oz) baby corn

2 chillies, seeded and chopped

60 mL soya sauce (low sodium)

100 g (4 cups) baby spinach, washed

Pepper

Method

1 Heat the oil in a wok until it starts smoking. Sauté the leeks, garlic and tofu for 3 minutes.

2 Add the carrots, stir-fry for 2 minutes.

3 Add the pepper, corn and chillies and stir-fry for 5 minutes.

4 Add the soya sauce and spinach and stir-fry until the spinach has wilted.

5 Serve while hot.

Nutrition analysis per portion

Energy	202 kcal (847 kJ)
Protein	11 g
Carbohydrate	7.5 g
Fat	12.5 g
Cholesterol	0 mg
Fibre	4 g

Food note: Tofu or soya bean curd is high in protein and low in fat, making it a good choice for healthy vegetarian meals.

CHAPTER 8

Fluid Balance

Key terms	
Water	Isotonic, hypotonic and hypertonic
Electrolytes	beverage
Water losses	Over-hydration
Dehydration	Water intoxication
Percentage body weight loss	Ratings of stomach fullness
Sweat loss	Osmotic imbalance
Sweat rate	Exercise-associated hyponatremia (EAH)
Fluid intake rates	Exercise-associated hyponatremic
Voluntary dehydration	encephalopathy (EAHE)
Ad libitum fluid ingestion	'Stitch' or 'side ache'
Serum sodium concentration	Exercise-related transient abdominal pain
Serum osmolality	(ETAP)
Isotonicity	Gastric emptying
Thirst	Carbohydrate oxidation
Metabolic water	Skin wetting ('sponging')
Carbohydrate-electrolyte beverage	Alcohol

Considering that the body weight is made up of 50–65% water, with no storage site for water, this nutrient is the second most essential nutrient to the human body, after oxygen.

Functions of water

- Component of lean muscle (~70% water)
- Component of fat and bone (~20–25% water)
- Transports nutrients, gases and waste products

Nutrition for Sport and Exercise: A Practical Guide, First Edition. Hayley Daries.
© 2012 Blackwell Publishing Ltd. Published 2012 by Blackwell Publishing Ltd.

- Regulates temperature, through sweating and in vapour from the lungs (for every litre perspired, heat loss through sweat equals around 600 kcal of energy) (Robinson et al, 1986)
- Lubrication of joints, eyes and cushioning of cells
- Main solvent; most substances dissolve in water
- Reactive medium for minerals and other chemicals in the body
- Component of many foods

Electrolytes are substances that, when dissolving in water, dissociate and carry an electrical change. Examples of positive ions (or *cations*) are sodium and potassium, whereas an example of a negative ion (or *anion*) is chloride. Concentrations of electrolytes in solutions are measured in milliequivalents, milligrams or millimoles per litre.

Functions of electrolytes

- Maintain osmotic pressure
- Control nervous irritability
- Control muscle contraction
- Regulate acid-balance
- Facilitate movement of nutrients into cells
- Facilitate movement of removal of waste products

A person can go without food for days, weeks, even months, but without water, humans can die within days. However, in very hot environments, death from heatstroke can occur within hours, but it precedes the risks associated with significant fluid losses. Humans merely stop exercising at dehydration rates of 7–10%, while the risk of organ failure or death occurs when dehydration reaches levels of 15–20% or more (Noakes, 2001).

Water losses

At rest, water losses in healthy people include urine output and faeces, sweat and water lost through breathing. This water requirement is met by an intake of 2.0–2.5 L of water daily, the need rises as calorie intake increases, and in hotter climates. Water is obtained from liquids, food and as a result of the metabolism of nutrients.

During exercise, water and electrolytes are lost through sweat, and as water losses exceed fluid intake, dehydration can occur. During *prolonged* exercise, the amount of sodium and potassium in the body determines the amount of water (in the body), therefore forcing water to be excreted as sodium is lost in sweat. This maintains the blood sodium concentration and prevents it from becoming diluted (Noakes, 2001).

Sweat loss is dependent on several factors, such as genetics, body size, gender, age, fitness level, metabolism and exercise intensity.

Sweat rates among athletes

Fluid loss during exercise is determined by the sweat rate, which is proportional to the athlete's metabolic rate (Wyndham et al, 1970; Davies et al, 1976; Costill, 1977; Davies, 1979; Greenhaff, 1989; Noakes et al, 1991). The athletes' metabolic rate is affected by their running speed (or rate of heat production) and body weight (Costill, 1977). Thus, faster or heavier athletes sweat more than slower or smaller (lighter) athletes. Other factors such as environmental temperature and humidity affect sweat rate.

There appears to be great individual variability in sweat rates and sweat losses of individuals differs also within activities. A review of the literature by the American College of Sports Medicine (ACSM) suggests that competitive athletes sweat at rates of between 0.3 and 2.4 L/h (Sawka et al, 2007). Typical sweat rates in runners during longer distance races are ~1.2 L/h (Noakes, 1993). Higher than 1.2 L/h sweat rates are usually recorded only when environmental temperatures are greater than 25°C or for elite athletes competing at very high exercise intensities.

Under both moderate (22°C) and hot (32–33°C) conditions cyclists are reported to sweat 1.2–1.4 L/h while riding at 62–70% VO_2max. (Hamilton et al, 1991; Montain and Coyle, 1992a, 1992b). In ultra-endurance cycling races such as the Tour de France, cyclists can sweat around 3 L/h and lose as much as 6% body weight or 4 kg per stage.

A note on football

Football (soccer) is characterised by intermittent high-intensity exercise lasting 90 minutes and competitive players experience a high heat load, especially in the hot environments. With core temperature rising to over 39°C during the course of a game (Ekblom, 1986), heat loss is achieved mainly through sweating. In a temperate environment (20–25°C), players can lose 1.0–2.5 L during a game and up to 3 L for international level players (Ekblom, 1986). In hotter environments (24–29°C), Maughan et al (2004) reported average sweat rates of over 2 L (2033 mL) in competitive players (English Premier League Football Team) during a pre-season training session. Similarly, on average, players did not match fluid intakes (~971 mL) with sweat losses, but clearly the range of intake (265–1661 mL) demonstrated individual variability and different behavioural practices among the same group. Shirreffs et al (2005) subsequently reported a "failure" of elite football players to match sweat losses during training. However, even in cool environments (6–8°C), average sweat losses of competitive footballers (English Premier League Reserve Football Team) have been reported to average 1.68 L with large variations between individuals (Maughan et al, 2007). This study also reported that fluid intakes (~0.85 L) did not match sweat losses. The question of whether *failure to match sweat rate* is an appropriate response is examined later in the chapter.

Awareness of sweat losses is important for elite players who report the highest sweat rates. Competitive players who have been identified in the literature as 'salty sweaters' (Montain et al, 2006), and who exercise at high exercise intensities in hot environments, often lose more fluid than they replace, leading to dehydration. Some argue that the effects of increasing dehydration causes fatigue and affects players' exercise performance (Mohr et al, 2010), while others report that no single metabolic factor (i.e. dehydration) causes fatigue in elite soccer (Edwards and Noakes, 2009).

Historical perspective of fluid intake during distance running

A case for dehydration and its 'detrimental effects on health and exercise performance', *as a means to encourage fluid intake during exercise,* has been favoured since the early studies with athletes in the 1960s (Pugh et al, 1967; Wyndham and Strydom, 1969). These early studies focused on the 'dangers of dehydration' and influenced sports governing bodies, athletic race rules and other exercise scientists in the field. The gap between theory and practice was eventually closed by the growth and development of the current beverage industry, which brought their interpretation of the 'science of fluid replacement' to the masses of athletes.

In fact, it was early 20th century industrial and military investigations of fluid balance in men working and exercising in hot (32–49°C) environments that first showed the effects of drinking on work and exercise performance, as well as on physiological functions (Talbott et al, 1933; Adolf and Dill, 1938; Pitts et al, 1944; Adolf, 1947). These findings included the following:

- Talbott et al (1933) found that although workmen had large sweat losses, their physiological functions remained within normal limits. They concluded that prolonged physical activity in the heat was not detrimental to an individual's health.
- Adolf and Dill (1938) found that the average fluid intake of construction workers was about 4 L/day in high environmental temperatures. Sweat rates varied from 04 L/h at rest to 1.5–1.7 L/h during 1–2 hours of exercise in the heat, but the workmen hardly drank during exercise. The workmen drank more fluid immediately after exercise and stopped

when they replaced 50% of their fluid losses. These findings led to the concept of 'voluntary dehydration', described later in the chapter.

- Pitts et al (1944) tested male subjects who ran on a treadmill for 4 hours in a hot environment (38°C and 35% humidity) with or without ingesting fluid. They found that the men had higher rectal temperatures and heart rates after 4 hours when fluid was withheld than when volunteers drank *ad libitum*. Furthermore, providing saline or glucose affected the subjects' heart rates but only marginally lowered their rectal temperature.
- Adolf (1947) studied soldiers who walked a distance of 33.6 km or until exhaustion in the heat (31–34°C). They found that rectal temperatures, pulse rates and levels of dehydration increased with exercise time, and that subjects became exhausted at dehydration levels of around ~8%.

The findings showed that the effect of *no fluid* ingestion during exercise led to dehydration that affected physiological function (i.e. reduced plasma volume, reduced skin blood flow, increased body (core) temperature, impaired temperature regulation, increased heart rate, reduced stroke volume, reduced cardiac output, increased plasma sodium (NA^+) concentration, increased plasma osmolality, reduced body weight and increased perception of effort).

However, athletes were unaware of these investigations and their need for fluid consumption during exercise. Rather, fluid ingestion during exercise was frowned upon at that time. As a test of their fitness, marathon runners of the early 1900s believed that drinking water was not beneficial, and therefore delayed or avoided drinking water during a race (Noakes, 1995). Furthermore, the International Amateur Athletic Federation (IAAF) rules governing the intake of fluids during prolonged exercise appeared not to oppose such fluid restrictions and, in fact, discouraged marathon runners from drinking during races.

It was only in their 1953 (IAAF) handbook that they made the first official reference to fluid replacement during long-distance running. It stated, *'refreshments shall only be provided by the organisers of a race after 15 km or 10 miles, and thereafter every 5 km or 3 miles. No refreshments may be carried or taken by a competitor other than that provided by the organisers'*. The IAAF rules evolved from 1953 to 1990 regarding fluid intake during marathon races as follows:

- *1953*: Water every 5 km after 15 km
- *1967*: Water every 5 km after 11 km
- *1977*: Water every 2.5 km after 5 km
- *1990*: Water with/without carbohydrate every 3 km

In the late 1960's some studies were conducted that created an interest in fluid replacement. In a study of competitive marathon runners, Pugh et al (1967) found that the fastest runner (race winner) of an English marathon had the highest fluid loss, sweat rate and post-race rectal temperature. These runners only drank ~400 mL of fluid and dehydrated by ~5.9% of body weight. The authors appeared more interested in the association between runners with the highest levels of dehydration and success in distance running. They neither appeared too alarmed by the effect of these marked levels of dehydration nor suggested a fluid regime. This study showed that there were no 'dangers of dehydration', only apparent advantages of being dehydrated as the most dehydrated/hot runners won the race.

The IAAF rules still appeared to discourage marathon runners from drinking during a race. At the time, the IAAF rule (1967) stated that marathon runners could drink water only after the 11-km mark of the 42-km standard marathon, and then every 5 km.

Later, the findings of a classic study by Wyndham and Strydom (1969) also demonstrated a benefit of dehydration during exercise. In their study, they observed two groups of athletes competing in a 20-mile (32 km) road-race, and found that the runners who became dehydrated during the race had elevated post-race rectal temperatures. The most dehydrated athletes (>3% of their body weight) had the highest rectal temperatures (~40°C).

Thus, the fastest runner was the hottest and most dehydrated, suggesting a benefit of dehydration similar to findings of Pugh et al (1967).

However, these were not the conclusions of Wyndham and Strydom, since their study was entitled 'The dangers of an inadequate water intake during marathon running'. While the study was a landmark in the field of fluid replacement, it did so for all the wrong reasons since it drew faulty conclusions. Their findings led Wyndham and Strydom to speculate that the athletes' level of dehydration and their elevated post-race temperatures were causally related (*not possible in a cross-sectional study*) and that dehydration alone was the most important factor determining rectal temperature during prolonged exercise (Wyndham and Strydom, 1969; Wyndham, 1977), and may predispose athletes to heatstroke. These researchers also failed to note that rectal temperatures are more a function of metabolic rate than of dehydration (Noakes et al, 1991). Furthermore, even though their athletes drank ~100 mL fluid/h, the authors suggested athletes' prevent body weight loss of >3%, by drinking at rates of 1 L fluid/h (250 mL every 15 minutes).

As a result of Wyndham and Strydom's (1969) study, the concept that fluid replacement alone was of primary importance for optimising performance during prolonged exercise was promoted. Costill and Saltin (1974) reinforced the notion that *water* was the optimum fluid replacement during prolonged exercise. Their study showed that drinks with a high (6.25 or 37.5 g/100 mL) carbohydrate content emptied more slowly from the stomach than water during exercise.

At this time the IAAF changed their rules that competitors during a marathon could now have *'refreshments provided by the organisers of the race after approximately 5 km or 3 miles'*. In addition they added that the *'organisers shall provide sponging points where water only shall be supplied midway between (two) refreshment stations'* (IAAF handbook, 1977, pp. 98).

Dehydration, fluid intake and exercise performance

Humans may dehydrate because they lose sodium chloride in sweat (Dill, 1938). As a result of sodium chloride losses in human sweat, serum osmolality rises less during exercise-induced dehydration than what would occur otherwise. Nose et al (1988a, 1988b, 1988c) have shown that human drinking behaviour is regulated by changes in both serum osmolality and plasma volume, although Dill (1938) thought that thirst was related primarily to plasma sodium concentration, not the plasma volume. Thus, dipsogenic drive in dehydrated humans ceases prematurely when serum osmolality is returned to isotonicity by the ingestion of plain water before either fluid or sodium losses are replaced. Ingestion of solutions containing sodium chloride also terminates drinking prematurely by restoring plasma and extracellular volumes before fluid losses are replaced. The result is whether dehydrated humans drink plain water or sodium chloride solutions they tend to stop drinking before they are fully rehydrated.

Early experiments demonstrated that in the absence of fluid replacement, progressive dehydration during prolonged exercise could adversely affect physiological function and exercise performance. The subjects in these experiments were working at relatively low rates for many hours in the dry heat.

Several studies have since reported that dehydration is detrimental to exercise performance and that athletes cannot 'toughen up' by repeated exposure to dehydration. Many studies report the benefit of fluid ingestion in improving performance, e.g. in extending endurance and delaying fatigue in moderate- to high-intensity exercise (McConnel et al, 1987; Maughan et al, 1989; Barr et al, 1991; Milliard-Stafford et al, 1997; Montain and Coyle, 1992a, 1992b; Fallowfield et al, 1996) and improving exercise performance in the heat (Walsh et al, 1994; Below et al, 1995; Milliard-Stafford et al, 1992; Carter et al, 2003). The ACSM's (1996) position stand on fluid replacement recommended that 'during exercise, athletes should start drinking early and at regular intervals in an attempt to consume fluid at a rate sufficient to replace all the water lost though sweating (body weight loss), or consume the maximal amount that can be tolerated' (Convertino et al, 1996). In 2007, ACSM reported that levels of dehydration of greater than 2% reduce performance during aerobic exercise, and more so in warm–hot weather. Their revised fluid guidelines advised athletes not to lose >2% of their starting body weight during any form of exercise (Sawka et al, 2007). Further reports of sports performed in the heat show that low (<2% of body mass) levels of dehydration may impair high-intensity exercise performance in high ambient temperatures (31–32°C). Edwards et al (2007) found that such levels of dehydration reduce soccer (football) performance, a high-intensity intermittent exercise. Even reports of resistance exercise show body water deficits negatively affected performance (Judelson et al, 2007).

Many of these studies form the collective group that subscribe to a linear relationship between dehydration (% body weight loss) and exercise performance, i.e. the level of dehydration determines the extent at which performance is affected or impaired. Some have gone as far as to suggest that fluid losses in excess of 5% of body weight can reduce exercise capacity by as much as 30%. This concept often demonstrated by a line graph showing the relationship between increasing dehydration and declining exercise performance has been used in many sport and exercise textbooks and classrooms.

However, irrespective of the level of dehydration that develops during exercise, performance is optimised by *ad libitum* fluid intake or drinking to prevent the development of thirst, and not by *preventing dehydration*. Sharwood et al, 2004 observed no apparent effect of body weight losses up to 12% on ironman performance (or body temperature), revealing that athletes who are top finishers in competitive endurance events (i.e. marathon, ultra-marathon and ironman race winners, or with the fastest times) are *distinctly* dehydrated (Figure 8.1).

As for dehydration and it's affect on health, it has been regarded as an 'illness' to be feared by athletes. However, over the last 20 years there has been no evidence in the literature of exercise-related death or serious illness due exclusively to 'dehydration' (Noakes, 2010).

Involuntary dehydration

Earlier studies suggested that some level of dehydration may actually be *unintentional* as sweat rates invariably exceed rates of fluid intake during competitive exercise. The concept that athletes fail to fully replace their body weight losses has been known for years as 'voluntary' dehydration and described by Rothstein et al (1947), and occurs because thirst does not appear to be a sufficient stimulus for drinking (Ladell, 1965) or maintaining body water. As dehydrated persons have no preference to rehydrate, the term *involuntary* dehydration was used subsequently (Nadel et al, 1990). Therefore, it was believed that thirst does not drive athletes

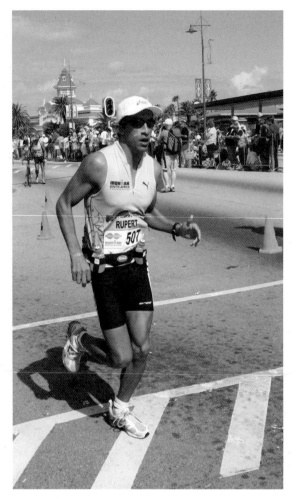

Figure 8.1 Performance is optimized by *ad libitum* fluid intake, not by *preventing dehydration*, as seen in competitive ironman triathletes who have the fastest race times despite a distinct body weight loss.

to match fluid intake with fluid losses, since it may only be perceived by athletes when water deficits are in the range of ~2% (Adolf, 1947) and plasma osmolality is above 295 milliosmoles (mOsmol)/kg (Hubbard et al, 1990; Armstrong et al, 1997). Hubbard et al (1990) concluded in their review that thirst was delayed not inadequate, a delay manifested by the body's osmotic control.

In an updated fluid recommendation position statement by Hew-Butler et al (2006), the International Marathon Medical Directors Association (IMMDA) regards 'voluntary' and 'involuntary' dehydration as terms that devalued thirst. Evidence suggests that it is thirst that primarily regulates fluid homeostasis during exercise. Thirst is affected by changes in plasma osmolality (serum sodium concentration reflects plasma osmolality).

Plasma osmolality is defended over body fluid volume, and is maintained with normal ranges until the accumulation of ∼4% body weight losses through sweating (Hew-Butler et al, 2006).

Thus, humans do not defend their weight by replacement of fluid losses during exercise. It is well known that voluntary fluid consumption does not fully replace body weight loss during exercise. In a review by Noakes (1993), voluntary rates of fluid ingestion and exercise-induced weight changes in runners, cyclists and triathletes competing over a wide range of distances were investigated. That review suggests that most endurance athletes voluntarily drink less than 0.5 L fluid/h and lose up to 1.0–1.5 L sweat/h in distance races conducted in 20–25°C (Noakes, 1993). Fluid ingestion rates may be as low as 0.27–0.45 L/h (Wilmore and Costill, 2004). When athletes attempt to drink fluid at rates closer to their 1.0–1.5 L sweat rates or more, they generally experience gastrointestinal (GI) discomfort (), or 'stitch' (side ache), especially in running (Costill et al, 1970; Brouns et al, 1987; Plunkett and Hopkins, 1999; Daries et al, 2000; Morton et al, 2004). Adolf and Dill (1938) found that after 1–2 hours of exercise in the heat, construction workers stopped re-hydrating when they had replaced 50% of their fluid losses. Nose et al (1988a) offered either water or saline to re-hydrate their dehydrated volunteers. Despite being able to drink *ad libitum*, the volunteers only restored 53% or 67% of the water lost, respectively. Szlyk et al (1989) reported that 13 of 33 men were classified as 'reluctant' drinkers during exercise in the heat because they did not maintain body weight loss below 2% despite the provision of water *ad libitum*.

Thus, despite access to fluids, many athletes do not replace fluid losses during exercise. Furthermore, in sedentary persons, the metabolism of nutrients releases metabolic water. The breakdown of glucose, protein and fat, as well as water released from stored glycogen contributes approximately 14% to the daily water requirement (McArdle et al, 2010). During prolonged exercise, it has been calculated that fluid is lost from oxidation of metabolic fuels, glycolysis and other metabolic water, which accounts for ∼1800–2000 g (Pastene et al, 1996) contributing to sweat loss and that does not require replacement.

Drinking no fluid, *ad libitum* or 'as much as tolerable' during exercise

Optimum hydration and thermoregulation are important considerations in any environment (hot or cool). Since we already know the importance of fluid ingestion during exercise (Noakes, 2003), what needs to be established is *how much* fluid is required to improve performance or what are *ad libitum* rates.

Studies examining the difference in dehydration and performance be-tween no fluid or full fluid replacement have been well documented, but without providing answers to any added benefit of drinking 'as much as tolerable' versus drinking *ad libitum*. In a review by Cheuvront et al (2003), several studies reporting the effects of dehydration on performance showed that ingesting *no fluid* during prolonged exercise in the heat re-duced exercise performance.

For example, Walsh et al (1994) compared full fluid versus no fluid in-gestion and found that a 'mild' level of dehydration (1.8% body mass loss), as a result of no fluid ingestion, limited cycling performance. However, when cyclists fully replaced their $\sim$1.1 L fluid losses during 1-hour rides at an exercise intensity of 70% VO_2max in the heat, they were able to cycle for 34% longer in subsequent exercise bout at 90% VO_2max.

To date, a few studies have reported on *ad libitum* rates of fluid in-take on weight-bearing (running) and non-weight bearing (cycling) exer-cise. Daries et al (2000) investigated whether the ACSM (1996) guidelines for fluid replacement presented any physiological or performance advan-tage over *ad libitum* fluid ingestion on 2-hour running performances in a thermo-neutral environment (25°C). During three trials, their highly trained runners ran on a treadmill at 65% VO_2max for 90 minutes and then 'as far as possible' in 30 minutes. In each trial, runners drank a 6.9% carbohydrate-electrolyte beverage either *ad libitum* or in set volumes of 150 or 350 mL/70 kg BW every 15–20 minutes. Plasma volume, serum sodium and osmolality, plasma glucose and lactate concentration, ratings of perceived exertion and stomach fullness and running performances were observed. Increasing fluid ingestion from $\sim$0.4 L/h in the *ad libitum* and 150 mL/70 kg trials to $\sim$0.9 L/h in the 350 mL/70 kg trial reduced subjects' loss of body mass and levels of dehydration (1.2% vs. 2.7–3.4%). However, this had no measurable effect on physiology or exercise perfor-mance in a 25°C environment. In fact, *ad libitum* drinking produced in-significantly faster performance in the 30-minute performance run than the other two trials. The only effect of the additional $\sim$1 L of fluid in the 350 mL/70 kg trial was on ratings of stomach fullness (RSF). The runners felt uncomfortably bloated, so much that two of the subjects failed to com-plete their performances runs.

Similarly, Dugas et al (2009) found no benefit to exercise performance when drinking more than *ad libitum*. Replacing either 66% or 100% of fluid did not have an added benefit beyond drinking *ad libitum* or replacing approximately $\sim$55% fluid losses. However, drinking less than *ad libitum* was associated with a 2% decrease in performance.

Perhaps the simplest *biological* explanation is that humans are delayed drinkers, one of the reasons explaining why we were such good hunters. And if drinking to thirst is an endogenous biological signal (Noakes, 2010), it could be that athletes' thirst does not develop because *their* bodies do not need fluid.

Unlike *ad libitum* drinking, drinking large volumes of fluid or 'as much as tolerable' or full fluid replacement (replacement of sweat losses or body mass losses) have practical disadvantages and potentially fatal consequences for athletes.

Practical disadvantages

It appears that irrespective of the sport participation or environmental conditions, athletes seldom match fluid intakes with their sweat rates – *this is the correct, biologically driven response.* 'Failure to match sweat rates' is not a failure, rather it is human nature to drink to thirst.

Athletes may associate drinking with slowing their pace or changing their streamlined position. Both runners (Costill et al, 1970) and cyclists (Mitchell and Voss, 1991) do not match fluid losses as they experience abdominal 'fullness' when they attempt to drink fluid at rates equal to or greater than 0.8 L/h. Indeed, some sports may reduce the desire to drink, such as running. Brouns et al (1991) showed that the rate of fluid ingestion of subjects encouraged to drink as much as possible during a simulated triathlon was two to three times higher during the cycle leg (0.6–0.8 L/h) than during the running leg (0.1–0.3 L/h). The discomfort of drinking large volumes of fluid is especially marked during running (Brouns et al, 1987, 1991; Daries et al, 2000).

Thus, studies show that when athletes drink large volumes of fluid during exercise they experience GI symptoms. Abdominal bloating, flatulence, stomach ache, stomach fullness, nausea, vomiting, diarrhoea, heartburn, side ache, intestinal cramping and GI bleeding may occur for various reasons during exercise and are commonly reported among athletes. Some evidence exist that over-training, intense exercise and prolonged exercise produce GI symptoms (for review see Gisolfi et al, 1990).

Clearly, clinical trials show that there is either no difference in exercise performance between full fluid replacement and *ad libitum* intake (for reviews see Noakes, 2007, 2010), or that large volumes actually impair performance (Daries et al, 2000).

Over-hydration

Over the last 20 years, a life-threatening condition began to develop and resulted directly from over-drinking during exercise. In 1985, the first cases of over-hydration were recognised in triathlons (Hiller et al, 1985) and ultra-marathons (Noakes et al, 1985). The latter report documented four athletes who developed water intoxication during prolonged exercise.

Their post-race serum sodium concentration ranged between 115–125 mmol/L, and included the first known case of water intoxication.

Drinking too much fluid can be detrimental to an athletes' health as it can lead to over-hydration, water intoxication or hyponatraemia (a low sodium concentration) (Noakes, 1992) that creates an osmotic imbalance. Slower endurance athletes who over-drink during/after a run, walk or triathlon are at risk, as well as athletes who consume large amounts of hypotonic fluids that draw sodium out of the cells.

The first known case was a 46-year-old female runner partaking in the 90-km Comrades ultra-marathon, who stopped after ~7 hours, was administered fluid and lapsed into a coma. At the hospital her serum sodium concentration was found to be 115 mmol/L and once diagnosed with EAHE, she was treated with normal saline and fully recovered with a few days (Noakes et al, 1985).

It has since been established that the development of EAH and EAHE during and after prolonged exercise is distinguished by three independent biological mechanisms, namely:
1 over-drinking;
2 inappropriate antidiuretic hormone (ADH) secretion (failing to suppress ADH when total body water is increasing); and
3 a failure to mobilise sodium from osmotically inactive, exchangeable sodium stores, or osmotic inactivation of sodium (lack of compensation for the sodium losses during exercise).

(Noakes et al, 2005)

Symptoms of hyponatremia

Headache, confusion, nausea or cramping to more severe seizures, coma, cardiac arrest and death.

Athletes at risk for hyponatremia
- Athletes partaking in prolonged exercise
- *Female athletes (lighter in weight)*: Athletes at risk of exercise-associated hyponatremia (EAH) or exercise-associated hyponatremic encephalopathy (EAHE) are female marathon runners who run 42-km races at slower speeds (<8–9 km/hr, ~5 mph) (Noakes, 2003b). These are non-elite female runners who drink more and run slower (Almond et al, 2005; Chorley et al, 2007).
- *Athletes with high fluid intake*: The reported fluid intake of fluid overloaded athletes who develop hyponatremia (serum sodium concentration of 122.4 ± 2.2 mmol/L) are in the range of 0.8–1.3 L/h compared with

fluid ingestion rates of 0.6 L/h in normonatremic runners (Noakes and Speedy, 2006).

- Slower athletes
- Less experienced athletes
- Athletes in extreme heat or humidity
- Athletes taking many opportunities to drink
- Athletes drinking just water without sodium

Furthermore, in symptomatic hyponatremia, the athlete is also likely to feel 'bloated' or 'swollen', may feel disorientated, confused and may have vomited clear fluid during the race (Noakes, 2001).

The current treatment for this condition in severe cases is to infuse hypertonic saline solutions (3–5%) (Hew-Butler et al, 2005).

Finally, *ad libitum* drinking (not drinking to stay ahead of thirst) is the naturally chosen human behaviour (Noakes, 2007), and it is common practice for athletes to drink sparingly during competition. A recent survey of runners found that 55.7% drink to thirst, while some 36.5% drink to a set schedule and a significant few drink as much as possible (8.9%) (Winger et al, 2011). The authors suggest over-hydration in mass running should be treated as a public health issue.

Carbohydrate and exercise performance

There is no argument that carbohydrate added to a fluid replacement drink has a performance-enhancing effect.

In a study by Hargreaves et al (1984), cyclists were fed repeated solid carbohydrate feedings containing 43 g of sucrose with 400 mL water at the start of exercise and every hour thereafter (at time 0, 1, 2 and 3 hours) during a 4-hour cycle ride. Compared with a non-nutritive (artificially sweetened) drink, when ingesting carbohydrate with water, cyclists were able to maintain blood glucose levels, reduce muscle glycogen depletion during prolonged exercise and enhance sprint performance at 100% VO_2max by 45% after the 4-hour cycle ride.

Coombes and Hamilton (2000) document the benefits of carbohydrate on performance during prolonged exercise of $\geq$2 hours at ~70% VO_2max by one or more of the following ways:

- It delays fatigue.
- It improves fuel substrate availability and oxidation rates.
- It improves performance times.

Below et al (1995) reported that carbohydrate was associated with a 6.3% improvement in time trial performance, compared with no carbohydrate replacement. When their subjects drank 1.3 L of fluid during a 50-minute ride at 80% VO_2max in the heat, they were able to complete a subsequent (~10 minutes) work bout faster than without fluid ingestion. The researchers observed no differences in physiological parameters between the two trials. Similarly, Carter et al (2003) showed a 13.5% increase in time to exhaustion when their cyclists ingested a 6% carbohydrate drink compared to a flavoured placebo. Cyclists rode at 73% VO_2max to exhaustion in the heat.

In contrast, not all studies have found physiological benefits or exercise performance effects of ingestion of water and/or a carbohydrate-electrolyte beverage. Robinson et al (1995) found that when cyclists in their trials drank 1.5 L of water, it had no measurable physiological benefit and impaired 1-hour cycling performances in a moderate ambient temperature of 20°C. Water ingestion at these temperatures only produced an uncomfortable abdominal fullness and a 2% reduction on the 'distances covered' in simulated cycle rides. Similarly, Marino et al (2010) found that neither full fluid or no fluid ingestion improved performance in self-paced cycling, nor was it affected by an ambient temperature that was either moderate (~19.8°C) or hot (~33.2°C).

Desbrow et al (2004) applied stricter dietary control of their subjects' pre-exercise diets in order to examine the performance benefits of a carbohydrate-electrolyte beverage. It appears that when an optimal amount of carbohydrate and fluid is ingested 24 hours before (energy ≈ 55 kcal/kg BW, carbohydrate ≈ 9 g/kg BW), as well as and including a pre-exercise meal 2–4 hours before (carbohydrate ≈ 2 g/kg BW), even a 6% carbohydrate-electrolyte beverage (at 14 mL/kg BW) taken during exercise has no significant effect on 1-hour cycling performance at ~65% VO_2max at a moderate temperature of 22°C.

Similarly, studies on high-intensity running of less than 1.5 hours have also found performance disparities between running in the heat compared with moderate and cool environments (<25°C). Milliard-Stafford et al (1997) stated that runners' performance in a time trial in the heat was improved by the ingestion of a 6% or 8% carbohydrate-electrolyte drink, compared with a flavoured placebo. In contrast, in a study of runners in 18-km road race, van Nieuwenhoven et al (2005) did not find any performance benefit of a 7% carbohydrate drink, compared with water ingestion.

From the latter findings, the purpose of fluid replacement in a thermoneutral environment has been raised (Coyle and Hamilton, 1990; Daries et al, 2000). According to Coyle and Hamilton (1990), the sole purpose of fluid replacement during prolonged exercise in a cool environment may be to prevent increase in body temperature that may impair performance or damage vital organs. While the Cheuvront et al (2003) review reports that dehydration of more than 2% during exercise lasting more than 90 minutes appears to reduce endurance performance in moderate environments (20–21°C), this is based on studies comparing no fluid inges-tion and some fluid or full fluid ingestion, rather than *ad libitum* drinking. Furthermore, Mündel (2011) argues that real life competition is a self-paced 'as fast as possible' situation, rather than 'as far as possible' and questions the validity of the latter model as a performance measure.

However, in the real world of athletic competition, where athletes are self-paced and racing as fast as possible, it still remains that athletes who drink to the dictates of thirst or *ad libitum*, are the fastest marathon, ultra-marathon and ironman triathletes and are reported to be amongst the most dehydrated athletes in the field (Cheuvront and Haymes, 2001; Sharwood et al, 2004; Kao et al, 2008; Zouhal et al 2009).

Fluid ingestion and 'stitch'

'Stitch' or 'side ache' is a symptom often associated with fluid ingestion that is experienced by some athletes, and is more common in activities that involve repetitive actions (i.e. running). Athletes may be less aware of its formal term, known as exercise-related transient abdominal pain (ETAP) (Morton et al, 2004). Likely causes of stitch are as follows:

- Tugging of the viscera on peritoneal ligaments
- Irritation of the parietal peritoneum (a sheath-like covering of the ab-dominal wall)
- Ischaemia caused by a reduction of blood flow to the diaphragm
- A neural irritation caused by the activity itself

Carbohydrate content and osmolality of the ingested beverage appear to affect the degree of stitch experienced. Although the addition of glucose to a solution can increase sodium absorption four-fold and water absorp-tion six-fold (Gisolfi et al, 1990), a high carbohydrate, hypertonic bev-erage slows gastric emptying (Murray et al, 1999; Plunkett and Hopkins, 1999) and reduces intestinal absorption (Ryan et al, 1984, 1998; Gisolfi, 1992). Ryan et al (1984) have shown that the intestinal absorption of water can decrease by 50% when a higher (8%) carbohydrate drink is ingested compared with a lower (6%) carbohydrate drink. Thus, reduced gastric emptying and lower rates of intestinal fluid absorption caused more retention of fluid in the GI tract that produces more symptoms of stitch than a beverage with less carbohydrate and osmolality. Isotonic bever-ages (i.e. 6% carbohydrate-electrolyte sports drink) or hypotonic bever-ages (i.e. water) have lower/no carbohydrate concentration and lower osmolality.

Studies have shown that high carbohydrate, hypertonic drinks affect both running and intermittent high-intensity exercise. Plunkett and Hop-kins (1999) suggested that isotonic beverages produced less symptoms of stitch than high carbohydrate, hypertonic beverages during running exercise, and that stitch was related to fluid ingestion. This was supported by Morton et al (2004) whose sample included recreational athletes who ran on a treadmill for 23 minutes at an average running speed of 10.3 km/h during four trials. Following a no-fluid trial, on the three remaining trials, subjects consumed very high volumes of either a hypotonic drink (flavoured water with no carbohydrate, osmolality 48 mOsmol/L), an isotonic drink (sports drink with 6% carbohydrate, 295 mOsmol/L) or a hypertonic drink (reconstituted fruit juice with 10.4% carbohydrate, 489 mOsmol/L). The average rate of fluid intake in the fluid trials was 2373 mL/h, much higher than current recommendations of ~400–800 mL/h (Noakes, 2003). Considering also that the maximum rates of intestinal fluid absorption at rest are about 0.8 L/h (Davis et al, 1980), it may be less during exercise. Furthermore, large volumes of fluid cause abdominal fullness leading to stomach distension affecting stretch receptors in the gut wall. This reduces the dipsogenic drive causing athletes to not drink. Such high volumes can also cause water intoxication.

However, although previous work by Morton and Callister (2000) reported that drinking provoked ETAP, the results by Morton et al (2004) show that even if *no fluid* is ingested during exercise, ETAP can be experienced to some measure. Clearly the highest carbohydrate concentration and osmolality beverage (fruit juice) produced the greatest severity of ETAP experienced, compared with the sports drink, flavoured water and no fluid.

Even athletes involved in intermittent high-intensity exercise may experience ETAP as a result of carbohydrate concentration and hypertonicity of beverages. In a study by Shi et al (2004), subjects took part in simulated training and performance of stop-and-go sports consisting of four circuits (4×12 minute quarters) of three exercise stations incorporating intermittent sprinting, lateral hops, shuttle runs and vertical jumps for a total time of 48 minutes. The average exercise intensity was 76% HR_{max}. Subjects drank volumes that approximated sweat losses. Two carbohydrate-electrolyte beverages were compared, that of a 6% carbohydrate, 305 mOsmol/kg beverage and an 8% carbohydrate, 434 mOsmol/kg beverage. The latter, hypertonic carbohydrate drink produced significantly more symptoms of side ache during high-intensity intermittent exercise than the isotonic beverage containing 6% carbohydrate. To avoid stitch, athletes could do the following:

- Avoid a large meal before exercise. Rather eat small, frequent meals.
- If susceptible to stitch, avoid drinking hypertonic drinks (e.g. soft drinks or reconstituted fruit juices) or beverages with similar high carbohydrate concentration and high osmolality before and during exercise.

- If susceptible to stitch, isotonic or hypotonic (sports) drinks with a lower carbohydrate concentration and lower osmolality may be better tolerated.
- Ensure adequate hydration before exercise, but avoid large volumes before starting exercise and during exercise.
- Practice drinking to thirst and determine *ad libitum* fluid ingestion during training to prevent over-drinking during competitive events.

Optimal hydration strategies

Determining the optimal hydration package that maintains physiological functions and enhances performance during exercise and sport is dependent on a number of factors including the type and amount (concentration) of nutrients, the addition of electrolytes, volume of the drink, gastric emptying rate of fluids, intestinal absorption of fluids, oxidation of nutrients, duration and intensity of exercise and individual taste and preference.

Gastric emptying

Even though gastric emptying rates of more than 1 L/h are possible (Convertino et al, 1996), athlete's fluid intakes of ~0.5 L/h do not match these rates.

Factors influencing gastric emptying rate

- *Gastric distension and drink volume*: Starting exercise fully hydrated assists gastric emptying during exercise. If hypo-hydrated before exercise, gastric emptying will be slowed. Although larger drink volumes lead to greater gastric emptying rates, it is only favourable up to ~600 mL. Thus, very large volumes and/or very small volumes are most likely to delay gastric emptying.
- *Caloric content of the drink*: Drinks with a high caloric content empty more slowly from the stomach than drinks with little caloric value.
- *The amount (if any) of protein, fat and/or fibre of the drink*: Fat slows gastric emptying, as does fibre.
- *Type and concentration of carbohydrate in the drink*: High carbohydrate drinks (>7–8%) delay gastric emptying. High drink volume also increases carbohydrate content and ingestion.
- *Temperature of the drink*: At rest, cooler drinks empty quicker from the stomach.
- *Electrolyte concentration and osmolality of the drink*: Hypertonic (higher osmolality) drinks slow gastric emptying, although the energy value

(caloric content) has greater control over gastric emptying than beverage osmolality.

- *pH*: The acidity of drink affects gastric emptying, which is lower after a meal/drink with high concentration of acid. Citric acid used to flavour some drinks slows gastric emptying.
- *Mental attitude*
- *Exercise intensity*: Gastric emptying rates are higher during exercise compared to rest, and higher in some sports (i.e. running) more than others (i.e. cycling) at the same moderate exercise intensity (70% VO_2max).
- *Heat stress*: Thermal strain delays gastric emptying.

(Costill, 1990)

Oxidation of carbohydrate

Studies have established that premature fatigue during exercise of moderate intensity is due to the effect of:

1 a low muscle glycogen content;
2 hypoglycaemia; or
3 a reduced rate of carbohydrate oxidation.

Muscle glycogen is the predominant fuel providing carbohydrate energy for exercise, and carbohydrate oxidation derived primarily from this source can reach 3.0–4.0 g/min (Angus et al, 2002). However, both liver and muscle glycogen stores become depleted after ~2 hours of continuous exercise. The ingestion of carbohydrate and the maintenance of blood glucose levels are imperative for performance in latter stages of prolonged exercise when liver glycogen stores are low. Carbohydrate fuels spare liver glycogen by reducing the rate of liver glycogen depletion, but does not affect the rate at which muscle glycogen is depleted, although it affects how lactate (a fuel for muscles) is used (Bosch et al, 1993). Carbohydrate intake during exercise, therefore, serves to delay fatigue by slowing liver glycogen depletion and preventing hypoglycaemia by ensuring blood glucose levels are maintained. Carbohydrate consumption is also helpful to athletes whose muscle and liver glycogen stores are low when starting exercise, i.e. those who exercise in a fasted state or who have not followed a glycogen-loading plan.

Previous literature has reported a threshold to how much carbohydrate can be ingested during exercise that is related to the oxidation of exogenous carbohydrate and the liver's release of glucose into the bloodstream. The heart's capacity to deliver oxygen does not match what the muscle can take up; similarly, there is a rate-limiting step for the oxidation of glucose and its subsequent delivery to, and uptake by, the muscles. It appears also that the liver's capacity to release glucose does not match the muscles' capacity to take up glucose. The liver can only release glucose at a rate of

1.0 g/min *under normal physiological conditions* (in the absence of illness or disease).

Therefore, exogenous carbohydrate oxidation rates for glucose remain at 1.0 g/min irrespective of the type of carbohydrate (with the exception of fructose and galactose). As early as 1992, Hawley et al, showed that during experimentally-induced *hyperglycemia* through glucose infusion, carbohydrate oxidation increased to 2.2 g/min, clearly indicating that the rate-limiting step, *under normal physiological conditions*, is the liver's capacity to oxidise exogenous carbohydrate and release glucose into the bloodstream.

Thus, the body can only oxidise exogenous carbohydrate at 1.0 g/min, with the exception of fructose and galactose, which are oxidised more slowly.

However, trials with carbohydrate mixtures have resulted in higher oxidation rates than previously thought. When combining glucose with fructose and sucrose (2.4 g/min ingested), the oxidation increased to 1.70 g/min, and when glucose was combined with fructose only (at 2.4 g/min ingested) the oxidation rates rose to 1.75 g/min. Clearly this showed a staggering increase in carbohydrate delivery and performance benefits (Jentjens et al, 2004; Jentjens and Jeukendrup, 2005). Later Currell and Jeukendrup (2008) showed how cycling performance increased by 8% by consuming a glucose + fructose mixture as compared with glucose only feedings. This carbohydrate mixture was later used by Dutch cyclists in the Tour de France.

Thus, the research suggests that if using glucose only, the amount of ingested carbohydrate that is recommended needs match the rate of exogenous carbohydrate oxidation and the liver's release of glucose (~1 g/min). However, carbohydrate mixtures of glucose and fructose can produce greater oxidation rates, increase delivery of carbohydrate during exercise and improve performances. The GI effects (i.e. diarrhoea) of high fructose drinks should be considered by athletes if choosing this route.

Recommendations for fluid intake before, during and after exercise or sport

To date there is *no ideal drink formula* for optimal hydration and sports performance, and the debates continue. Fluid ingestion before, during and after exercise serves the primary need for water, and a dual purpose of providing water *and* carbohydrate when required. The intake of electrolytes is not essential during short or moderate duration exercise, but sodium *may* be beneficial during very prolonged exercise in the heat and/or for athletes who drink and retain abnormally large volumes of fluid.

What we know

During exercise

- *No fluid ingestion*: It leads to dehydration, reduces physiological functions and impairs exercise performance.
- *Drinking as much as tolerable*: It encourages over-drinking, may impair performance, affects fluid homeostasis, can lead to serious consequences such as EAH and EAHE, even death.
- *Ad libitum drinking (drinking to the dictates or thirst)*: A biologically driven response, it reduces physiological stress, improves exercise performance and maintains health.

In the author's opinion, the 2007 ACSM revised fluid guidelines advising athletes against over-drinking but not to lose >2% of their starting body weight during any form of exercise (Sawka et al, 2007) could still promote over-drinking in some athletes.

While there are a multitude of sports, drinking to thirst is the recommended hydration strategy. Guidelines set by the International Marathon Medical Directors Association (IMMDA) (Noakes, 2002, 2003), and their hydration position stand (Hew-Butler et al, 2006) and the EAH consensus document (Hew-Butler et al, 2007) provide the current evidence-base for the drinking to thirst practice. These guidelines have also been adopted by United States of America Track and Field (USATF).

Suggested guidelines: 'First Do No Harm'

Heed physiologic cues during exercise
Perception of thirst: Increase fluid intake.
Increased urination, bloating and weight gain: Decrease fluid intake.
Weight gain with signs of headache, confusion, nausea and vomiting clear fluid: Stop fluid intake, seek medical attention.

During exercise lasting 1 hour or more

- Aim to drink to thirst
- *Drink type*: Water is the primary requirement. Beverages containing carbohydrate, with or without sodium, can also be used as exercise duration increases.
- *Amount of carbohydrate*: Ideally 30–60 g/h, and up to 70 g/h (i.e. ~0.7–1.0 g carbohydrate per minute) if using glucose. Higher rates of carbohydrate intake (2.4 g/min, ~144 g CHO/hr) are reported to increase exogenous carbohydrate oxidation, when combining glucose with fructose, or glucose, fructose and sucrose.
- *Drink volume*: During prolonged exercise, 400 mL/h (smaller athletes) to up to no more than 800 mL/h (heavier athletes). Athletes are cautioned

not to drink excessively as this could lead to fluid overload and hypona-tremia. A survey of drinking behaviour of runners revealed that many of the 'at risk' runners (non-elite female runners with slower times) did not know that over-drinking causes EAH (Winger et al, 2011).

- *Timing of fluid intake*: Drink to thirst or ~150–200 mL every ~15–20 minutes depending on body weight and speed of running. Slower runners should be cautious of over-drinking.

  A note on osmolality:

  ○ Osmolality is the number of osmotically active particles in a kilogram of solvent and is measured in milliosmoles (mOsmol). Although osmolarity represents the number of osmotically active particles in a litre of solution, often osmolality is the preferred term when referring to solutions, when actually osmolarity is stated. Water-soluble nutrients and minerals increase the osmolality of a solution, drink or supplement (liquid meal) (Thomas and BDA, 2001).

  ○ The osmolality of blood plasma is usually ~280–290 mOsmol/kg. When there is a deficit in body water at rest (termed 'hypohydration'), the concentration of electrolytes increase causing osmolality to increase from ~283 mOsmol/kg (a state of 'euhydration') to over 300 mOsmol/kg (Sawka and Pandolf, 1990). Sports drink solutions are categorised according to their osmolality compared to plasma. Isotonic solutions have the same osmolality as that of plasma. Hypotonic solutions have a lower osmolality than plasma (i.e. sweat is hypotonic to blood plasma). Hypertonic solutions have a higher osmolality than plasma.

- *Drink concentration*: 5–10% carbohydrate drink (5–10 g CHO/100 mL fluid) depending on intensity and duration of exercise. Some athletes prone to stitch may be better off with a carbohydrate concentration drink of <8%, ideally 4–8% (4–8 g CHO/100 mL fluid).

- *Sodium concentration in drink*: Beverages and snacks with sodium stimulate thirst and encourage drinking. However, sodium replacement is not essential during exercise, although serum sodium concentration can become diluted during over-drinking. Sodium deficiency has been linked with muscle cramping or weakness, but this is not proven. Neither is it clear whether sports drinks with low sodium content can minimise EAH (Noakes, 2007). Athletes, as the public, should be guided by individual requirements, their state of health and dietary reference values. In the United Kingdom, the recommended salt intake is 6 g (2.4 g sodium/day) for adults aged 19–50 years.

- *Monitoring*:

  ○ *Body weight*: In longer ultra-endurance events athletes could monitor body weight changes (some events provide body weight scales *en route* and at the finish line).

○ *Urine*: Check urine colour for hydration status. A very light urine colour is the best measure that fluid ingestion is optimal. Dark colour urine is an indication of dehydration (or high supplement use can also concentrate urine). Familiarisation with a urine colour chart will also help identify optimal fluid balance.

- *Other beneficial hydration practices*: In hot environments, skin wetting (sponging) is advised to lower skin temperature and maintain skin blood flow (Noakes, 2001).

For exercise lasting <1 hour (30–60 minutes)
- The need for fluid is very small in exercise lasting less than 1 hour.
- Drink to thirst.
- No more than ~400–600 mL/h.
- Water is the primary need. Beverages containing 2–6 g CHO/100 mL of fluid may be tolerated and provide a nutritional advantage for some athletes.

After exercise
- Combine fluid and food to replace sweat and sodium losses.
- After prolonged exercise, check for signs of over-hydration, stop drinking and report for *medical care*.
- Check for signs of dehydration, replace lost fluids *under medical supervision*.
- Post-race recovery fluids and snacks should provide the first 50 g carbohydrate in 30 minutes, repeated after 30-minutes and then every 2 hours, adding protein-rich foods/fluids at later meals.
- Protein (amino acids) added to a drink may help to retain fluid, although it may be more useful after an exercise bout.
- Aim for a rate of ~5 g or more CHO/kg BW over 24 hours. Larger carbohydrate feedings are common in ultra-endurance athletes following races lasting longer than 6 hours.
- High glycaemic index carbohydrates encourage glycogen storage.
  Refer also to Chapter 4 for post-exercise recovery.

Alcohol and sport

Alcohol consumption is typically associated with certain sports, especially team sports. Beverage companies have long been sponsors of competitive events of rugby, cricket and other popular sports. Studies have provided evidence of higher consumption of alcohol in team sports, even by elite athletes, compared with athletes in endurance and strength sports categories. Van Erp-Baart et al (1989) found that team sport athletes consume roughly 5% energy from alcohol.

Alcohol is also a concentrated source of energy and yields 7 kcal (29 kJ)/g. It has a diuretic action and stimulates urine production, which may lead to body water deficits and affect re-hydration during recovery after exercise. It is not suitable for fluid replacement as after exercise water losses need to be replaced, and alcohol consumption delays full re-hydration by increasing urine output (Sawka et al, 2007). Nor is alcohol a useful fuel for exercising muscles. In fact, alcohol is converted to acetaldehyde (in the liver), which is a very inferior fuel (Noakes, 1992). The ingestion of alcohol should be avoided immediately before and after competition, especially those athletes who are injured. Harmful effects of alcohol consumption include the following:

- Impaired motor and intellectual performance
- Depressant effect
- Diuretic effect, causing fluid loss through urine
- Dehydration
- Poor fuel stores
- Impaired skills
- Heat losses (vasodilation effects)
- Hypoglycaemia
- (Indirect) interference with glycogen re-synthesis

After strenuous exercise, liver glycogen stores are low and often depleted. Gluconeogenesis (liver glucose production) restores glycogen stores in the liver, but alcohol can inhibit gluconeogenesis by blocking the conversion of lactate to glucose and causing lactate accumulation or lactic acidosis. The result is hypoglycaemia, which can cause irreparable damage to the central nervous system.

Furthermore, in the recovery phase after exercise, focus needs to be on carbohydrate ingestion and other nutrients that enhance glycogen recovery. Alcohol indirectly affects glycogen re-synthesis by interfering with the athlete's interest to follow these optimal post-exercise nutrition guidelines (Burke et al, 2004).

For guidelines on the sensible intake of alcohol please refer to Chapter 3 and Table 3.3.

Chapter summary

- Water is the second most essential nutrient, following oxygen, and makes up 50–65% of the body.
- There is great individual variability in sweat rates amongst athletes, ranging from 0.3 to 2.4 L/h and ~1.2 L/h in runners.
- The absence of fluid ingestion during exercise leads to dehydration and reduced physiological function.
- At dehydration rates of 7–10% humans stop exercising. And when dehydration reaches levels of 15–20%, there is a risk of organ failure and death.

- Exercise performance is optimised by *ad libitum* fluid intake or drinking to prevent the development of thirst.

- Thirst is an endogenous biological signal that regulates fluid homeostasis during exercise.

- Athletes voluntarily drink ~500 mL fluid/h.

- Athletes who drink large volumes of fluid during exercise may experience gastrointestinal (GI) symptoms, i.e. abdominal bloating, flatulence, stomach ache, stomach fullness, nausea, vomiting, diarrhoea, heartburn, side ache, intestinal cramping and GI bleeding.

- Over-drinking can cause water intoxication leading to exercise-associated hyponatremia (EAH) and/or exercise-associated hyponatremic encephalopathy (EAHE).

- Recreational, amateur or non-elite female marathon or ultra-marathon runners who run at slower speeds (<8–9 km/h, ~5 mph) and who drink more fluids are at risk of EAH.

- The addition of carbohydrate to a fluid replacement drink has a performance-enhancing effect. It maintains blood glucose levels, reduces muscle glycogen depletion during prolonged exercise, delays fatigue, improves fuel substrate availability and oxidation rates and enhances sprint performance.

- To avoid 'stitch' or exercise-related transient abdominal pain (ETAP), avoid large volumes of fluid, especially hypertonic drinks (e.g. soft drinks or reconstituted fruit juices) or beverages with similar high carbohydrate concentration and high osmolality, before and during exercise.

- Gastric emptying rate is affected by the drink's volume, nutrient content, caloric value, electrolytes and osmolality, temperature, pH, as well as thermal strain, the exercise intensity and mental attitude of the athlete.

- Exogenous carbohydrate oxidation rates differ between carbohydrate mixtures. Glucose is oxidised at a rate of ~1 g/min, compared with glucose, sucrose and fructose at 1.70 g/min and glucose and fructose at 1.75 g/min.

- While there is *no ideal drink formula*, the optimal hydration practice is to drink to thirst. Water is the primary need. The addition of carbohydrate, with or without sodium, to a fluid replacement drink is of benefit during longer duration exercise.

- Alcohol is a very inferior fuel that should be avoided immediately before and after competition, especially those athletes who suffer from injuries.

CHAPTER 9

Performance-Enhancing (Ergogenic) Aids

Key terms

Nutritional supplement
Nutritional ergogenic aid
Banned substance
Doping
Anti-doping code
Caffeine
Caffeine-habituated users (responders)
Caffeine-naïve users (non-responders)
Dietary creatine
Endogenous creatine

Free creatine
Phosphocreatine (PCr)
Creatine monohydrate
Creatine loading
Bicarbonate
Buffering agent
Sodium bicarbonate ($NaHCO_3$)
Sodium citrate
Bicarbonate loading

The ancient Olympic ideal that an athlete should win through his or her own attempt, that is, independent of any aid, is echoed by today's sporting authorities around the world.

The supplement industry is a lucrative industry often associated with high costs, false claims and health risks. In a highly competitive environment, athletes want the edge, and teamed with a lack of knowledge of nutrition fundamentals this fuels their drive to use what is marketed as 'sport supplements'. Surveys of athletes show a high prevalence of supplement use, with nearly 100% use in certain sports such as swimming, triathlon and bodybuilding.

There is a plethora of information regarding supplements out there in the sports domain, however, two distinct categories exist that can help athletes differentiate between what is useful towards their athletic goals and what is not.

Nutrition for Sport and Exercise: A Practical Guide, First Edition. Hayley Daries.
© 2012 Blackwell Publishing Ltd. Published 2012 by Blackwell Publishing Ltd.

Nutritional supplements

Nutritional supplements contain a dietary component such as a nutrient (i.e. vitamin) in similar amounts as those found in food. Its use in sport is to treat a suboptimal nutrient level or a nutrient deficiency, such as treating iron deficiency or iron-deficiency anaemia with an iron supplement that provides a prescribed dose of iron in a pill or liquid form. Furthermore, nutritional supplements have a role in nutrition and metabolism, and can enhance exercise performance. Foods and fluids containing energy-dense forms of carbohydrate and/or protein in drinks, gels, energy bars or powders and liquid meal supplements are just a few known supplements that are used by athletes with high energy and nutrient requirements. These supplements conveniently provide amounts of energy and nutrients in concentrated and convenient forms, which can be taken before, during and after exercise, or added to meals to increase the energy and/or nutrient content.

Nutritional ergogenic aids

Nutritional ergogenic aids, also known as performance-enhancing aids, may or may not be a dietary component of food and usually occur in amounts greater than those found in food or food components. Initially defined by its pharmacological effect, its role in nutrition, metabolism and exercise performance has been explored and its use is either supported by scientific evidence, refuted or banned in competitive environments by sporting authorities.

Nutritional ergogenic aids aim to improve performance in one or more of the following ways:

- Affecting energy metabolism (e.g. creatine serves to increase the availability of a limited fuel).
- Affecting the central nervous system (CNS) (e.g. caffeine is a stimulant of the CNS and peripheral nervous system (PNS)).
- Stimulating protein synthesis and increasing lean body mass (e.g. protein and amino acids).
- Affecting metabolic by-products during exercise performance (e.g. sodium bicarbonate ($NaHCO_3$) and sodium citrate neutralizes and buffers acid during maximal anaerobic exercise).
- Reducing body fat content.

(Maughan, 2002; McArdle et al, 2010)

Leading authorities in sport, i.e. both national governing bodies in sport in the United Kingdom, and international authorities, advise athletes against the use of nutritional ergogenic aids to avoid the associated risks. Although many 'sport supplements' have been marketed specifically for use in sport and exercise, only a few are supported by sound scientific evidence. Athletes could rely on a comprehensively researched supplement programme that delivers up to date and current evidence-based research on sports supplements. Such programmes should be supported by a panel of experts in sports nutrition, medicine and science, be unbiased and have long-standing credibility in the sports supplement field. Ideally, it could provide a ranking system of *unbranded* supplements, sports foods and fluids, based on an evidence base for benefit and risk of each product, and which is updated regularly. Table 9.1 categorises the supplements in tiers by the following:

- Nutritional supplements
- Nutritional ergogenic aids with proven benefits

Nutritional ergogenic aids with unproven claims and banned supplements are not listed here. Athletes and those supporting them, including the sport and exercise specialists, need to consider the validity and reliability of the science supporting any nutrition-related ergogenic. They could start with the following few questions before making a decision to take it:

- Is it based on an anecdote or scientific theory, or is it based on rigorous scientific study?
- Are there effects of health and well-being in the short-term or long-term?
- If it is not banned, what dose (per kg BW) is safe and legal?
- How can one be sure that it is not contaminated by other harmful or banned substances?
- What measurable and proven advantage will it have for well-being and exercise performance, apart from what an optimal diet, training programme, recovery and sleep can provide?

The role players in clean sport

Many supplements fail to be approved since they are based on testimonials of other athletes or unsupported claims by manufacturers. Athletes competing in a national and international level are advised to be aware of banned supplements and doping regulations/codes. *The International Olympic Committee (IOC)* defines doping as: 'the administration or the use by a competing athlete of any substance foreign to the body or of any physiological substance taken in abnormal quantity or taken by an abnormal route of entry into the body, with the sole intention of increasing in an artificial or unfair manner his performance in competition.'

Table 9.1 Nutritional supplements and ergogenic aids.

Group	Examples
Nutritional supplements (covered in Chapters 4,5,6,7 and 8)	Carbohydrate-containing drinks, energy bars, gels and powders Protein-containing powders, energy bars and drinks Liquid meal supplement containing carbohydrate, protein, fat, vitamins and minerals Multi- or single vitamin supplement Multi- or single mineral supplement Electrolyte replacement Oral rehydration solution Fatty acids supplement and/or fish oils Iron supplement Calcium supplement Antioxidants supplements Trace elements
Nutritional ergogenic aids with proven benefits	*Caffeine* Caffeine is a stimulant found naturally in nuts, seeds, plants, coffee and tea, and added to over-the-counter medications, colas, energy bars and drinks. It affects muscle tissue, the central nervous system and adrenalin. Caffeine improves reaction time, increases mental alertness and concentration. It increases fat breakdown and oxidation, may reduce carbohydrate use and spare glycogen during exercise. It enhances endurance capacity and delays fatigue, increasing power output and prolonging time to exhaustion. It reduces perception of effort/fatigue/pain. It also improves short-term, high-intensity exercise. Dose administered: • 2–6 mg/kg before exercise, or • 0.75–2 mg/kg during exercise. *Creatine* Creatine is a non-essential nutrient replenished endogenously, and through the diet from meat and fish. Creatine maintains ATP levels in the muscle cells, supports muscle contraction, delays fatigue and can increase lean body mass. Creatine is best for single-effort or repeated bouts of short duration and very powerful exercise that involve short recovery periods. Dose administered: • *rapid loading*: 20–25 g creatine monohydrate/day taken as 5 g × 4–5 doses for 5–7 consecutive days. Maintenance dose of 2–3 g/day. • *slow loading*: 2–3 g creatine monohydrate/day for 1 month. Maintenance dose of 2–3 g/day. *Bicarbonate* Bicarbonate (HCO_3^-), a base, is a major chemical buffer in blood. Sodium bicarbonate and sodium citrate are buffering agents, providing an alkaline environment that favours high-intensity exercise performance of more than 30 seconds. Its benefits include delaying fatigue during high-intensity exercise, increasing performance in maximal anaerobic exercise lasting 1–7 minutes, improving repeated-sprint ability by contributing to an increased anaerobic energy production and improving lactate threshold and endurance performance. Dose administered: • 300 mg/kg BW taken with 1 L water, 1–2 hours prior to high-intensity exercise. • 300–500 mg/kg BW/day in 5-day loading protocols.

The *World Anti-doping Agency (WADA)* is an independent international agency committed to doping-free sport through scientific research, education development and monitoring of the World Anti-Doping Code (Code). The Code is a core document that aims to harmonise anti-doping effects worldwide. Since its inception in January 2004, it has since been reviewed and the revised code took effect in January 2009. WADA recently updated its prohibited list (January 2011), which includes substances and methods prohibited at all times, in competition and in particular sports (see Internet Resources on page 259). *UK Anti-Doping* ensures that UK sports agencies comply with the national and international (WADA) code.

There is a plethora of information available on the hundreds of sport supplements in use by athletes. For further reading on this subject, the recent (2009, 2010, 2011 and current) *British Journal of Sports Medicine* 'Nutritional supplement series' is a set of monthly reviews entitled: 'A–Z of nutritional supplements: dietary supplements, sports nutrition foods and ergogenic aids for health and performance.'

All *nutritional supplements* are covered in previous chapters. In this chapter only certain *nutritional ergogenic aids* will be discussed, namely those that are proven to enhance the athlete's exercise performance, i.e. caffeine, creatine, $NaHCO_3$ and sodium citrate.

Caffeine

Qualities of caffeine
- It is a stimulant (drug) affecting muscle tissue, the CNS and adrenalin.
- It is naturally found in nuts, seeds, plants, coffee and tea.
- In the diet, athletes may obtain it from coffee, tea, colas, chocolate and cocoa-rich food and drinks, novel drinks and energy bars with added caffeine, as well as some over-the-counter medications (e.g. cold and flu medication).

Benefits for exercise
- Since caffeine improves reaction time (Duvnjak-Zaknich et al, 2011), it increases mental alertness (Goldstein et al, 2010) and concentration (Hogervorst et al, 2008).
- Caffeine mobilises fat from adipose tissue (free fatty acids) and muscle cell (intramuscular triglyceride). Subsequently, this action may reduce carbohydrate use and spare glycogen during exercise. The ability to mobilise fat may be reduced in athletes who are carbohydrate loaded (Weir et al, 1987).
- Caffeine can improve endurance performance by delaying fatigue, increasing power output and prolonging time to exhaustion.

- It can reduce perception of effort/fatigue at a given exercise intensity (measured as rating of perceived exertion or RPE), thus enhancing endurance capacity. This may allow athletes to exercise at a higher exercise intensity and yet experience the same perceived effort.
- Caffeine can improve short-term, high-intensity exercise, and reduce the perception of pain.
- It stimulates release and activity of adrenaline.

Scientific evidence

Some of the earliest, well-controlled studies used caffeine as a performance-enhancing aid in cycling trials (Costill et al, 1978; Ivy et al. 1979). In these landmark trials, caffeine ingested 1 hour before exercise may not have significantly increased fatty acid concentration but significantly improved endurance performance/capacity. Costill et al (1978) showed that a dose of 330 mg caffeine prior to exercise increases time to exhaustion (90 minutes compared with 75 minutes). When (250 mg) caffeine is consumed before exercise and (250 mg) during exercise, power output increases (Ivy et al, 1979).

Subsequent studies have also shown enhanced performance in cycling (51%) and running (44%) (Graham and Spriet, 1991), and improvement in other endurance-type exercise such as swimming. Doses of more than 3 mg caffeine/kg BW to as much as 13 mg/kg BW have showed improved endurance capacity (Costill et al, 1978; Clarkson, 1993; Graham and Spriet, 1996), although some studies have observed that higher doses, >9 mg caffeine/kg BW, appear to show no greater gains in cycling performance (Pasman et al, 1995) or in some cases, the least effect on endurance running performance, compared with smaller doses (Graham and Spriet, 1995). The ergogenic effect of caffeine does not appear to be gender-specific, since performance effects are seen in both male and female athletes (Anselme et al, 1992; McIntosh and Wright, 1995; Jackman et al, 1996; Anderson et al, 2000; Bruce et al, 2000; Bell et al, 2002; McLellan and Bell, 2004).

Exercise of higher intensity and shorter duration may also benefit from caffeine intake. Wiles et al (1992) demonstrated that a moderate caffeine dose of 150–200 mg improved well-trained runners' 1500-m run time by 4 minutes and increased the speed of their 'finishing burst'. Performance increased by 19% in repeated cycling sprints (Jackman et al, 1996). Furthermore, other types of exercise, i.e. involving repeated bouts of high-intensity exercise such as team sports, may be substantially enhanced by caffeine intake (Stuart et al, 2005). A recent review of studies showed that caffeine ingestion significantly improved performance in short-term high-intensity exercise. Elite team-sport and power-based (sprint) athletes, who do not habitually consume caffeine, and resistance-trained athletes can benefit considerably from caffeine consumption (Astorino and Roberson, 2010).

Not all studies have found that caffeine has one or more of the following effects: increased fatty acid concentrations, increased fat oxidation, improved performance, in endurance exercise (Hunter et al, 2002), during shorter, high-intensity exercise (Gastin et al, 1990; Dodd et al, 1991) or during sprint performance (Greer et al, 1998). Graham et al (2008) recently found no glycogen-sparing effect of caffeine after prolonged endurance exercise.

In some studies, differences in performance effects of caffeine were observed between caffeine responders (or 'caffeine-habituated' users) and non-responders (or 'caffeine-naïve' users), which may also be due to other individual variations and/or factors such as exercise type, duration, intensity and dose of caffeine ingested. An analysis of 40 well-controlled performance-based caffeine studies since 1975 found that caffeine improved endurance exercise, and to a lesser extent, high-intensity exercise. They concluded that although many of the potential moderating factors (such as dietary caffeine consumption, fitness or training status, caffeine dosage, period of withdrawal from caffeine, exercise mode) will have no major influence on the effects of caffeine on performance, two factors have been marked as requiring further investigation, i.e. (1) the mode and pattern of caffeine administration (single versus repeated doses) and (2) habitual intake of caffeine (Doherty and Smith, 2004).

Application

Predominantly, investigations of the effects of caffeine have concentrated on prolonged exercise. However, some studies have shown a positive performance effect on team-sport and/or anaerobic high-intensity exercise. Stuart et al (2005) found that caffeine enhances sprint speed during high-intensity team sport performance.

Dose administered

Previously, urinary levels of 12 µg caffeine/mL (achieved by consuming ≥500 mg caffeine) was regarded as over the limit or 'doping' by international sports organisations. Since 2004, caffeine could again be used by athletes in competitive sport since it was removed from WADA's Prohibited List and the IOC's list of banned substances. Both small (1–3 mg/kg BW, ~70–150 mg caffeine) and larger doses (6–9 mg/kg BW, ~400–600 mg caffeine) appear to enhance endurance performance and power output, although higher doses (≥9 mg/kg BW) will not necessarily increase performance (Goldstein et al, 2010). Rather, due to individual variation in response to caffeine, the smallest dose required for a performance effect should be sort. Recent reviews of the scientific literature suggests that a caffeine consumption of ~2 or 3–6 mg/kg before exercise, or 0.75–2 mg/kg during exercise will improve endurance exercise (Ganio et al, 2009; Tarnopolsky, 2010). Caffeine taken in a capsule, pill or powder form is more potent than coffee (Goldstein et al, 2010). Furthermore, Ganio et al (2009) observed that withdrawing caffeine consumption for 7 days before use may be the most effective way to optimise its ergogenic benefits. However, these findings are in contrast to a recent study by Irwin et al (2011), who imposed a 4-day caffeine withdrawal on habitual caffeine users. They found that 3 mg caffeine/kg BW significantly improved high-intensity endurance cycling performance in a time trial irrespective of a withdrawal period.

Since most research so far has centred around a few types of sport (e.g. cycling and running), dose-specific caffeine ingestion protocols are further required to determine the performance benefit of caffeine across a *wider* range of exercise and sport activities.

Side effects

- Elevated heart rate and ventilatory response in caffeine-naïve athletes (Dodd et al, 1991).
- Diuretic effect, gastrointestinal distress, decreased motor control, shivering, headache, dizziness and small elevations in blood pressure and resting heart rate (van Loon and Saris, 2005)
- High doses ($\geq$6–9 mg/kg BW) can cause tremors, headaches and impaired sleep (Burke et al, 2006; Stear et al, 2010). Caffeine has been removed from the AIS Sports Supplement Programme, and is no longer available to their athletes.
- Caffeine increases calcium excretion in the urine and can accelerate the loss of minerals from bone tissue. Its intake is one of the risk factors for fractures relating to osteoporosis. A cohort study found that women with low calcium intake who consume four or more cups of coffee daily are particularly at risk for osteoporotic fractures (Hallström et al, 2006).

Creatine (refer also to Chapter 1)

Qualities of creatine

- Creatine is not an essential nutrient as it is replenished daily at a rate of ~2 g/day by endogenous synthesis, and through dietary intake of animal food sources.
- The amino acids, namely, arginine, glycine and methionine are used to make creatine in the liver, kidneys, pancreas and other tissues, and then transport it to the muscle for uptake.

- The main source of creatine in the diet is primarily meat, especially lean beef, but it also occurs in fish, especially oil-rich varieties like herring and salmon. A serving size (225 g/8 oz) of herring may contain more creatine (2.5–4.0 g) than lean beef (1.5–2.5 g), pork (1.5–2.5 g) or salmon (1.5–2.5 g), and a serving of low-fat milk contains only 0.05 g creatine (Tarnopolsky, 2010).
- Compared with the total adenosine triphosphate (ATP) pool (80–100 g), the total quantity of endogenous creatine in the body is around 120–140 g for the average 70 kg man. Most creatine is found in skeletal muscle, which holds 95% of the body's creatine stores (~40% as free creatine and ~60% of *phosphocreatine* (PCr)) (Bemben and Lamont, 2005).
- Creatine phosphate (CP) or PCr is a high-energy phosphate compound and muscle fuel in the cell.
- Whereas the amount of intramuscular ATP is limited (5 mmol/kg wet weight (WW) of muscle) and can provide rapid energy for only a few seconds of maximal exercise, creatine is stored in greater amounts in skeletal muscle (intramuscular stores of PCr ~20 mmol/kg WW of muscle) and broken down quickly during exercise to provide energy for ATP re-synthesis.
- Since CP concentration within the cell is three or more times greater than ATP, it is known as the high-energy phosphate 'reservoir' (McArdle et al, 2010).
- Non-meat eaters, i.e. those who consume a vegetarian diet, have been shown to have lower skeletal muscle total creatine content (Lukaszuk et al, 2002; Watt et al, 2004).
- While high dietary creatine intake reduces endogenous creatine production, low dietary creatine intake in vegetarians/vegans decreases urinary excretion of creatine (as creatinine). Since no meat is consumed, creatine intake in these groups is dependant on their egg/fish intake (if any).

Benefits for exercise
- Creatine is involved in anaerobic production of ATP and thus maintains ATP levels in the muscle cells.
- It supports muscle contraction during repeated bouts of high-intensity exercise of short duration (i.e. weight lifting, cycling, sprints and jumps in football/soccer and other intense interval-type sports such as ball and racquet sports). Single-effort or repetitive sprint performance is improved with creatine supplementation (Earnest et al, 1995; Kreider et al, 1998).
- As creatine is a high-energy phosphate buffer in the cell, it buffers hydrogen ions (of lactic acid) likely delaying fatigue during high-intensity exercise.

- Creatine monohydrate is widely used as an oral creatine supplement and is known to increase both free creatine by 10–30% and CP (PCr) by 10–40% (Kreider, 2003).
- When combined with resistance exercise, creatine supplementation increases lean body mass (Volek et al, 1997; Williams et al, 1999; Branch, 2003).

Scientific evidence

Various creatine-loading regimes have been used in studies in an attempt to maximise increases in total muscle creatine levels. Although individual variation exists between subjects on the same loading regime, it appears that athletes with very low creatine concentration 'respond' the most to supplementation. Daily ingestion of 30 g of creatine monohydrate (consumed as 5 g × 4–6 doses/day) for more than 2 days increase muscle creatine content by up to 50% (Harris et al, 1992), although on average, a 20% increase in muscle creatine content (from ~70–90 to ~85–105 mmol/kg dry weight) is more common (Harris et al, 1992; Hultman et al, 1996). A creatine upper limit of ~160 mmol/kg dry weight (~40 mmol/kg WW of muscle) can be attained through creatine monohydrate supplementation, independent of whether supplementation is by rapid loading (2–6 days) using larger doses or by slow loading (28–30 days) with a smaller dose. Maintenance would be same for both regimes, at a rate of 2–3 g/day (Hultman et al, 1996).

Furthermore, both exercise and carbohydrate may enhance creatine uptake (Terjung et al, 2000). Consuming a ~100 g simple carbohydrate solution with each dose of creatine supplement *after exercise* may enhance creatine accumulation in the muscle up to 60% (Green et al, 1996), although it may not be practical or healthy for athletes to consume this amount of carbohydrate or calories for long periods of time (Terjung et al, 2000).

It is evident from the literature that creatine supplementation causes weight gain (~1 kg) (Greenhaff et al, 1994; Volek et al, 1997; Kreider et al, 1998; Eichner et al, 1999; Williams et al, 1999), although there appears to be differences in opinion around the primary and secondary effects thereof. Most speculate that the weight gain is largely due to water retention (Hultman et al, 1996; Williams and Branch, 1998) during creatine loading and uptake in the muscle, leading to protein synthesis and a reduction in protein breakdown (Haussinger et al, 1993). Others attribute protein synthesis as the leading cause (Kreider et al, 1998). Long-term gains in muscle mass can be achieved by combining creatine supplementation with resistance training (Williams et al, 1999; Branch, 2003).

The performance effects of creatine have been studied extensively since Harris et al's (1992) study showed that large doses of creatine monohydrate increased muscle creatine levels. A review of a majority of studies of creatine supplementation and high-intensity exercise show enhanced high-intensity performance (Williams et al, 1999), especially short-term exercise tasks lasting less than 30 seconds that are dependent on the phosphagen (ATP-PCr) system for PCr (Williams and Branch, 1998). Singe effort or repetitive bouts of high-intensity short-duration activities, interval training such as high-intensity sprint cycling (Balsom et al, 1995; Casey et al, 1996; Van der Berrie et al, 1998), short treadmill run performances (Balsom et al, 1993; Harris et al, 1993; Earnest et al, 1997), football/soccer-specific vertical jumps and sprint performance (Mujika et al, 1998; Stout et al, 1999; Cox et al, 2002; Ostojic, 2004), swimming velocity (Peyreburne et al, 1998), gross and/or propelling efficiency in swimming (Silva et al, 2007) and resistance exercise (Volek et al, 1997; Law et al, 2009), all benefit from creatine loading. Some racquet sport athletes also benefit from creatine supplementation, such as competitive squash players (Romer et al, 2001), but not tennis players (Op't Eijnde et al, 2001; Pluim et al, 2006). Small (but not significant) improvements in performance may benefit rugby players using creatine supplements (Ahmun et al, 2005).

Some studies show that creatine supplementation improves aerobic endurance of *short duration* (for reviews see Williams et al, 1999; Kreider, 2003) and is beneficial for aerobic–anaerobic trained athletes (Chwalbinska-Moneta, 2003). It may also enhance muscle glycogen storage (Burke et al, 2006). Kendall et al (2009) found that creatine supplementation improved the effects of high-intensity interval endurance training on endurance (cycling) performance.

However, endurance running performance is not enhanced by creatine supplementation. Balsom et al, 1993 found that run time decreased during a 6-km terrain run after creatine supplementation. Similarly, Astorino et al (2005) found no effect on 5-km run time, despite using a serum form of creatine, which is marketed specifically for endurance athletes. Furthermore, Glaister et al (2006) also found no performance benefits for runners after creatine loading for multiple sprint runs.

Application

Creatine is best for single-effort or repeated bouts of short duration and very powerful exercise that involve short recovery periods.

Not all athletes respond to creatine supplementation, in fact some are non-responders (Greenhaff et al, 1994). Failure to distinguish between those who respond to creatine uptake and non-responders may mask any effect of creatine supplementation (Kilduff et al, 2004).

Dose administered

Typical doses are:
- *Rapid loading*: 20–25 g creatine monohydrate/day taken as 5 g × 4–5 doses for 5–7 consecutive days. Maintenance dose of 2–3 g/day.

- *Slow loading*: 2–3 g creatine monohydrate/day for 1 month. Maintenance dose of 2–3 g/day.

Side effects

Previously, oral creatine supplementation for up to 8 weeks appeared safe and was not associated with any health risks (Williams and Branch, 1998). Further investigation has showed the creatine supplementation by healthy individuals over short-term (5 days), medium-term (4–9 weeks) and long-term (up to 5 years) do not damage their kidneys or liver (Poortmans and Francaux, 2000). Recently, a placebo-controlled study on top-level male soccer-players investigated gastrointestinal effects of creatine loading (Ostojic and Ahmetovic, 2008). They found the incidence of diarrhoea to be related to the dose, and concluded that the risk of diarrhoea may be increased when 10 g creatine is ingested *per single serving*.

Although not all studies report significant ergogenic effects of creatine supplementation, it seems that few studies to this point have reported that creatine supplementation *impairs* exercise performance (Balsom et al, 1993).

The following areas in creatine research warrant further investigation:

- Individual variability in creatine stores
- Gender and age effects
- Effect of exercise training
- Safety of long-term, high-dose creatine supplementation
- Contamination of supplements

Creatine has never been banned and is not on WADA's Prohibited List.

Sodium bicarbonate

Qualities of sodium bicarbonate

- Bicarbonate (HCO_3^-), a base, is a major chemical buffer in blood.
- Lactic acid, a metabolic by-product of anaerobic metabolism, accumulates in muscles during near-maximal anaerobic exercise, causing a build-up of hydrogen ions [H^+]. The drop in pH is associated with muscle fatigue and can be offset by bicarbonate (Applegate, 1999).
- $NaHCO_3$ (ingested as *baking soda or antacid*) is a buffering agent, providing an alkaline environment that favours high-intensity exercise performance of more than 30 seconds.

Benefits for exercise

- Intense muscular activity, such as sprinting, often produces large amounts of H^+ that can inhibit muscle contraction and reduce the activity of enzymes involved in energy production. Muscular pain and fatigue sets in, impairing the ability to maintain exercise intensity for a more prolonged period (Geissler and Powers, 2005).

- Bicarbonate loading is the process of ingesting bicarbonate to increase the blood's bicarbonate concentrations and elevate blood pH. Increasing the capacity to buffer acids may delay fatigue during high-intensity exercise (Wilmore and Costill, 2004).
- $NaHCO_3$ increases performance in maximal anaerobic exercise lasting 1–7 minutes.
- $NaHCO_3$ improves repeated-sprint ability by contributing to an increased anaerobic energy production (Bishop et al, 2004).
- $NaHCO_3$ improves lactate threshold and endurance performance, likely due to less metabolic acidosis during training and augmented muscle oxidative capacity (Edge et al, 2006).

Scientific evidence

Several controlled studies have been carried out using $NaHCO_3$ and sodium citrate pre-exercise loading regimes on well-trained athletes partaking in specific sports. For the most part, performance has been tested during anaerobic components of cycling, swimming, running, rowing and team sport simulated exercise.

Improvement in time trial performance in well-trained cyclists can be achieved with bicarbonate (McNaughton et al, 1999) or citrate loading (Potteiger et al, 1996). Running time for the 400 m, 800 m and 1500 m distances can be enhanced by bicarbonate loading (Wilkes et al, 1983; Goldfinch et al, 1988; Bird et al, 1995) and citrate loading improves 3000-m and 5000-m performance (Shave et al, 2001; Oopik et al, 2003). $NaHCO_3$ improves single-bout 200-m freestyle swim performance (Lindh et al, 2008). Furthermore, adding $NaHCO_3$ has been combined with other ergogenic aids to promote performance, especially swim performance. $NaHCO_3$ added to caffeine reverses the negative effects of caffeine (i.e. lower blood pH and slower recovery of blood bicarbonate after exercise) on repeated maximal exercise performance (Pruscino et al, 2008). Similarly, $NaHCO_3$ combined with creatine improves consecutive maximal swims (Mero et al, 2004).

Team sport athletes may also benefit from bicarbonate loading, as shown in team sports simulation trials (Price et al, 2003; Bishop and Claudius, 2005).

Majority studies appear to be in agreement that $NaHCO_3$ and sodium citrate raise and maintain pH levels during exercise, providing an ergogenic benefit, although individual variability exists. The level of physical conditioning of the athlete and their tolerance of the buffer substance may explain why there are differences in the ergogenic benefit of bicarbonate and citrate (Requena et al, 2005). Furthermore, McClung and Collins (2007) proved how the impact of 'expectancy' of bicarbonate's ergogenic effect influences performance. During a series of 1000-m time trials, elite runners who *believed* that they had been given NaHCO$_3$ (even though they had actually received a placebo) ran almost as fast as those associated with consuming the drug itself. Conversely, when they *were* given NaHCO$_3$ but were not told, their performance did not improve significantly.

Application

Best for 1–7-minute exercise bouts, i.e. repeated sprints and interval-style exercise involving maximal anaerobic exercise.

Dose administered

300 mg/kg BW taken with 1 L water, 1–2 hours prior to high-intensity exercise. Recently Stellingwerff et al (2007) reviewed the performance benefits of NaHCO$_3$ on middle-distance race performance and found a small but significant effect of 0.3 g NaHCO$_3$ /kg BW (in solution) taken 1–2 hours before exercise.

Some studies report that improvements in anaerobic performance may be dose dependent. Douroudos et al (2006) found that 5 days of supplementation with 500 mg NaHCO$_3$/kg BW/day had a greater performance effect in the Wingate (cycle) test than 300 mg NaHCO$_3$/kg BW/day. Doses of 300–500 mg sodium citrate/kg BW are typically used in loading protocols.

Side effects

However, ingesting >300 mg NaHCO$_3$ may lead to gastrointestinal distress such as cramping, bloating and diarrhoea. Similar gastrointestinal symptoms may be experienced when ingesting excessive doses of sodium citrate.

Chapter summary

- Nutritional supplements contain a dietary component such as a nutrient (i.e. vitamin) in similar amounts as those found in food.
- Nutritional supplements treat a suboptimal nutrient level or a nutrient deficiency, have a role in nutrition and metabolism and can enhance exercise performance.
- Nutritional ergogenic aids, also known as performance-enhancing aids, may or may not be a dietary component of food and usually occur in amounts greater than those found in food or food components.
- Known for its pharmacological effect, some nutritional ergogenic aids have a role in nutrition, metabolism and exercise performance.

- The rigorous science, its effects of health and well-being, the safe and legal dose, risk of contamination and proven advantages for exercise performance are just some of the areas that need to be investigated for each ergogenic aid and its claim.
- Caffeine is a stimulant that affects muscle tissue, the central nervous system and adrenalin.
- Caffeine is found naturally in nuts, seeds, plants, coffee and tea, and added to over-the-counter medications, colas, energy bars and drinks.
- Its benefits for performance include improved reaction time, increased mental alertness and concentration.
- Caffeine increases fat breakdown and oxidation, and may reduce carbohydrate use and spare glycogen during exercise.
- It enhances endurance capacity and delays fatigue, increasing power output and prolonging time to exhaustion.
- It improves short-term, high-intensity exercise, and reduces the perception of pain.
- The dose administered is either 2–6 mg/kg before exercise or 0.75–2 mg/kg during exercise.
- Creatine is a non-essential nutrient replenished endogenously at a rate of ~2 g/day, and obtained through the diet from meat and fish.
- The total quantity of endogenous creatine in the body is around 120–140 g mostly found in skeletal muscle, which holds 95% of the body's creatine stores (~40% as free creatine and ~60% of phosphocreatine).
- Creatine maintains ATP levels in the muscle cells, supports muscle contraction, delays fatigue and can increases lean body mass.
- Creatine is best for single-effort or repeated bouts of short duration and very powerful exercise that involve short recovery periods.
- Dose administered is either for rapid loading: 20–25 g creatine monohydrate/day taken as 5 g × 4–5 doses for 5–7 consecutive days, followed by a maintenance dose of 2–3 g/day; or for slow loading: 2–3 g creatine monohydrate/day for 1 month, followed by a maintenance dose of 2–3 g/day.
- Bicarbonate (HCO_3^-), a base, is a major chemical buffer in blood.
- Sodium bicarbonate and sodium citrate are buffering agents, providing an alkaline environment that favours high-intensity exercise performance or intermittent type exercise of more than 30 seconds.
- It increases the capacity to buffer acids, thereby delaying fatigue during high-intensity exercise, increasing performance in maximal anaerobic exercise lasting 1–7-minutes, improving repeated-sprint ability by contributing to an increased anaerobic energy production and improving lactate threshold and endurance performance.
- Dose administered is either once-off 300 mg/kg BW taken with 1 L water, 1–2 hours prior to high-intensity exercise, or as part of a 5-day loading protocol of 300–500 mg/kg BW/day.

APPENDIX

Reference Values for Estimated Energy Expenditure

Reference table for basal metabolic rate (BMR)

Gender	Body weight	Energy (kcal/day)				
		10–17	18–29	30–59	60–74–	74+
Women	40	1228	1079	1178	1055	1016
	45	1295	1153	1220	1101	1065
	50	1362	1227	1261	1147	1114
	55	1429	1301	1303	1193	1163
	60	1496	1375	1344	1239	1212
	65	1563	1449	1386	1285	1261
	70	1630	1523	1427	1331	1310
	75	1697	1597	1469	1377	1359
Men	50	1542	1447	1448	1295	1241
	55	1631	1523	1506	1355	1283
	60	1719	1598	1563	1414	1325
	65	1808	1674	1621	1474	1367
	70	1896	1749	1678	1533	1409
	75	1985	1825	1736	1593	1451
	80	2073	1900	1793	1652	1493
	85	2162	1976	1851	1712	1535
	90	2250	2051	1908	1771	1577

Source: Adapted from Thomas and Bishop (2007).

Energy

1 kcal = 4.2 kJ
1 g carbohydrate = 17 kJ (4 kcal)
1 g protein = 16 kJ (4 kcal)

Nutrition for Sport and Exercise: A Practical Guide, First Edition. Hayley Daries.
© 2012 Blackwell Publishing Ltd. Published 2012 by Blackwell Publishing Ltd.

1 g fat = 37 kJ (9 kcal)
1 g alcohol = 29 kJ (7 kcal)

Protein

1 g nitrogen = 6.35 g protein

Glossary

adenosine triphosphate (ATP) A high-energy compound that is required for cellular work. It provides kinetic energy for skeletal muscles to do mechanical work.

adenosine triphosphatase (ATPase) An enzyme that releases energy by reducing ATP to adenosine diphosphate (ADP) and inorganic phosphate (P_i).

aerobic metabolism Producing energy (ATP) in the presence of oxygen.

ad libitum **(fluid ingestion)** During exercise – drinking to the dictates of one's own thirst.

allergen Usually a protein-type substance that causes an allergic response.

amenorrhoea The absence of menstrual cycle in women.

amino acids (AA) Building blocks of protein.

anaerobic metabolism Producing energy (ATP) when oxygen supply is limited.

antioxidant A compound that can stop free radicals from causing damage to body tissues.

basal metabolic rate (BMR) The minimal energy expended that can support life in a fasted state at rest at ambient room temperature.

basic energy expenditure (BEE) The energy expended in a fasted state at rest at ambient room temperature, excluding the energy expended through the thermic effect of food, activity or exercise.

bicarbonate HCO_3^-, a base, is a major chemical buffer in blood. Used as a nutritional ergogenic aid to offset the drop in pH that results from the build-up of lactic acid, a metabolic by-product of anaerobic metabolism associated with muscle fatigue.

bicarbonate loading The process of ingesting bicarbonate to increase the blood's bicarbonate concentrations and elevate blood pH. Increasing the capacity to buffer acids may delay fatigue during high-intensity exercise.

biologic value (BV) A measure of the effectiveness of food protein in living tissues. Factor 100 denotes the percentage of nitrogen (from protein) absorbed that is retained by the body.

body composition Measures body fatness, and fat-free mass, including lean body mass and body water.

body mass index (BMI) It is a height-for-weight index used to assess degree of obesity (body fatness). Weight (kg) divided by height (m) squared (kg/m^2).

caffeine A stimulant (drug) affecting muscle tissue, the central nervous system and adrenalin. It is found naturally in nuts, seeds, plants, coffee and tea, and used as a nutritional ergogenic aid.

calorie (cal) The unit of energy, where 1 cal is the heat energy required to raise the temperature of 1 g water by $1°C$.

carbohydrate (CHO) A compound containing carbon, hydrogen and oxygen atoms. Includes sugars, starches and fibre.

carbohydrate loading or glycogen loading A plan involving tapered training and a diet high in carbohydrates to enhance the glycogen stores above normal levels.

creatine Made from amino acids and found in skeletal muscle. Phosphocreatine (PCr) – a high-energy phosphate compound serves as muscle fuel for anaerobic production and maintenance of ATP. Used as a nutritional ergogenic aid to support muscle contraction during repeated bouts of high-intensity exercise of short duration.

dehydration Loss of body water.

delayed onset muscle soreness (DOMS) Muscle soreness that usually occurs within 24–48 hours of severe exercise in trained athletes, or within 4–6 days of unaccustomed exercise in untrained individuals. Causes include free radical damage, muscle enzyme leakage, breakdown of protein and muscle cells and accumulation of phosphate.

dietary reference values (DRV) Defined as a series of estimates of the amount of energy and nutrients required by different groups of healthy people.

electrolytes Electrically charged ions that function as minerals essential for body water balance and chemical reactions.

energy Various forms of energy exist to do work in the body including light, chemical, mechanical, osmotic, electrical and heat (thermal) energy.

energy balance When the sum of energy intake from food, fluids and supplements is equal to energy expended through exercise, basal metabolism and the thermic effect of food.

essential amino acids (EAA) Amino acids that are needed for human growth and survival that cannot be made in the body and need to be obtained from dietary sources.

essential fatty acids (EFA) Fatty acids that cannot be synthesised by the body and has to come from dietary sources. Alpha-linolenic acid and linoleic acid are the two essential fatty acids in the diet.

estimated average requirement (EAR) The estimated average requirement for energy or nutrients of a population.

estimated energy cost of activity Measure the intensity of physical activity and expressed as energy consumption over time, or kilocalorie per minute (kcal/min).

exercise-associated hyponatremia (EAH) Hyponatremia in athletes engaged in prolonged exercise, defined as a serum or plasma sodium concentration below reference range, <135 mmol/L.

exercise-associated hyponatremic encephalopathy (EAHE) Symptomatic EAH, defined by the presence of specific central nervous system symptoms regardless of actual serum sodium concentration.

exercise-related transient abdominal pain (ETAP) Abdominal pain experienced during exercise, informally referred to as *'stitch'* or *'side ache'*.

fat Organic compounds made up of carbon, hydrogen and oxygen. Also known as lipids, a group of organic compounds that are do not dissolve in water. Occurs in various forms including free fatty acids, triglycerides, sterols (like cholesterol) and phospholipids.

fibre Known as a non-starch polysaccharide (NSP), it is an indigestible carbohydrate that has many health benefits.

food allergy An adverse reaction to a food substance mediated by the immune system.

free fatty acids (FFAs) The components of fat made available to the cells for energy.

free radical An atom or molecule with one or more unpaired electrons causing damage to body tissues.

gastric emptying The movement of gastric contents (foods, fluids) from the stomach into the small intestine.

glycaemic index (GI) A ranking of carbohydrate foods according to how quickly the food is converted to glucose and is absorbed into the bloodstream. Foods are ranked according to high, intermediate (moderate) or low GI and usually indicated by a number (0–100), where 100 is the highest GI (white bread or glucose).

glycaemic load (GL) Takes into account the amount of available carbohydrate in the food and its blood glucose response. GL values range from low to high GL <5, <10, <15, <20.

glycogen The storage form of carbohydrate in the body, found in liver and muscles.

guideline daily amount (GDA) Guidelines that appear on nutritional labels about the approximate amount of particular nutrients and the calories required for a healthy diet.

intramuscular triacylglycerol (IMTG) A small amount of fat stored in muscle tissue and found between muscle fibres, and as fat droplets within muscle cells.

kilocalorie (kcal) A kilocalorie is the heat energy required to raise the temperature of 1 kg of water by 1°C. 1kcal = 1000 cal.

kilojoule (kJ) A unit of energy (metric system). 1 kJ = 0.239 kcal.

mineral An inorganic substance incorporated into structural components of the body tissues and present in body fluids.

muscle hypertrophy An increase in muscle mass or size.

nitrogen balance When the intake of nitrogen (protein intake from the diet) is equal to nitrogen excretion (protein from urine, faeces, sweat and other secretions (skin, hair, nails)), a state of nitrogen balance or nitrogen equilibrium is achieved.

non-essential amino acids (NEAA) Amino acids that can be made in a healthy body in sufficient amounts.

nutritional ergogenic aid Also known as performance-enhancing aids, they may or may not be a dietary component of food, and usually occur in amounts greater than those found in food or food components.

nutritional supplement Contain a dietary component such as a nutrient (i.e. vitamin), in similar amounts as those found in food.

oxidative stress Disturbance in the pro-oxidant–antioxidant balance in favour of oxidants with the imbalance leading to oxidative damage in cells.

physical activity levels (PAL) The ratio of overall daily energy expenditure (from occupational and non-occupational activities) to basal metabolic rate.

protein A compound formed by amino acids and containing nitrogen.

reactive oxygen species (ROS) Refers not only to oxygen-centred radicals but also includes reactive derivatives of oxygen such as hydrogen peroxide.

reference nutrient intake (RNI) Defined as an estimate of the amount of a nutrient (protein, vitamins and minerals) that is required to meet the needs of more than 97.5% of healthy persons, including someone who has high needs for it.

skinfold fat thickness Measurements of body fat at skinfold sites on the body, used to estimate body fatness and fat-free mass.

sports anaemia An increase in plasma volume in the blood that is associated with endurance exercise and/or intense training. It can also 'dilute' free iron concentration, causing low levels of haemoglobin.

thermic effect of food (TEF) or diet-induced thermogenesis (DIT) The energy expended through digestion, absorption and metabolism of energy-giving nutrients.

triglyceride or triacylglycerol (TG) A simple lipid that consists of 1 unit of glycerol and 3 units of fatty acids. It is the storage form of fat, abundant in adipose tissue.

vitamin A potent organic substance required from the diet in small quantities for highly specific physiologic functions in the body that is essential to life.

water intoxication During exercise – a result of voluntarily drinking too much fluid.

Student Exercises

Chapter 1

Michelle is a 28-year old masters swimmer, who trains competitively with a squad twice a week. Each session lasts 1 hour. In addition to this, 3 mornings per week she does long distance freestyle swims (1.5–3 km) with a friend and afterwards she grabs a cup of coffee at the gym's breakfast bar. She takes part in monthly Club Galas over long course of 50 m within the county, and aims to compete in the National Championships later this year that will involve lengthy travel by coach. On the advice of a fellow swimmer and to lose body fat, Michelle has been following a low-calorie diet for a number of weeks and has also excluded all bread from her diet. She regularly eats a couple of sandwiches at lunch, but since starting the diet she has quickly run out of meal ideas for lunchtime and has resorted to 'healthy' ready meals to get her through the day. She hardly prepares any cooked meals most evenings after work as she finds it time-consuming and would rather pick on 'whatever is in the fridge' while working on her post-graduate thesis. She complains of sluggishness, says she needs more energy and does not know how to prepare quick and healthy low-calorie meals.

1 What could be the physical demands of swimming?

2 Are Michelle's existing dietary practices in line with the goals of an adequate sports diet?

3 What factors affect her food choices? What can she do to overcome any challenges?

4 What are some immediate effects of excluding bread from her diet? Could there be short-term consequences to her health and performance?

Nutrition for Sport and Exercise: A Practical Guide, First Edition. Hayley Daries.
© 2012 Blackwell Publishing Ltd. Published 2012 by Blackwell Publishing Ltd.

5 Is there any information, knowledge or skills that may help her achieve her goals? What practical tips regarding preparing and planning of food may she need to achieve her goals?

6 What nutrition issues will she face when travelling long distances?

Chapter 2

The local triathlon club has asked you to give a pre-season talk to some of their new members who have joined the club with a previous sports background, mostly in swimming and running. The athletes are a fairly homogenous group of recreational triathletes (similar ages, BMI, training load) and spend an average of 10 hours per week training (4.5 km swimming, 110 km cycling and 25 km running). The time allocated for each discipline is on average:

- ~1 hour 45 minutes swimming
- ~6 hours cycling
- ~2 hours 15 minutes running

The coach is concerned as these athletes have high-energy demands. One triathlete has been complaining of cold intolerance, and the coach has observed that another has lost power. Some find it hard to do the 'brick' (back-to-back training) or consecutive daily sessions and their recovery between sessions is beginning to waver.

1 What factors of energy metabolism during exercise are important for determining the energy cost of exercise?

2 What impact could participation in a sprint, standard (Olympic distance) or ironman triathlon have on fuel use? What practical challenges could the athlete face during training?

3 What investigations could help explain the symptoms experienced by the two athletes (cold intolerance and loss of power)?

4 Regarding the physical demands of exercise, the group wants to know the average energy cost of training. Suppose the energy cost of freestyle swimming is 10 kcal/min, cycling is 11.8 kcal/min and running 16.2 kcal/min, calculate the total cost of their training per week and per day. What may they expect to expend in a standard triathlon (1.5 km swim, 40 km bike, 10 km run) if they aim to complete the race in 2 hours 20 minutes?

5 At the end of the talk, Simon, a 30-year-old triathlete weighing 65 kg asks you to calculate his energy and nutrient requirements. Of particular concern to him is whether he is getting enough protein in

the diet and wants to know the amount of protein that is sufficient to meet the needs of an endurance athlete. He loves sardines on toast and wants to know if sardines are a good source of protein compared to chicken or beef. His is concerned about the oil content of the fish.

Calculate daily energy requirements, total energy expenditure, and determine individual nutrient needs expressed as percentage contribution to total energy intake and gram of nutrient per kilogram body weight per day (g/kg BW/day).

Chapter 3

A Food quiz

1 The major nutrient in cereal, bread, rice, pasta and potato is:
   A Essential fats
   B Amino Acids
   C Carbohydrates

2 A type of 'heart healthy fat' of the following food sources is:
   A Saturated fat in butter
   B Trans fats in margarine
   C Monounsaturated fat in avocado

3 Of the following, the highest source of dietary cholesterol is:
   A 1 large egg
   B 100 g shelled prawns
   C 100 g Lamb's liver

4 Orange-fleshed fruit and vegetables are the best source of which antioxidant:
   A Linoleic acid
   B Beta-carotene
   C Trytophan

5 Which of the following food is a good source of omega-3 polyunsaturated fatty acid, and calcium?
   A Sardines
   B Olive Oil
   C Steak

6 The energy (and fat) content is lowest in 50 g of:
   A Mozzarella cheese
   B Feta cheese
   C Edam cheese

7 The protein content is greater in 100 g of which plant food:

   A Soya beans

   B Quinoa

   C Bamboo shoots

8 **True or False**

   a Protein is the primary source of energy for the working muscles.

   b Taking dietary supplements before competition is an essential practice for athletes.

   c The following fruits provide a good source of Vitamin C: guava, kiwi fruit and papaya.

   d A good source of soluble fibre in the diet is from oats, apples and beans.

   e Drinking alcohol after exercise can delay an athlete's recovery from a sports injury.

9 What the main nutrients supplied by the following foods?

   a Streaky bacon

   b Baked beans

   c Avocado

   d Raisins

   e Muesli

   f Cheese and tomato pizza

   g Quorn

B Menus

1 Rio is at a sports college and plays league football. Since starting at the new high school he has been eating meals and snacks regularly at the school's dining hall. He has shown an interest in nutrition and wants to know from the menu below which of the following meals are:

   a High in carbohydrate

   b High in fat

   c A good source of fibre

   d Rich in vitamins and minerals

   e High in amino acids

   f A good vegetarian option

   g A low Glycemic Index food

   h A high Glycemic Index food

MENU

Grated carrot and orange

Couscous

Jacket potato

Cole slaw

Vegetable rice with sunflower seeds

Baked beans on wholemeal toast

Steamed fish in parsley sauce

Pasta and lentil bolognaise

A bowl of oats with cinnamon and apple

2 Assess Rio's 6-day breakfast menu and answer the questions below.

Day	Rio's Menu
Monday (home)	1 cereal bar
Tuesday (home)	Toast (white), cheddar cheese, butter, tea with whole milk and sugar
Wednesday (School Breakfast Club)	Fortified cereal (high-fibre flakes) with whole milk and sugar, bread, butter and jam
Thursday	*No breakfast*
Friday (home)	Fruit juice and a short-bread biscuit
Saturday (football pitch)	Breakfast roll with fried egg and sausage

a How is breakfast consumption viewed as a healthy lifestyle factor? What are the benefits for young athletes?

b How does skipping breakfast affect his nutritional status in the short-term (day-to-day) and long-term (through the life cycle)?

c With reference to the healthy eating messages, list the changes he can make to his current menu? Make suggestions for healthier options, keeping in mind that he is a fussy eater and wants to keep things as they are.

Chapter 4

1 Describe how carbohydrates are classified?

2 Why is carbohydrate the preferred energy source during exercise? How does intensity and duration of exercise affect how fuel is used?

3 Name 3 factors that affect glycogen repletion. What method is used by endurance athletes to optimise glycogen stores?

4 What are the recommended guidelines for carbohydrate intake in athletes? How many of the food groups in *the eatwell plate* contain carbohydrate-rich foods?

5 Describe all aspects to consider for the ideal pre-exercise meal.

6 A cyclist consumes a glucose drink and a packet of raisins (supplying a total of 50 g CHO) 40 minutes before a cycling race in which he cycles

at ~69% VO_2max. Shortly into the race he experiences trembling, dizziness and feels so weak that he has to stop by the side of the road. Explain the possible causes that led to his symptoms. Is there anything he could have done to prevent it?

7 Explain the use of fructose in sports drinks.

8 What are the nutrition considerations after exercise? Which nutrients play a role in the post-exercise menu and why?

Chapter 5

1 What are essential amino acids and their role in the diet?

2 What is biologic value of protein? Which food sources are high biologic value proteins? Explain complementary proteins.

3 Name the functions of proteins and its role during endurance exercise and high-intensity team sports.

4 In what form is protein stored in the body? How many kilograms of protein does the average male of ~70 kg body weight have?

5 Does protein have a role during and after exercise? Would this information change fluid replacement guidelines in the future? For which group of athletes may it be relevant?

6 How do an athlete's nitrogen losses affect their protein status?

7 Could the RNI for protein (for adults) meet the needs of a bodybuilder in the 'bulking up' phase who wishes to increase muscle size? Provide recommendations for daily rates of protein intake and list the consequences of excessive protein intake above recommended levels.

8 Name 3 common food allergens that could possibly be present in the following recipe: *Vegetarian lasagne*.

9 What practical and healthy food preparation tips could athletes who wish to increase their consumption of meat and meat products, poultry, fish and eggs follow?

Chapter 6

Cricket, the 'gentleman's game' is a major international sport played commonly by the British Commonwealth nations. Although strictly a non-contact sport, physical demands of the game are high. For example, the bowling action involves repetitive twisting, extension, and rotation of the trunk at the same time as absorption of large ground reaction forces over a short period of time.

Philip is hearing-impaired and works as a skilled cabinet maker for a small business. He is a bowler in his mid-20s and plays for his cricket club's special needs team.

During the cricket season, the team meets once a week for a training session and on match-day Saturdays. Every training session usually lasts 90 minutes and includes fitness drills, running and skilled components such as batting, bowling and fielding.

Over the winter, many players stop training. Some continue jogging a few days a week and may take part in another sport until pre-season. Philip's job keeps him busy and during the off-season he works over-time and takes on extra jobs in the evenings and Saturdays. This leaves him with little time to exercise, even though he enjoys mountain biking on weekends.

Over the past winter Philip has been recovering from an injury and could not mountain-bike. Furthermore, his long hours at work resulted in erratic eating behaviours involving take-away and ready meals such as pizza, meat burgers, and fried chicken. His favourite take-away meal is Indian curry and he regularly stops at the local curry take-away shop for tikka masala with pilau rice and naan bread.

As the seasons changed Philip noticed that he could not fit into some of his old cricket trousers. On a visit to his GP he was told he had gained weight, and that his BMI and waist circumference are 'concerning'. His GP spoke to him about his weight issue, advising him to lose some weight since he had other risk factors that included a family history of Hyperlipidemia (familial hyperlipidemia, resulting in high blood lipid levels).

He presently weighs 112 kg and is 1.85 m tall, has a waist circumference of 103 cm and a skinfold sum of 96 mm.

A sample of his usual daily dietary intake follows:

Breakfast

3 slices of bread
Thickly spread butter
2 large eggs, fried in butter
3 beef sausages
2 mugs of coffee (strong, black)
2 t Sugar
(He takes a flask of coffee and a couple of sandwiches to work.)

Mid-morning

2 mugs of coffee
2 × 2 t Sugar
1 sandwich (2 slices of white bread with butter & sliced ham)
Cream doughnut

Lunch

500 ml bottle of cola
Pastry (e.g. a chicken pie, or 2 x sausage rolls)
1 (30 g) packet of salted crisps

Afternoon

1 bottle of water

Evening meal

(Usually a take-away)
1 × large serving of:
Tikka masala
Pilau rice
Naan bread
1 × pot of chocolate mousse

Evening snack

1 mug of coffee
2 t sugar
2–3 shortbread biscuits

1   Calculate Philip's BMI and interpret his results for BMI and waist circumference.

2   Identify the key factors in Philip's diet that may be the cause of his weight issue.

3 Using the key healthy eating messages in chapter 3 and recommendations from this chapter, suggest changes to improve his usual food choices, diet-associated behaviours and lifestyle habits.

4 Explore how Philip can increase his intake of essential fatty acids. Which dietary fats can be replaced or reduced, and which included in the 'new' pattern? Discuss the benefits he may gain from a diet rich in EFAs.

Chapter 7

Kathy is a 20-year-old ultra-distance runner who turned vegetarian 3 months ago. Since then she has completely changed her diet by avoiding all meat and meat products, chicken and fish. She is trying to exclude eggs but still consumes milk, yoghurt and cheese. She prefers rye and oats to wheat. Her favourite drink is black tea especially English breakfast tea and she drinks several cups a day.

She has since lost 9 kg but complains of fatigue and poor performance. She is also expressing low moods.

Upon assessment, her haematology report shows sub-optimal serum ferritin levels. Results from the biochemical lab test show that she also has lowered zinc levels. She was prescribed two supplements, one of which is a zinc supplement.

1 What may Kathy's diagnosis be, and what evidence supports it? What dietary intervention is needed? Describe in full detail.

2 Is the RNI for the deficient nutrients different for Kathy as compared with other females of the same age? Substantiate your answer.

3 What zinc-rich food sources are lacking from her diet? How will zinc supplementation affect her nutritional status considering the presence of other dietary factors?

4 Name the factors that have put Kathy 'at risk'? What would the long-term problems be for her if no dietary intervention is followed?

Chapter 8

1 How did early studies of fluid replacement in prolonged exercise shape race rules in marathons?

2 What challenges do team sport athletes face regarding hydration during a game?

3 Is dehydration during exercise a health and performance threat? Explain.

4 What are the risks related to over-drinking? What is exercise-associated hyponatremia (EAH) and exercise-associated hyponatremic encephalopathy (EAHE)?

5 Describe the typical profile of an athlete at risk of EAH, or EAHE.

6 What are the likely causes of exercise-related transient abdominal pain (ETAP) and how is it avoided?

7 How, and which athletes could benefit from carbohydrate ingestion during exercise?

8 What factors need to be considered for optimal hydration during exercise.

9 What sensible advice should athletes follow regarding alcohol consumption for health and sport?

Chapter 9

1 Differentiate between nutritional supplements and nutritional ergogenic aids? Provide examples to support your answer.

2 What information could athletes consider about a nutritional ergogenic aid they wish to consume?

3 Name the role players involved in keeping sport 'clean'.

4 Name the natural and artificial sources of caffeine?

5 What are the benefits of caffeine ingestion in sport? List the dosage administered and side effects of caffeine.

6 What foods sources contain high amounts of creatine?

7 What are the benefits of creatine supplementation in sport? Could all athletes benefit from creatine loading? Explain.

8 Which common household product contains sodium bicarbonate?

9 What are the benefits of sodium bicarbonate or sodium citrate ingestion in sport? List the dosage administered. Are there any side effects of sodium bicarbonate or sodium citrate ingestion?

Answers to Student Exercises

Leading words to Student Exercises

Chapter 1

1 Aerobic and anaerobic. Explosive movements, starts, dives, pulsing, strokes, pulling, pushing, lunging, kicks, flips and turns, tumbles, etc.

2 Food exclusion, irregular pattern, stimulant use, fad diet. Evaluate energy and nutrient value, physical symptoms, etc.

3 Assess knowledge, cooking skills, access and selection of food, motivation, training schedule and free time, travel, etc.

4 Nutrient value of bread, contribution to health and exercise performance. Evaluate alternatives used. Check reported symptoms, demands of training load and impact on recovery.

5 Address dietary extremism and issues identified at Question 3. Check budget, cooking facilities and support structures. Use pictorial food guide, serving suggestions, food labels, recipes, etc.

6 Fatigue, food supply, preparation, cooking facilities, restaurant and take-away choices, etc.

Chapter 2

1 Intensity, duration, body weight, etc.

2 Assess intensity and duration. Refer to aerobic and anaerobic metabolism, substrate partitioning and the 'cross-over' concept. Training load, nutrient needs, preparation time, etc.

3 Nutritional assessment: anthropometry (i.e. skinfolds, BMI, weight) and clinical/physical investigation (i.e. micronutrient status, signs of deficiency). Assess weight, body fat and fat free mass.

Nutrition for Sport and Exercise: A Practical Guide, First Edition. Hayley Daries.
© 2012 Blackwell Publishing Ltd. Published 2012 by Blackwell Publishing Ltd.

4 Assume 65 kg (average) body weight, and a moderately active PAL (1.7): refer to Table 2.2 for calculations.

5 Refer to Table 2.2 for calculation of EAR. Suggest nutrient contribution (i.e. 60% carbohydrate, 12–15% protein, 20–35% fats). Convert to gram nutrient/kg BW/day. Determine nutrient value of sardines – check food composition tables or food label per average portion. Consider fresh, frozen and canned variety, and benefits of this source of protein. Compare with same portion of chicken and beef.

Chapter 3
Answers to Multiple Choice Questions
A.

1 C

2 C

3 C

4 B

5 A

6 A

7 A

Answers to True/False Questions

8(a) F

8(b) F

8(c) T

8(d) T

8(e) T

Answers to Short Questions

9(a) Fat, protein, B vitamins

9(b) Carbohydrate, protein, fibre

9(c) Fat (monounsaturated), vitamin E, potassium

9(d) Carbohydrate, potassium, iron

9(e) Carbohydrate, protein, fibre

9(f) Carbohydrate, fat, lycopene, calcium

9(g) Protein, fibre, zinc

B. Menus

1(a) Couscous (also jacket potato)

1(b) Vegetable rice (if fried) with sunflower seeds, cole slaw (heavy dressing of regular mayonnaise)

1(c) Baked beans on wholemeal toast

1(d) Grated carrot and orange, Cole slaw (plain)

1(e) Steamed fish in parsley sauce

1(f) Pasta and lentil bolognaise

1(g) A bowl of oats with cinnamon and apple

1(h) Baked potato

2(a) Affects health, weight and mood. Benefits mental, creative and physical performance at school and sports field, etc.

2(b) Evaluate energy and nutrient contribution of breakfast. Determine vital nutrient contribution for his age group. Determine long-term risk factors of avoiding these nutrients through the life cycle, considering disease and performance.

2(c) Suggest regular pattern. Improve nutrient value of daily menu (use pictorial food guide to achieve balance). Consider adding fruit, vegetables and fibre. Provide alternatives for white bread, shortbread biscuit. Suggest healthy cooking methods.

Chapter 4

1 Previously simple and complex. Now refer to GI and GL

2 Energy conversion, consider oxygen availability. Refer to Chapter 2 for substrate partitioning and the 'cross-over' concept.

3 Consider amount, timing and super-compensation of stores.

4 Determine by level of participation, consider health and risk factors. Bread, cereals, milk and dairy, fruit and vegetables, sugary foods, beans, etc.

5 GI, amount and type of nutrients, timing, etc.

6 Investigate hypoglycaemia (rebound). Evaluate symptoms, confirm by blood glucose test. Consider effect of GI, timing, in susceptible athletes.

7 Explore carbohydrate oxidation rates compared with other sugars.

8 Regard carbohydrate, protein, amount, timing, etc.

Chapter 5

1 Indispensible, obtained from food sources only.

2 Explore quality of proteins (retained nitrogen by body). Score of 100 denotes high quality (i.e. egg-white). Combination of plant foods sources useful for vegetarians and vegans.

3 Consider structural and functional roles at rest. Consider fuel source, increases in lean body mass, strength and power, tissue maintenance, etc.

4 Explore many different forms and storage sites. Consider skeletal muscle. Refer also to Chapter 3 (mass of protein stores in body).

5 Consider glycogen depleting exercise and endurance athletes.

6 Explore losses through sweat. Consider positive and negative nitrogen balance, carbohydrate depletion and training adaptations.

7 Determine RNI for protein, and explore requirement for a highly positive nitrogen balance for muscle hypertrophy. Consider training phase.

8 Wheat (in lasagne pasta sheets), milk in the white sauce and soy (vegetable protein).

9 Provide examples of lower fat, lower salt versions, and explore cooking styles that use less fat. Give vegetarian, or plant sources of proteins as alternatives or 'meal fillers'.

Chapter 6

1 BMI (kg/m^2) = weight (kg)/height^2 (m) (refer also to Chapter 2). Obese, increased health risk.

2 Explore his current diet, physical activity, eating habits, work conditions, injury. Consider energy value of meals, SFA, processed foods, take-away meals, drinks and overall nutrients lacking in the diet.

3 Use eight key messages (refer also to Chapter 3). Comb through diet, modify behaviour and suggest lifestyle changes. Refer to Table 6.3 for better choices when dining out or explore the healthy recipes provided in the book.

4 Determine sources of omega-3 and 6. Explore link between omega-3 fatty acids and muscle loss related to immobilisation after an injury.

Further benefits: protect against inflammation, helps depression, lower lipid levels, etc.

Chapter 7

1 Iron depletion. Dilution of blood measure of iron status. Consider symptoms and diet history/food record. Address vegetarianism and identify iron-rich foods to include. Consider dietary iron intake, add factors to enhance iron absorption, identify and remove or reduce factors that inhibit absorption (i.e. tannins (in tea), phytates (fibre), etc.). Address iron supplementation.

2 Consider effect of vegetarianism, and iron losses (in ultra-distance running) on iron balance.

3 Vegetarian source: wheatgerm, quorn, seeds and nuts, etc. Zinc supplementation inhibits iron absorption.

4 Determine if 'at risk athlete' (refer to Table 7.3) and explore the dietary factors that inhibits iron and zinc absorption in her diet. Examine effects of deficiency of both minerals (Table 7.2).

Chapter 8

1 Explore 'dangers of dehydration', physiological functions and perception of effort. Evolution of IAAF race rules.

2 Consider level of participation (i.e. competitive), opportunities to drink, hot environments, etc.

3 Consider exercise performance and physiological indices measured in dehydrated elite endurance athletes. Examine *ad libitum* intake on exercise performance, perception of effort and stomach fullness.

4 Osmotic imbalance, water intoxication and hyponatremia. Refer to serum sodium concentration and associated symptoms.

5 Slower, less experienced athletes, lighter weight (perhaps female), taking many opportunities to drink, drinking just water, etc. Explore symptomatic hyponatremia.

6 Fluid ingestion, repetitive motion. Consider carbohydrate concentration and osmolality of solution.

7 Explore prolonged exercise, late stages of glycogen depletion. Examine use of carbohydrate mixtures.

8 Consider physiological cues and monitor perception of thirst, or bloating and weight gain or additional symptoms (i.e. confusion, nausea, vomiting, etc.). Further evaluate use of drink type, volume,

nutrient composition, etc. Individual considerations: body weight, level of participation and experience, environment, fluid availability, etc.

9 Address harmful effects of alcohol consumption. Refer also to Chapter 3 and Table 3.3 for sensible intake and unit equivalents of various alcoholic beverages.

Chapter 9

1 Consider similarity to food compared with excessive amounts of a single nutrient or non-food substance. Evaluate effect of health and exercise performance, and safe practice.

2 Measurable scientific proof, short- and long-term effects, safety, etc.

3 Explore IOC, WADA, etc.

4 Nuts, seeds, plants, coffee, tea, colas, chocolate and cocoa-rich food and drinks, novel drinks, energy bars with added caffeine, as well as some over-the-counter medications.

5 Investigate reaction time, concentration, endurance performance, perception of effort/fatigue, etc. Consider small to large doses, timing of intake and method of administration. Elevated heart rate, headaches, etc.

6 Lean beef, herring, salmon.

7 Maintains ATP levels, benefits high-intensity exercise of short duration (i.e. sprints), buffers hydrogen ions, increases lean body mass, etc. Consider athletes' creatine levels, intensity and duration of exercise, etc.

8 Baking soda.

9 A chemical buffer in the blood, delays fatigue, etc. Consider units (in mg) and volume of water accompanying intake. Gastrointestinal distress.

References

Adolf, E.F. (1947) *Physiology of man in the desert*. New York: Interscience Publishers.

Adolf, E.F. & Dill, D.B. (1938) Observation on water metabolism in the desert. *American Journal of Physiology*, 123: 369–378.

Ahlborg, B., Bergstrom, J., Brohult, J., Ekelund, L.G., Hultman, E. & Maschio, G. (1967) Human muscle glycogen content and capacity for prolonged exercise after different diets. *Forvarsmedicin*, 3: 85–89.

Ahmun, R.P., Tong, R.J., Alexy, U., Sichert-Hellert, W. & Kersting, M. (2002) Fifteen year time trends in energy and macronutrient intake in German children and adolescents: results of the DONALD study. *British Journal of Nutrition*, 87: 595–604.

Ahmun, R.P., Tong, R.J. & Grimshaw, P.N. (2005) The effects of acute creatine supplementation on multiple sprint cycling and running performance in rugby players. *Journal of Strength and Conditioning Research*, 19: 92–97.

Almond, C.S., et al (2005) Hyponatremia among runners in the Boston marathon. *New England Journal of Medicine*, 352: 1550–1556.

Alway, S.E., Grumbt, W.H., Stray-Gundersen, J. & Gonyea, W.J. (1992) Effects of resistance training on elbow flexors of highly competitive bodybuilders. *Journal of Applied Physiology*, 72: 1512–1521.

American College of Sports Medicine (1996) Position stand on exercise and fluid replacement. *Medicine and Science in Sports and Exercise*, 28: i–vii.

American College of Sports Medicine (2001) Appropriate intervention strategies for weight loss and prevention of weight regain for adults. *Medicine and Science in Sports and Exercise*, 33(12): 2145–2156.

Anderson, J.W., Konz, E.C., Frederich, R.C. & Wood, C.L. (2001) Long-term weight loss maintenance: a meta-analysis of US studies. *American Journal of Clinical Nutrition*, 74: 579–584.

Anderson, M.E., Bruce, C.R., Fraser, S.F., Stepto, N.K., Klein, R., Hopkins, W.G. & Hawley, J.A. (2000) Improved 2000-meter rowing performance in competitive oarswomen after caffeine ingestion. *International Journal of Sports Nutrition*, 10: 464–475.

Angus, D.J., Febbraio, M.A. & Hargreaves, M. (2002) Plasma glucose kinetics during prolonged exercise in trained humans when fed carbohydrate. *American Journal of Physiology*, 283: E573–E577.

Anselme, F., Collomp, K., Mercier, B., Ahmadi, S. & Prefaut, C. (1992) Caffeine increases maximal anaerobic power and blood lactate concentration. *European Journal of Applied Physiology*, 65: 188–191.

Applegate, E. (1999) Effective nutritional ergogenic aids. *International Journal of Sports Nutrition*, 9: 229–239.

Armstrong, L.E., Maresh, C.M., Gabaree, C.V., Hoffman, J.R., Kavouras, S.A., Kenefick, R.W., Castellani, J.W. & Ahlquist, L.E. (1997) Thermal and circulatory responses during exercise: effects of hypohydration, dehydration, and water intake. *Journal of Applied Physiology*, 82: 2028–2035.

Ashwell, M. (1992) Obesity in middle aged women. In: Nutrition, Social Status and Health. Proceedings of a Conference held in 1991. London: National Dairy Council.

Astorino, T.A. & Roberson, D.W. (2010) Efficacy of acute caffeine ingestion for short-term high-intensity exercise performance: a systematic review. *Journal of Strength and Conditioning Research*, 24(1): 257–265.

Astorino, T., Marrocco, A.C., Gross, S.M., Johnson, D.L., Brazil, C.M., Icenhower, M.E. & Kneessi, R.J. (2005) Is running performance enhanced with creatine serum ingestion? *Journal of Strength and Conditioning Research*, 19: 730–734.

Astrand, P.O. (1967) Diet and athletic performance. *Federation Proceedings*, 26: 1772–1777.

Balsom, P.D., Harridge, S.D.R., Soderlund, K., Sjodin, B. & Ekblom, B. (1993) Creatine supplementation per se does not enhance endurance exercise performance. *Acta Physiologica Scandinavica*, 149: 521–523.

Balsom, P.D., Soderlund, K., Sjodin, B. & Ekblom, B. (1995) Skeletal muscle metabolism during short duration high-intensity exercise: influence of creatine supplementation. *Acta Physiologica Scandinavica*, 1154: 303–310.

Bangsbo, J. (1994) The physiology of soccer – with special reference to intense intermittent exercise. *Acta Physiologica Scandinavica*, 619: 1–155.

Bangsbo, J. Norregaard, L. & Thorso, F. (1991) Activity profile of competition soccer. *Canadian Journal of Sport Sciences*, 16: 110–116.

Barr, S.I. (1987) Nutrition knowledge of female varsity athletes and university students. *Journal of the American Dietetic Association* 87: 1660–1664.

Barr, S.I., Costill, D.L. & Fink, W.J. (1991) Fluid replacement during prolonged exercise: effects of water, saline, or no fluid. *Medicine and Science in Sports and Exercise*, 23: 811–817.

Barry, D.W. & Kohrt, W.M. (2008) BMD decreases over the course of a year in competitive male cyclists. *Journal of Bone Mineral Research*, 23(4): 484–491.

Beaton, L.J., Allan, D.A., Tarnapolsky, M.A., Tiidus, P.M. & Phillips, S.M. (2002) Contraction-induced muscle damage is unaffected by vitamin E supplementation. *Medicine and Science in Sports and Exercise*, 34: 798–805.

Bell, D.G., McLellan, T.M. & Sabiston, C.M. (2002) Effect of ingesting caffeine and ephedrine on 10-km run performance. *Medicine and Science in Sports and Exercise*, 34: 344–349.

Below, P.R., Mora-Rodriguez, R. Gonzalez-Alonso, J. & Coyle, E.F. (1995) Fluid and carbohydrate ingestion independently improve performance during 1 hour of intense exercise. *Medicine and Science in Sports and Exercise*, 27: 2001–2010.

Bemben, M.G. & Lamont, H.S. (2005) Creatine supplementation and exercise performance: recent findings. *Sports Medicine*, 35(2): 107–125.

Bergstrom, J. & Hultman, E. (1966) Muscle glycogen synthesis after exercise: an enhancing factor localised in muscle cells in man. *Nature*, 210: 309–310.

Bergstrom, J., Hermansen, L., Hultman, E. & Saltin, B. (1967) Diet, muscle glycogen and physical performance. *Acta Physiologica Scandanavica*, 71: 140–150.

Binkley, J.K., Eales, J. & Jekanowski, M. (2000) The relation between dietary change and rising U.S. obesity. *International Journal of Obesity and Related Metabolic Disorders*, 24: 1032–1039.

Bird, S.R., Wiles, J. & Robbins, J. (1995) The effect of sodium bicarbonate ingestion on 1500-m racing time. *Journal of Sports Science*, 13: 399–403.

Bishop, D. & Claudius, B. (2005) Effects of induced metabolic alkalosis on prolonged intermittent sprint performance. *Medicine and Science in Sports and Exercise*, 37: 759–767.

Bishop, D., Edge, J. & Goodman, C. (2004) Induced metabolic alkalosis affects muscle metabolism and repeated-sprint ability. *Medicine and Science in Sports and Exercise*, 36(5): 807–813.

Blair, S.N. & Church, T.S. (2004) The fitness, obesity and health equation. Is physical activity the common denominator? *Journal of the American Medical Association*, 292: 1232–1234.

Bloomer, R.J., Goldfarb, A.H., McKenzie, M.J., You, T. & Nguyen, L. (2004) Effects of antioxidant therapy in women exposed to eccentric exercise. *International Journal of Sport Nutrition and Exercise Metabolism*, 14: 377–388.

Bock, L. & Lambert, E.V. (1990) Nutrition for exercise: finding the balance. In: *Food, what's in it for you?* J. Husskisson (ed). Cape Town, South Africa: Don Nelson.

Bolanowski, M. & Nilsson, B.E. (2001) Assessment of human body composition using dual-energy x-ray absorptiometry and bioelectrical impedance analysis. *Medical Science Monitor*, 7(5): 1029–1033.

Børsheim, E., Aarsland, A. & Wolfe, R.R. (2004) Effect of an amino acid, protein, and carbohydrate mixture on net muscle protein balance after resistance exercise. *International Journal of Sport Nutrition and Exercise Metabolism*, 14: 255–271.

Børsheim, E., Tipton, K.D., Klein, S. & Wolfe, R.R. (2002) An abundant supply of amino acids enhances the metabolic effect of exercise on muscle protein. *American Journal of Physiology –Endocrinology and Metabolism*, 273: E122–E129.

Bosch, A.N., Dennis, S.C. & Noakes, T.D. (1993) Influence of carbohydrate loading on fuel substrate turnover and oxidation during prolonged exercise. *Journal of Applied Physiology*, 74(4): 1921–1927.

Bourque, S.P., Pate, R.R. & Branch, J.D. (1997) Twelve weeks of endurance exercise training does not affect iron status measures in women. *Journal of American Dietetic Association*, 7: 1116–1121.

Branch, J.D. (2003) Effect of creatine supplementation on body composition and performance: a meta-analysis. *International Journal of Sport Nutrition and Exercise Metabolism*, 13: 198–226.

Brookes, G.A. & Mercier, J. (1994) Balance of carbohydrate and lipid utilization during exercise: the crossover concept. *Journal of Applied Physiology*, 76: 2253–2261.

Brotherhood, J.R. (1984) Nutrition and sports performance. *Sports Medicine*, 1: 350–389.

Brownell, K.D. (1984) The psychology and physiology of obesity: implications for screening and treatment. *Journal of the American Dietetic Association*, 84: 406–414.

Brownlie, T., Utermohlen, V., Hinton, P.S., Giordano, C. & Haas, J.D. (2002) Marginal iron deficiency without anemia impairs aerobic adaptation among previously untrained women. *American Journal of Clinical Nutrition*, 75(4): 734–742.

Brownlie, T., Utermohlen, V., Hinton, P.S. & Haas, J.D. (2004) Tissue iron deficiency without anemia impairs adaptation in endurance capacity after aerobic training in previously untrained women. *American Journal of Clinical Nutrition*, 79(3): 437–443.

Brouns, F., Becker, E., Knopfli, B., Villager, B. & Saris, W. (1991) Rehydration during exercise effect of electrolyte supplementation on selection blood parameters. *Medicine and Science in Sports and Exercise*, 23: S84.

Brouns, F., Saris, W.H.M. & Rehrer, N.J. (1987) Abdominal complaints and gastrointestinal function during long-lasting exercise. *International Journal of Sports Medicine*, 8: 175–189.

Bruce, C.R., Anderson, M.E., Fraser, S.F., Stepto, N.K., Klein, R., Hopkins, W.G. & Hawley, J.A. (2000) Enhancement of 2000-m rowing performance after caffeine ingestion. *Medicine and Science in Sports and Exercise*, 32: 1958–1963.

Bryer, S. & Goldfarb, A.H. (2001) The effects of vitamin C supplementation on blood glutathione status, DOMS, and creatine kinase. *Medicine and Science in Sports and Exercise*, 33(5): S122.

Burd, N.A., Tang, J.E., Moore, D.R. & Phillips, S.M. (2009) Exercise training and protein metabolism: influences of contraction, protein intake, and sex-based differences. *Journal of Applied Physiology*, 106: 1692–1701.

Burke, L. & Deakin, V. (eds) (2000) *Clinical Sports Nutrition*, 2nd edn. Sydney, Australia: McGraw-Hill.

Burke, L. & Deakin, V. (eds) (2006) *Clinical Sports Nutrition*, 3rd edn. Sydney, Australia: McGraw-Hill.

Burke, L. & Read, R.S. (1987) A study of carbohydrate loading techniques used by marathon runners. *Canadian Journal of Sport Science*, 12: 6–10.

Burke, L.M., Angus, D.J., Cox, G.R. Cummings, M. Febbraio, M.A., Gawthorn, K., Hawley, J. A., Minehan, M., Martin, D. T. & Hargreaves, M. (2000) Effect of fat adaptation and carbohydrate restoration on metabolism and performance during prolonged cycling. *Journal of Applied Physiology*, 89: 2413–2421

Burke, L.M., Claassen, A., Hawley, J.A. & Noakes, T.D. (1998) Carbohydrate intake during prolonged cycling minimizes effect of glycemic index of pre-exercise meal. *Journal of Applied Physiology*, 85: 2220–2226.

Burke, L.M., Collier, G.R. & Hargreaves, M. (1993) Muscle glycogen storage after prolonged exercise: the effect of the glycemic index of carbohydrate feedings. *Journal of Applied Physiology*, 75: 1019–1023.

Burke, L.M., Hawley, J.A., Angus, D.J., Cox, G.R., Clark, S.A., Cummings, N.K., Desbrow, B. & Hargreaves, M. (2002) Adaptations to short-term high-fat diet persist during exercise despite high carbohydrate availability. *Medicine Science Sports Exercise*, 34: 83–91.

Burke, L.M., Kiens, B. & Ivy, J.L. (2004) Carbohydrates and fat for training and recovery. *Journal of Sports Sciences*, 22: 15–30.

Burke, L., Shaw, N. & Warnes, O. (2006) Supplements and sports foods. In: *Clinical Sports Nutrition*, 3rd edn, L. Burke & V. Deakin (eds). Sydney, Australia: McGraw-Hill, pp. 485–579.

Bussau, V.A., Fairchild, T.J., Rao, A., Steele, P. & Fournier, P.A. (2002) Carbohydrate loading in human muscle: an improved 1 day protocol. *European Journal of Applied Physiology*, 87: 290–295.

Butterfield, G.E. (1987) Whole-body protein utilization in humans. *Medicine and Science in Sports and Exercise*, 19(Suppl. 5): S157–S165.

Buttriss, J. (ed) (2002) Adverse reactions to food. In: *The Report of a British Nutrition Foundation Task Force*. Oxford, England: Blackwell Science, pp. 77–103.

Cann, C.E., Martin, M.C., Genant, H.K. & Jaffe, R.B. (1984) Decreased spinal mineral content in amennorheic women. *Journal of the American Medical Association*, 251: 626–629.

Carey, A.L., Staudacher, H.M., Cummings, N.K., Stepto, N.K., Nikolopoulos, V., Burke, L.M. & Hawley, J.H. (2001) Effects of fat adaptation and carbohydrate restoration on prolonged endurance exercise. *Journal Applied Physiology*, 91: 115–122.

Carter, J., Jeukendrup, A.E., Mundel, T. & Jones, D.A. (2003) Carbohydrate supplementation improves moderate and high-intensity exercise in the heat. *Pflügers Archiv – European Journal of Physiology*, 446(2): 211–219.

Casey, A., Constantin-Teodosiu, D., Howell, S., Hultman, E. & Greenhaff, P.L. (1996) Creatine ingestion favourably affects performance and muscle metabolism during maximal exercise in humans. *American Journal of Physiology*, 271: E31–E37.

Caspersen, C.J., Powell, K.E. & Christensen, G.M. (1985) Physical activity, exercise, and physical fitness: definitions and distinctions for health-related research. *Public Health Reports*, 100: 126–131.

Castell, L.M., Burke, L.M., Stear, S.J. & Maughan, R.J. (2010) BJSM reviews: A–Z of nutritional supplements: dietary supplements, sports nutrition foods and ergogenic aids for health and performance Part 8. *British Journal of Sports Medicine*, 44: 486–470.

Cheuvront, S.N. & Haymes, E.M. (2001) Thermoregulation and marathon running: biological and environmental influences. *Sports Medicine*, 31: 743–762.

Cheuvront, S.N., Carter, R., III & Sawka, M.N. (2003) Fluid balance and endurance exercise performance. *Current Sports Medicine Reports*, 2: 202–208.

Chorley, J., Cianca, J. & Divine, J. (2007) Risk factors for exercise-associated hyponatremia in non-elite marathon runners. *Clinical Journal of Sports Medicine*, 17: 471–477.

Chwalbinska-Moneta, J. (2003) Effect of creatine supplementation on aerobic performance and anaerobic capacity in elite rowers in the course of endurance training. *International Journal of Sports Nutrition and Exercise Metabolism*, 13: 173–183.

Clarkson, P.M. (1993) Nutritional ergogenic aids: caffeine. *International Journal of Sport Nutrition*, 3: 103–111.

Clarkson, P.M. (1995) Antioxidants and physical performance. *Critical Reviews in Food Science and Nutrition*, 35: 131–141.

Clarkson, P.M. & Thompson, H.S. (2000) Antioxidants: what role do they play in physical activity and health? *American Journal of Clinical Nutrition*, 72: 637S–646S.

Clement, D. & Sawchuk, L. (1984) Iron status and sports performance. *Sports Medicine*, 1: 65–74.

Coetzer, P., Noakes, T.D., Sanders, B., Lambert, M.I., Bosch, A.N., Wiggins, T. & Dennis, S.C. (1993) Superior fatigue resistance in elite black South African distance runners. *Journal of Applied Physiology*, 75: 1822–1827.

Coggan, A.R. & Coyle, E.F. (1991) Effects on metabolism and performance. In: *Exercise and Sport Science Reviews*, Vol. 19, J.O. Holloszy (ed). Baltimore: Williams & Wilkins.

Combes, G.F. (1998) *The Vitamins. Fundamental Aspects in Nutrition and Health*, 2nd edn. San Diego, CA: Academic Press.

Condon, E.M., Dube, K.A. & Herbold, N.H. (2007) The influence of the low-carbohydrate trend on collegiate athletes' knowledge, attitudes, and dietary intake of carbohydrates. *Topics in Clinical Nutrition*, 22(2): 175–184.

Consolazio, C.F. (1983) Nutrition and performance. Sweat losses. *Progress in Food and Nutrition Science*, 7: 113–128.

Convertino, V., Armstrong, L., Coyle, E., Mack, G. Sawka, M. & Sherman, W. (1996) American College of Sports Medicine position stand: exercise and fluid replacement. *Medicine and Science in Sports Exercise*, 28: i–vii.

Cook, J.D., Dessenko, S.A. & Whittaker, P. (1991) Calcium supplementation effect on iron absorption. *American Journal of Clinical Nutrition*, 53: 106–111.

Coombes, J.S. & Hamilton, K.L. (2000) The effectiveness of commercially available sports drinks. *Sports Medicine*, 29(3): 181–209.

Córdova, A., Navas, F.J. & Villa, G. (2002) Status and metabolism of iron in elite sportsmen during a period of professional competition. *Biological Trace Element Research*, 89: 205–213.

Costill, D.L. (1977) Sweating: its composition and effects on body fluids. In: *The Marathon: Physiological, Medical, Epidemiological and Psychological Studies*, Vol. 301, P. Milvy (ed). New York: New York Academy of Sciences.

Costill, D. (1990) Gastric emptying of fluids during exercise. In: *Fluid Homeostasis During Exercise*, Vol. 3, C.V. Gisolphi & D.R. Lamb (eds). Carmel, IN: WCB Brown and Benchmark, pp. 97–197.

Costill, D.L., Dalsky, G.P. & Fink, W.J. (1978) Effects of caffeine ingestion on metabolism and exercise performance. *Medicine and Science in Sports*, 10: 155–158.

Costill, D.L., Krammer, W.F. & Fisher, A. (1970) Fluid ingestion during distance running. *Archives of Environmental Health*, 21: 520–525.

Costill, D. & Miller, J. (1980) Nutrition for endurance sport: carbohydrate and fluid balance. *International Journal of Sports Medicine*, 1: 2–14.

Costill, D.L. & Saltin, B. (1974) Factors limiting gastric emptying during rest and exercise. *Journal of Applied Physiology*, 37: 679–683.

Cox, G.R., Broad, E.M., Riley, M.D. & Burke, L.M. (2002) Body mass changes and voluntary fluid intakes of elite level water polo players and swimmers. *Journal of Science and Medicine in Sport*, 5: 183–193.

Coyle, E.F. (1991) Timing and method of increased carbohydrate intake to cope with heavy training, competition and recovery. *Journal of Sport Sciences*, 9: 29–52.

Coyle, E.F. (2004) Fluid and fuel intake during exercise. *Journal of Sport Sciences*, 22: 39–55.

Coyle, E.F., Coggan, A.R., Hemmert, M.K., Lowe, R.C. & Walters, T.J. (1985) Substrate usage during prolonged exercise following a pre-exercise meal. *Journal of Applied Physiology*, 61: 165–172.

Coyle, E.F. & Hamilton, M. (1990) Fluid replacement during exercise: effects on physiological homeostasis and performance. In: *Perspective in Exercise Science and Sports Medicine, Fluid Homeostasis During Exercise*, Vol. 3, C.V. Gisolfi & D.R. Lamb (eds). Carmel, IN: Benchmark Press, pp. 281–303.

Craig, R. & Hirani, V. (eds) (2009) *Health Survey of England 2009: Health and Lifestyles*, Vol. 1. Leeds, England: The NHS Information Centre.

Cupisti, A., D'Alessandro, C., Castrogiovanni, S., Barale, A. & Morelli, E. (2002) Nutrition knowledge and dietary composition in Italian adolescent female athletes and non-athletes. *International Journal of Sport Nutrition and Exercise Metabolism*, 12(2): 207–219.

Curioni, C.C. & Lourenço, P.M. (2006) Long-term weight loss after diet and exercise: a systematic review. *Evidence-Based Nursing*, 9(2): 46–47.

Currell, K. & Jeukendrup, A.E. (2008) Superior performance with glucose and fructose ingestion during exercise. *Medicine and Science in Sports and Exercise*, 40(2): 275–281.

Daries, H.N., Noakes, T.D. & Dennis, S.C. (2000) Effect of fluid intake volume on 2-h running performances in a 25°C environment. *Medicine and Science in Sports and Exercise*, 32(10): 1783–1789.

Davies, C.T.M. (1979) Influence of skin temperature on sweating ad aerobic performance during severe work. *Journal of Applied Physiology*, 47: 770–777.

Davies, C.T.M., Botherhood, J.R. & Zeidifard, E. (1976) Temperature regulation during severe exercise with some observations on effects of skin wetting. *Journal Applied of Physiology*, 41: 772–776.

Davis, G.R., Santa Ana, C.A., Morawski, S.G. & Fordtran, J.S. (1980) Development of a lavage solution associated with minimal water and electrolyte absorption or secretion. *Gastroenterology*, 78: 991–995.

DeMarco, H.M., Sucher, K.P., Cisar, C.J. & Butterfiled, G.E. (1999) Pre-exercise carbohydrate meals: application of glycemic index. *Medicine and Science in Sports and Exercise*, 31(1): 164–170.

Department for Environment, Food, and Rural Affairs (DEFRA) (2000) *National Food Survey.* London: The Stationery Office.

Department of Health (1991) *Dietary Reference Values for Food Energy and Nutrients for the United Kingdom. Report of the Committee on the Medical Aspects of Food and Nutrition Policy on Health and Social Subjects,* Vol. 41. London: HMSO.

Department of Health (1994) *Nutritional Aspects of Cardiovascular Disease. Report of the Cardiovascular Review Group Committee on Medical Aspects of Food and Nutrition Policy. Report on Health and Social Subjects,* Vol. 46. London: HMSO.

Department of Health (1999) *Health Survey for England 1998.* London: The Stationary Office.

Department of Health (2004) *Health Survey for England 2003.* London: The Stationary Office.

Department of Health (2011). The eatwell plate. http://www.dh.gov.uk/en/Publichealth/Nutrition/DH_126493 (accessed 31 July 2011).

Department of Health (2011) Physical activity guidelines for adults (19–64 years). http://www.dh.gov.uk/en/Publicationsandstatistics/Publications/PublicationsPolicyAnd Guidance/DH_127931(accessed 11 July 2011).

Desbrow, B., Anderson, S., Barrett, J., Rao, E. & Hargreaves, M. (2004) Carbohydrate-electrolyte feedings and 1h time trial cycling performance. *International Journal of Sport Nutrition and exercise Metabolism,* 14: 541–549.

Dill, D.B. (1938) *Life, heat and altitude: Physiological Effects of Hot Climates and Great heights.* Cambridge, England: Harvard University Press.

Dodd, S.L., Brooks, E., Powers, S.K. & Tulley, R. (1991) The effects of caffeine on graded exercise performance in caffeine naive versus habituated subjects. *European Journal of Applied Physiology,* 62: 424–429.

Doherty, M. & Smith, P.M. (2004) Effects of caffeine ingestion on exercise testing. *International Journal of Sport Nutrition and Exercise Metabolism,* 14: 626–646.

Douroudos, I.I., Fatouros, I.G., Gourgoulis, V., Jamurtas, A.Z., Tsitsios, T., Hatzinikolaou, A., Margonis, K., Mavromatidis, K. & Taxildaris, K. (2006) Dose-related effects of prolonged NaHCO3 ingestion during high-intensity exercise. *Medicine and Science in Sports and Exercise,* 38(10): 1746–1753.

Drinkwater, B.L., Bruemmer, B.B. & Chesnut, C.H. (1990) Menstrual history as a determinant of current bone density in young athletes. *Journal of the American Medical Association,* 263: 545–548.

Dubnov, G. & Constantini, N.W. (2004) Prevalence of iron depletion and anemia in top-level basketball players. *International Journal of Sport Nutrition and Exercise Metabolism,* 14(1): 30–37.

Dugas, J.P., Oosthuizen, U., Tucker, R. & Noakes, T.D. (2009) Rates of fluid ingestion alter pacing but not thermoregulatory responses during prolonged exercise in hot and humid conditions with appropriate convective cooling. *European Journal of Applied Physiology,* 105: 69–80.

Duncan, C.S., Blimkie, C.J., Cowell, C.T., Burke, S.T., Briody, J.N. & Howman-Giles, R. (2002) Bone mineral density in adolescent female athletes: relationship to exercise type and muscle strength. *Medicine and Science in Sports and Exercise,* 34(2): 286–294.

Dunn, D., Turner, L.W. & Denny, G. (2007) Nutrition knowledge and attitudes of college athletes. *The Sport Journal,* 10(4): 45.

Duvnjak-Zaknich, D.M., Dawson, B.T., Wallman, K.E. & Henry, G. (2011) Effect of caffeine on reactive agility time when fresh and fatigued. *Medicine and Science in Sports and Exercise,* 43(8): 1523–1530.

Earnest, C., Snell, P., Rodriguez, R., Almada, A.L. & Mitchell, T.L. (1995) The effect of creatine monohydrate ingestion on anaerobic power indices, muscular strength and body composition. *Acta Physiologica Scandinavica*, 153: 207–209.

Earnest, C.P., Almada, A.L. & Mitchell, T.L. (1997) Effects of creatine monohydrate ingestion on intermediate duration anaerobic treadmill running to exhaustion. *Journal of Strength and Conditioning Research*, 11: 234–238.

Ebbeling, C.B., Leidig, M.M., Feldman, H.A., Lovesky, M.M. & Ludwig, D.S. (2007) Effect of low-glycemic load vs low-fat diet in obese young adults: a randomized trial. *Journal of the American Medical Association*, 297(19): 2092–2102.

Eckerson, J.M., Stout, J.R., Housh, T.J. & Johnson, G.O. (1996) Validity of bioelectrical impedance equations for estimating percent fat in males. *Medicine and Science in Sports and Exercise*, 28(4): 523–530.

Edge, J., Bishop, D. & Goodman, C. (2006) Effects of chronic NaHCO3 ingestion during interval training on changes to muscle buffer capacity, metabolism, and short-term endurance performance. *Journal of Applied Physiology*, 101(3): 918–925.

Edwards, A.M., Mann, M.E., Marfell-Jones, M.J., Rankin, D.M., Noakes, T.D. & Shillington, D.P. (2007) Influence of moderate dehydration on soccer performance: physiological responses to 45-min of outdoor match-play and the immediate subsequent performance of sport-specific and mental concentration tasks. *British Journal of Sports Medicine*, 41: 385–391.

Edwards, A.M. & Noakes, T.D. (2009) Dehydration: cause of fatigue or sign of pacing in elite soccer? *Sports Medicine*, 39: 1–13.

Eichner, E., King, D., Myhal, M., Prentice, B. & Ziegenfuss, T. (1999) Muscle builder supplements. *Sports Science Exchange Roundtable*, 10: 1–5.

Eisenkölbl, J., Kartasurya, M. & Widhalm, K. (2001) Underestimation of percentage fat mass measured by bioelectrical impedance analysis compared to dual energy X-ray absorptiometry method in obese children. *European Journal of Clinical Nutrition*, 55(6): 423–429.

Ekblom, B. (1986) Applied physiology of soccer. *Sports Medicine*, 2: 50–60.

Escott-Stump, S. (2002) *Nutrition and Diagnosis-Related Care*, 5th edn. London: Lippincott Williams & Wilkins.

Fallowfield, J.L., Williams, C. & Singh, R. (1995) The influence of ingesting a carbohydrate-electrolyte beverage during 4 hours of recovery on subsequent endurance capacity. *International Journal of Sports Nutrition*, 5: 285–299.

Fallowfield, J.L., Williams, C., Booth, W.J., Choo, B.H. & Growns, S. (1996) Effect of water ingestion on endurance capacity during prolonged running. *Journal of Sport Science*, 14: 497–502.

Farajian, P., Kavouras, S.A., Yannakoulia, M. & Sidossis, L.S. (2004) Dietary intake and nutritional practices of elite Greek aquatic athletes. *International Journal of Sport Nutrition and Exercise Metabolism*, 14: 574–585.

Felder, J.M., Burke, B.J., Lowdon, B.J., Cameron-Smith, D. & Collier, G.R. (1998) Nutritional practices of elite female surfers during training and competition. *International Journal of Sports Nutrition*, 8: 36–48.

Fogelholm, M. & Kukkonen-Harjula, K. (2000) Does physical activity prevent weight gain–a systematic review. *Obesity Research*, 1(2): 95–111.

Food Standards Agency (2003) *Expert Group on Vitamins and Minerals: Safe Upper Levels for Vitamins and Minerals*. London: HMSO.

Foresight (2007) *Tackling Obesities: Future Choices – Modelling Future Trends in Obesity and the Impact on Health*, 2nd edn. Government Office for Science. http://www.bis.gov.uk/foresight/our-work/projects/published-projects/tackling-obesities/reports-and-publications (online)

Foskett, A., Williams, C., Boobis, L. & Tsintzas, K. (2008) Carbohydrate availability and muscle energy metabolism during intermittent running. *Medicine & Science in Sports & Exercise*, 40(1): 96–103.

Freidman, B., Weller, E., Mairbaurl, H. & Bartsch, P. (2001) Effects of iron repletion on blood volume and performance capacity in young athletes. *Medicine and Science in Sports and Exercise*, 33: 741–746.

Friden, J. & Lieber, R.L. (2001) Eccentric exercise-induced injuries to contractile and cytoskeletal muscle fibre components. *Acta Physiologica Scandinavica*, 171: 321–326.

Fudge, B., Easton, C., Kingsmore, D., Kiplamai, F., Onywera, V., Westererp, K., Kayser, B., Naokes, T. & Pitsiladis, Y. (2008) Elite Kenyan endurance runners are hydrated day-to-day with *ad libitum* fluid intake. *Medicine and Science in Sports and Exercise*, 40(6): 1171–1179.

Gábor, A., Kovács, V.A., Fajcsák, Z. & Martos, É. (2010) From guidelines to practice – Nutritional habits of Hungarian elite athletes compared with the data from the 3rd National Dietary Survey. *Acta Alimentaria*, 39(1): 27–34.

Ganio, M.S., Klau, J.F., Casa, D.J., Armstrong, L.E. & Maresh, C.M. (2009) Effect of caffeine on sport-specific endurance performance: a systematic review. *Journal of Strength and Conditioning Research*, 23(1): 315–324.

Garn, S.M. & Clark, D.C. (1976) Trends in fatness and the origins of obesity. *Pediatrics*, 57: 443–456.

Garrow, J.S. (1988) *Obesity and Related Diseases*. London: Churchill Livingstone.

Gastin, P.B. (2001) Energy system interaction and relative contribution during maximal exercise. *Sports Medicine*, 31: 725–741.

Gastin, P.B., Misner, J.E., Boileau, R.A. & Slaughter, M.H. (1990) Failure of caffeine to enhance exercise performance in incremental treadmill running. *Australian Journal of Science and Medicine in Sport*, 22: 23–27.

Geissler, C.A. & Powers, H.J. (2005) *Human Nutrition*, 11th edn. London: Churchill Livingstone Elsevier.

Gisolfi, C.V., Summers, R.W. & Schedl, H.P. (1990) Intestinal absorption of fluids during rest and exercise. In: *Perspectives in Exercise Science and Sports Medicine, Fluid Homeostasis During Exercise*, Vol. 3, C.V. Gisolfi, & D.R. Lamb (eds). Carmel, IN: Benchmark Press, pp. 129–180.

Gisolfi, C.V., Summers, R.W., Schedl, H.P. & Bleiler, T.L. (1992) Intestinal water absorption from select carbohydrate solutions in humans. *Journal of Applied Physiology*, 73: 2142–2150.

Glaister, M., Lockey, R.A., Abraham, C.S., Staerck, A., Goodwin, J.E. & McInnes, G. (2006) Creatine supplementation and multiple sprint running performance. *Journal of Strength and Conditioning Research*, 20(2): 245–455.

Gleeson, M. (2005) Exercise, nutrition and immune function II. Micronutrient, antioxidants and other supplements. In: *Immune Function in Sport and Exercise*. Edinburgh, Scotland: Churchill Livingstone Elsevier, pp. 183–203.

Goldfinch, J., McNaughton, L. & Davies, P. (1998) Induced metabolic alkalosis and its effects on 400-m racing time. *European Journal of Applied Physiology*, 57: 45–48.

Goldstein, E.R., Ziegenfuss, T., Kalman, D., Kreider, R., Campbell, B., Wilborn, C., Taylor, L., Willoughby, D., Stout, J., Graves, B.S., Wildman, R., Ivy, J.L., Spano, M., Smith, A.E. & Antonio, J. (2010) International society of sports nutrition position stand: caffeine and performance. *Journal of the International Society of Sports Nutrition*, 7: 5.

Gontzea, I. Suzuki, M. & Dumitrache, S. (1975) The influence of adaptation to physical effort on nitrogen balance in man. *Nutrition Reports International*, 11: 231–236.

Graham, T.E. & Spriet, L.L. (1991) Performance and metabolic responses to a high caffeine dose during prolonged exercise. *Journal of Applied Physiology*, 71: 2292–2298.

Graham, T.E. & Spriet, L.L. (1995) Metabolic, catecholamine, and exercise performance responses to various doses of caffeine. *Journal of Applied Physiology*, 78: 867–874.

Graham, T.E. & Spriet, L.L. (1996). Caffeine and exercise performance. In *Sports Science Exchange*, Vol. 9 (1). Barrington, IL: Gaterade Sports Science Exchange, pp. 1–6.

Graham, T.E., Battram, D.S., Dela, F., El-Sohemy, A. & Thong, F.S.L. (2008) Does caffeine alter muscle carbohydrate and fat metabolism during exercise? *Applied Physiology, Nutrition, and Metabolism*, 33: 1311–1318.

Green, A.L., Hultman, E., Macdonald, I.A., Sewell, D.A. & Greenhaff, P.L. (1996) Carbohydrate feeding augments skeletal muscle creatine accumulation during creatine supplementation in man. *American Journal of Physiology*, 271: E821–E826.

Green, H.J., et al (1987) Training induced hypervolemia: lack of an effect on oxygen utilization during exercise. *Medicine and Science in Sports and Exercise*, 19: 202.

Green, R., Charlton, R. & Seftel, H. (1968) Body iron excretion in man: a collaborative study. *American Journal of Medicine*, 45: 336–353.

Greenhaff, P.L. (1989) Cardiovascular fitness and thermoregulation during prolonged exercise in man. *British Journal of Sports Medicine*, 23: 109–114.

Greenhaff, P.L., Bodin, K., Soderlund, K. & Hultman, E. (1994) The effect of oral creatine supplementation on skeletal muscle phosphocreatine resynthesis. *American Journal of Physiology*, 266: E725–E730.

Greer, F.C., McLean, C. & Graham, T. (1998) Caffeine, performance, and metabolism during repeated Wingate exercise tests. *Journal of Applied Physiology*, 85: 1502–1508.

Grimshaw, P.N. (2005) The effects of acute creatine supplementation on multiple sprint cycling and running performance in rugby players. *Journal of Strength and Conditioning Research*, 19(1): 92–97.

Guyton, A.G. (1984) *Physiology of the Human Body*, 6th edn. Philadelphia: Saunders College Publishing.

Gwinup, G. (1987) Weight loss without dietary restriction: efficacy of different forms of aerobic exercise. *American Journal of Sports Medicine*, 15(93): 275–279.

Haas, J.D. & Brownlie, T. (2001) Iron deficiency and reduced work capacity: a critical review of the research to determine a causal relationship. *Journal of Nutrition*, 131: 676S–690S.

Hadjiolova, I. Mintcheva, L. Dunev, S., Daleva, M., Handjiev, S. & Balabanski, L. (1982) Physical working capacity in obese women after an exercise programme for body weight reduction. *International Journal of Obesity*, 6: 405–410.

Hallström, H. Wolk, A., Glynn, A. & Michaëlsson, K. (2006) Coffee, tea and caffeine consumption in relation to osteoporotic fracture risk in a cohort of Swedish women. *Osteoporosis International*, 17(7): 1055–1064.

Hamilton, M.C., Gonzalez-Alonso, J., Montain, S. & Coyle, E.F. (1991) Fluid replacement and glucose infusion during exercise prevent cardiovascular drift. *Journal of Applied Physiology*, 71: 871–877.

Hargreaves, M., Costill, D.L., Coggan, A., Fink, W.J. & Nishibata, I. (1984) Effect of carbohydrate feedings on muscle glycogen utilization and exercise performance. *Medicine and Science in Sports and Exercise*, 16(3): 219–222.

Hargreaves, M. Hawley, J.A. & Jeukendrup, A. (2004) Pre-exercise carbohydrate and fat ingestion: effects on metabolism and performance. *Journal of Sports Sciences*, 22: 31–38.

Harris, R.C., Soderlund, K. & Hultman, E. (1992) Elevation of creatine in resting and exercised muscle of normal subjects by creatine supplementation. *Clinical Science*, 83: 367–374.

Harris, R.C., Viru, M., Greenhaff, P.L. & Hultman, E. (1993) The effects of oral creatine supplementation on running performance during short term exercise in man. *Journal of Physiology*, 467: 74P.

Haussinger, D., et al (1993) Cellular hydration state: an important determination of protein catabolism in health and disease. *Lancet*, 341: 1330–1332.

Hawley, J.A., Dennis, S.C., Lindsay, F.H. & Noakes, T.D. (1995) Nutritional practices of athletes: are they sub-optimal? *Journal of Sports Sciences*, 13: S75–S81.

Hawley, J.A., Dennis, S.C., Nowitz, A., Brouns, F. & Noakes, T.D. (1992) Exogenous carbohydrate oxidation from maltose and glucose ingested during prolonged exercise. *European Journal of Applied Physiology*, 64: 523–527.

Hawley, J.A., Palmer, G.S. & Noakes, T.D. (1997) Effects of 3 days of carbohydrate supplementation on muscle glycogen content and utilisation during a 1-h cycling performance. *European Journal of Applied Physiology*, 75: 407–412.

Heikkinen, A., Alaranta, A., Helenius, I. & Vasankari, T. (2011) Use of dietary supplements in Olympic athletes is decreasing: a follow-up study between 2002 and 2009. *Journal of the International Society of Sports Nutrition*, 8: 1.

Helge, J.W. (2002) Long-term fat diet adaptation effects on performance, training capacity, and fat utilization. *Medicine and Science in Sports and Exercise*, 34(9): 1499–1504.

Henderson, L., Gregory, J., Irving, K. & Swan, G. (2003) *The National Diet and Nutrition Survey: Adults Aged 19–64 years. Energy, Protein, Carbohydrate, Fat and Alcohol Intake*, Vol. 2. London: HMSO.

Henderson, L., Irving, K., Gregory, J., Bates, C.J., Prentice, A., Perks, J., Swan, G. & Farron, M. (2003) *The National Diet and Nutrition Survey: Adults Aged 19–64 Years. Vitamin and Mineral Intake and Urinary Analysis*, Vol. 3. London: HMSO.

Hew-Butler, T.D., et al (2005) Consensus document of the 1st International Exercise-Associate Hyponatremia (EAH) Consensus Symposium, Cape Town, South Africa 2005. *Clinical Journal of Sports Medicine*, 15: 207–213.

Hew-Butler, T.D., Verbalis, J.G. & Noakes, T.D. (2006) Defending plasma osmolality and plasma volume: updated fluid recommendations from the International Marathon Medical Directors Association. *Clinical Journal of Sports Medicine*, 16: 283–292.

Higgens, L. & Gray, W. (1999) What do anti-dieting programs achieve? *Australian. Journal of Nutrition and Dietetics*, 56: 128.

Hiller, W.D.B., et al (1985) Plasma and glucose changes during the Hawaiian ironman Triathlon. *Medicine and Science in Sports and Exercise*, 17: 219.

Hinton, P.S., Giordano, C., Brownlie IV, T. & Haas, J. (2000) Iron supplementation improves endurance after training in iron-depleted, non-anaemic women. *Journal of Applied Physiology*, 99: 1103–1111.

Hinton, P.S., Sanford, T.C., Davidson, M.M., Yakushko, O.F. & Beck, N.C. (2004) Nutrient intakes and dietary behaviours of male and female collegiate athletes. *International Journal of Sport Nutrition and Exercise Metabolism*, 14(6): 389–405.

Hogervorst, E., Bandelow, S., Schmitt, J., Jentjens, R., Oliveira, M., Aallgrove, J., Carter, T. & Gleeson, M. (2008) Caffeine improves physical and cognitive performance during exhaustive exercise. *Medicine and Science in Sports and Exercise*, 40(10): 1841–1851.

Howarth, K.R., Moreau, N.A., Phillips, S.M. & Gibala, M.J. (2009) Co-ingestion of protein with carbohydrate during recovery from endurance exercise stimulates skeletal muscle protein synthesis in humans. *Journal of Applied Physiology*, 106: 1394–1402.

Howarth, K.R., Phillips, S.M., MacDonald, M.J., Richards, D., Moreau, N.A. & Gibala, M.J. (2010) Effect of glycogen availability on human skeletal muscle protein turnover during exercise and recovery. *Journal of Applied Physiology*, 109: 431–438.

Huang, S.H., Johnson, K. & Pipe, A.L. (2006) The use of dietary supplements and medications by Canadian athletes at the Atlanta and Sydney Olympic Games. *Clinical Journal of Sport Medicine*, 16: 27–33.

Hubbard, R.W., Szlyk, P.C. & Armstrong, L.E. (1990) Influence of thirst and fluid palatability on fluid ingestion during exercise. In: *Perspectives in Exercise Science and Sports Medicine: Fluid Homeostasis During Exercise*, Vol. 3, C.V. Gisolphi & D.R. Lamb (eds). Carmel, IN: Benchmark Press, pp. 39–95.

Hulston, C., Wolsk, E., Grøndahl, T., Yfanti, C., & van Hall, G. (2010) Protein ingestion increases muscle protein synthesis after, but not during, endurance exercise. *British Journal of Sports Medicine*, 44: i6–i7.

Hultman, E., Soderlund, K., Timmons, J.A., Cederblad, G. & Greenhaff, P.L. (1996) Muscle creatine loading in men. *Journal of Applied Physiology*, 81: 232–237.

Hunter, A.M., St Clair Gibson, A., Collins, M., Lambert, M. & Noakes, T.D. (2002) Caffeine ingestion does not alter performance during a 100-km cycling time-trial performance. *International Journal of Sport Nutrition and Exercise Metabolism*, 12: 438–452.

Ivy, J.L., Costill, D.L. Fink, W.J. & Lower, R.W. (1979) Influence of caffeine and carbohydrate feeding on endurance performance. *Medicine and Science in Sports and Exercise*, 11: 6–11.

Ivy, J.L., Goforth, H.W., Damon, B.M., McCauley, T.R., Parsons, E.C. & Price, T.B. (2002) Early post-exercise muscle glycogen recovery is enhanced with a carbohydrate-protein supplement. *Journal of Applied Physiology*, 93: 1337.

Ivy, J.L., Katz, A.L., Cutler, C.L., Sherman, W.M. & Coyle, E.F. (1988) Muscle glycogen synthesis after exercise: effect of time of carbohydrate ingestion. *Journal of Applied Physiology*, 64: 1480–1485.

Ivy, J.L., Lee, M.C., Brozinick, J.T. and Reed, M.J. (1988) Muscle glycogen storage after different amounts of carbohydrate ingestion. *Journal of Applied Physiology*, 65: 2018–2023.

Irwin, C., Desbrow, B., Ellis, A., O'Keeffe, B., Grant, G. & Leveritt, M. (2011) Caffeine withdrawal and high-intensity endurance cycling performance. *Journal of Sports Sciences*, 29(5): 509–515.

Jackman, M., Wendling, P., Friars, D. & Graham, T.E. (1996) Metabolic, catecholamine and endurance responses to caffeine during intense exercise. *Journal of Applied Physiology*, 81: 1658–1663.

Jacobs, K.A., Paul, D.R., Geor, R.J., Hinchcliff, K.W. & Sherman, W.M. (2004) Dietary composition influences short-term endurance training-induced adaptations of substrate portioning during exercise. *International Journal of Sports Nutrition*, 14: 38–61.

Jacobson, B.H. & Aldana, S.G. (1992) Current nutrition practice and knowledge of varsity athletes. *Journal of Applied Sport Science Research*, 6(4): 232–238.

Jenkins, D.A., Wolever, M.S., Taylor, R.H., Barker, H., Fielden, H., Baldwin, J.M., Bowling, A.C., Newman, H.C., Jenkins, A.L. & Goff, D.V. (1981) Glycemic index of foods: a physiological basis for carbohydrate exchange. *The American Journal of Clinical Nutrition*, 34: 362–366.

Jentjens, R.L.P.G., Achten, J. & Jeukendrup, A.E. (2004) High rates of exogenous carbohydrate oxidation from multiple transportable carbohydrates ingested during prolonged exercise. *Medicine and Science in Sport and Exercise*, 36(9): 1551–1558.

Jentjens, R.L.P.G. & Jeukendrup, A.E. (2005) High exogenous carbohydrate oxidation rates from a mixture of glucose and fructose ingested during prolonged cycling exercise. *British Journal of Nutrition*, 93(4): 485–492.

Jeukendrup, A. & Gleeson, M. (2004) *Sports Nutrition: An Introduction to Energy Production and Performance*. Leeds, England: Human Kinetics.

Jeukendrup, A.E. & Jentjens, L.P.G. (2000) Efficacy of carbohydrate feedings during prolonged exercise: current thoughts, guidelines and directions for future research. *Sports Medicine*, 29(6): 407–424.

Jeukendrup, A.E. & Killer, S.C. (2010) The myths surrounding pre-exercise carbohydrate feeding. *Annals of Nutrition and Metabolism*, 57(Suppl. 2): 18–25.

Jonnalagadda, S.S., Ziegler, P.J. & Nelson, J.A. (2004) Food preferences, dieting behaviours and body image perceptions of elite figure skaters. *International Journal of Sport Nutrition and Exercise Metabolism*, 14(5): 594–606.

Judelson, D.A., Maresh, C.M., Farrell, M.J., Yamamoto, L.M., Armstrong, L.E., Kraemer, W.J., Volek, J., Spiering, B.A., Casa, D.J. & Anderson, J.M. (2007) Effect of hydration state on strength, power and resistance exercise performance. *Medicine and Science in Sports and Exercise*, 39: 1817–1824.

Kanter, M.M. (1998) Nutritional antioxidants and physical activity. In: *Nutrition in Exercise and Sport*, I. Wolinsky (ed). Boca Raton, FL: CRC Press, pp. 245–255.

Kao, W.F., et al (2008) Athletic performance and serial weight changes during 12- and 24- hour ultra- marathons. *Clinical Journal of Sports Medicine*, 18: 155–158.

Kavouras, S.A., Troup, J.P. & Berning, J.R. (2004) The influence of low carbohydrate diet on a 45-min strenuous cycling exercise. *International Journal of Sport Nutrition and Exercise Metabolism*, 14(1): 62–72.

Kendall, K.L. Smith, A.E., Graef, J.L., Fukuda, D.H., Moon, J.R., Beck, T.W., Cramer, J.T. & Stout, J.R. (2009) Effects of four weeks of high-intensity interval training and creatine supplementation on critical power and anaerobic working capacity in college-aged men. *Journal of Strength and Conditioning Research*, 23(6): 1663–1669.

Kennedy, E.T., et al (2001) Popular diets: correlation of health, nutrition, and obesity. *Journal of the American Dietetic Association*, 101: 411–420.

Kiens, B., Esen-Gustavsson, B., Christiansen, N.J. & Saltin, B. (1993) Skeletal muscle substrate utilization during sub-maximal exercise in man: effect of endurance training. *Journal of Physiology (London)*, 469: 459–478.

Kiens, B. & Richter, E.A. (1996) Types of carbs in a ordinary diet effect insulin action and muscle substrates in humans. *American Journal of Clinical Nutrition*, 63: 47–53.

Kilduff, L.P., Georgiades, E., James, N., Minnion, R.H., Mitchell, M., Kingsmore, D., Hadjicharlambous, M. & Pitsladis, Y.P. (2004) The effects of creatine supplementation on cardiovascular, metabolic, and thermoregulatory responses during exercise in the heat in endurance-trained humans. *International Journal of Sport Nutrition and Exercise Metabolism*, 14(4): 443–460.

Kleiner, S.M., Bazzarre, T.L. & Litchford, M.D. (1990) Metabolic profiles, diet and health practices of championship male and female bodybuilders. *Journal of the American Dietetic Association*, 90: 962–967.

Klem, M.L., Wing, R.R., McGuire, M.T., Seagle, H.M. & Hill, J.O. (1997) A descriptive study of individuals successful at long-term maintenance of substantial weight loss. *American Journal of Clinical Nutrition*, 66: 239–246.

Klingshirn, L.A., Pate, R.R., Bourque, S.P., Davis, J.M. & Sargent, R.G. (1992) Effect of iron supplementation on endurance capacity in iron-depleted female runners. *Medicine and Science in Sports and Exercise*, 24: 819–824.

Knight, I.B. (1984) *The Heights and Weights of Adults in Great Britain*. London: OPCS.

Kramer, F.M., Jeffrey, R.W., Forster, J.L. & Snell, M.K. (1987) Long-term follow-up of behavioral treatment for obesity: patterns of weight regain among men and women. *International Journal of Obesity*, 13: 123–136.

Kreider, R.B. (2003) Effects of creatine supplementation on performance and training adaptations. *Molecular and Cellular Biochemistry*, 244(1–2): 89–94.

Kreider, R., Ferreira, M., Wilson, M., Grindstaff, P., Plisk, S., Reinardy, J., Cantler, E. & Almada, A.L. (1998) Effects of creatine supplementation on body composition, strength and sprint performance. *Medicine and Science in Sports and Exercise*, 30: 73–82.

Kumar, V., Atherton, P., Smith, K. & Rennie, M.J. (2009) Human muscle protein synthesis and breakdown during and after exercise. *Journal of Applied Physiology*, 106: 2026–2039.

Ladell, W.S.S. (1965) Water and salt (sodium chloride) intakes. In: *The Physiology of Human Survival*, O. Edholm & A. Bacharach (eds). New York: Academic Press, pp. 235–299.

LaManca, J.J. & Haymes, E.M. (1993) Effects of iron repletion on VO$_2$max, endurance, and blood lactate in women. *Medicine and Science in Sports and Exercise*, 25(12): 1386–1392.

Law, Y.L.L., Ong, W.S., GillianYap, T.L., Lim, S.C.J. & Chia, E.V. (2009) Effects of two and five days of creatine loading on muscular strength and anaerobic power in trained athletes. *Journal of Strength and Conditioning Research*, 23(3): 906–914.

Lemon, P.W.R. (1995) Do athletes need more dietary protein and amino acids? *International Journal of Sports Nutrition*, 5: S39–S61.

Lemon, P.W.R. & Nagle, F.J. (1981) Effects of exercise on protein and amino acid metabolism. *Medicine and Science in Sports and Exercise*, 13: 141–149.

Lindh, A.M., Peyrebrune, M.C., Ingham, S.A., Bailey, D.M. & Folland, J.P. (2008) Sodium bicarbonate improves swimming performance. *International Journal of Sports Medicine*, 29(6): 519–523.

Luden, N.D., Saunders, M.J. & Todd, M.K. (2007) Post-exercise carbohydrate-protein-antioxidant ingestion decreases plasma creatine kinase and muscle soreness. *International Journal of Sport Nutrition and Exercise Metabolism*, 17(1): 109–123.

Lukaszuk, J.M., et al (2002) Effect of creatine supplementation and a lacto-ovo-vegetarian diet on muscle creatine concentration. *International Journal of Sports Nutrition and Exercise Metabolism*, 12: 336–348.

Lun, V., Erdman, K. & Reimer, R. (2009) Evaluation of nutritional intake in Canadian high-performance athletes. *Clinical Journal of Sport Medicine*, 19(5): 405–411.

Macdemid, P.W. & Stannard, S.R. (2006) A whey supplemented, high protein diet versus a high-carbohydrate diet: effects on endurance cycling performance. *International Journal of Sport Nutrition and Exercise Metabolism*, 16: 65–77.

Magazanik, A., Weinstein, Y., Dlin, R.A., Derin, M., Schwartzman, S. & Allalouf, D. (1988) Iron deficiency caused by 7 weeks of intensive physical exercise. *European Journal of Applied Physiology and Occupational Physiology*, 57(2): 198–202.

Mahan, L.K. & Arlin, M.T. (1992) *Krause's Food, Nutrition and Diet Therapy*, 8th edn. Philadelphia: W.B. Saunders Company.

Main, F.A. & Wise, A. (2002) Relationship between knowledge and claimed compliance with genuine and false nutrition messages. *The British Dietetic Association*, 15: 349–353.

Malczewska, J., Raczynski, G. & Stupnicki, R. (2000) Iron status in female endurance athletes and in non-athletes. *International Journal of Sport Nutrition and Exercise Metabolism*, 10(3): 260–276.

Marino, F.E., Cannon, J. and Kay, D. (2010) Neuromuscular responses to hydration in moderate to warm ambient conditions during self-paced high-intensity exercise. *British Journal of Sports Medicine*, 44: 961–967.

Marquart, L.F., Cohen, E.A. & Short, S.H. (1997) Nutrition knowledge of athletes and their coaches and surveys of dietary intake. In: *Nutrition in Exercise and Sport*, 3rd edn, I. Wolinsky (ed). Boca Raton, FL: CRC Press, pp. 559–595.

Mastaloudis, A., Traber, M.G., Carstensen, K. & Widrick, J.J. (2006) Antioxidants did not prevent muscle damage in response to an ultramarathon run. *Medicine and Science in Sports and Exercise*, 38(1): 72–80.

Maughan, R. (2002) The athlete's diet: nutritional goals and dietary strategies. *Proceedings of the Nutrition Society*, 61: 87–96.

Maughan, R.J., Fenn, C.E. & Leiper, J.B. (1989) Effects of fluid, electrolyte and substrate ingestion on endurance capacity. *European Journal of Applied Physiology*, 58: 481–486.

Maughan, R.J., Merson, S.J., Broad, N.P. & Shirreffs, S.M. (2004) Fluid and electrolyte intake and loss in elite soccer players during training. *International Journal of Sport Nutrition and Exercise Metabolism*, 14: 333–346.

Maughan, R.J., Watson, P., Evans, G.H., Broad, N. & Shirreffs, S.M. (2007) Water balance and salt losses in competitive football. *International Journal of Sport Nutrition and Exercise Metabolism*, 17: 583–594.

McArdle, W.D., Katch, F.I. & Katch, V.L. (1991) *Exercise Physiology. Energy, Nutrition and Human Performance*, 3rd edn. Philadelphia: Lea & Febiger.

McArdle, W.D., Katch, F.I. & Katch, V.L. (2006) *Essentials of Exercise Physiology*, 3rd edn. Philapdelphia: Lippincott Williams & Wilkins.

McArdle, W.D., Katch, F.I. & Katch, V.L. (2010) *Exercise Physiology. Nutrition, Energy and Human Performance*, 7th edn. Philapdelphia: Lippincott Williams & Wilkins.

McClung, M. & Collins, D. (2007) "Because I know it will!" : placebo effects of an ergogenic aid on athletic performance. *Journal of Sport and Exercise Psychology*, 29(3): 382–394.

McConnel, G.K., Burge, C.M., Skinner, S.L. & Hargreaves, M. (1987) Influence of ingested fluid volume on physiology responses during prolonged exercise. *Acta Physiologica Scandanavica*, 160: 149–156.

McIntosh, B.R. & Wright, B.M. (1995) Caffeine ingestion and performance of a 1500 m swim. *Canadian Journal of Applied Physiology*, 20: 168–177.

McLellan, T.M. & Bell, D.G. (2004) The impact of prior coffee consumption on the subsequent ergogenic effect of anhydrous caffeine. *International Journal of Sport Nutrition and Exercise Metabolism*, 14: 698–708.

McNaughton, L., Dalton, B. & Palmer, G. (1999). Sodium bicarbonate can be used as an ergogenic aid in high-intensity, competitive cycle ergometry of 1 h duration. *European Journal of Applied Physiology*, 80: 64–69.

McRae, M.P. (2010) Male and female differences in variability with estimating body fat composition using skinfold calipers. *Journal of Chiropractic Medicine*, 9(4): 157–161.

Mehlenbeck, R.S., Ward, K.D., Klesges, R.C. & Vukadinovich, C.M. (2004) A pilot intervention to increase calcium intake in female collegiate athletes. *International Journal of Sports Nutrition*, 14(1): 18–29.

Mero, A.A., Keskinen, K.L., Malvela, M.T. & Sallinen, J.M. (2004) Combined creatine and sodium bicarbonate supplementation enhances interval swimming. *Journal of Strength and Conditioning Research*, 18(2): 306–310.

Miller, J.B. (1996) *The GI Factor: The Glycemic Index Solution*. Sydney, Australia: Hodder and Stoughton.

Milliard-Stafford, M., Rosskopf, L.B., Snow, T.K. & Hinson, B.T. (1997) Water versus carbohydrate-electrolyte ingestion before and during a 15-km run in the heat. *International Journal of Sports Nutrition*, 7: 26–38.

Millard-Stafford, M., Sparling, P.B., Rosskopf, L.B. & Dicarlo, L.J. (1992) Carbohydrate-electrolyte replacement improves distance running performance in the heat. *Medicine and Science in Sports and Exercise*, 24: 934–940.

Mohr, M., Ellingsgaard, H., Anderson, H., Bangsbo, J. & Krustrup, P. (2004) Physical demands in high-level female soccer: application of fitness tests to evaluate match performance. *Journal of Sport Sciences*, 22(6): 552–523.

Mohr, M., et al (2010) Examination of fatigue patterns in elite soccer – a multi-experimental approach. *Scandinavian Journal of Medicine and Science in Sports*, 20(Suppl. 3): 125–132.

Montain, S.J., Cheuvront, S.N. & Sawka, M.N. (2006) Exercise associated hyponatraemia: quantitative analysis to understand the aetiology. *British Journal of Sports Medicine*, 40: 98–105.

Montain, S.J. & Coyle, E.F. (1992a) Fluid ingestion during exercise increases skin blood flow independent of increases in blood volume. *Journal Applied Physiology*, 73: 903–910.

Montain, S.J. & Coyle, E.F. (1992b) The influence of graded dehydration on hyperthermia and cardiovascular drift during exercise. *Journal Applied Physiology*, 73: 1340–1350.

Morton, D.P., Aragon-Vargas, L.F. & Callister, R. (2004) Effect of ingested fluid composition on exercise related transient abdominal pain. *International Journal of Sport Nutrition and Exercise Metabolism*, 14(2): 197–208.

Morton, D.P. & Callister, R. (2000) Characteristics and etiology of exercise-related transient abdominal pain. *Medicine and Science in Sports and Exercise*, 32: 432–438.

Mujika, I., Padilla, S., Ibanez, J., Izquierdo, M. & Gorostiaga, E. (1998) Creatine supplementation and sprint performance in soccer players. *Medicine and Science in Sports and Exercise*, 30: S141.

Mündel, T. (2011) To drink of not to drink? Explaining "contradictory findings" in fluid replacement and exercise performance: evidence from a more valid model for real-life competition. Editorial. *British Journal of Sports Medicine*, 45: 2.

Murray, R., Bartoli, W.P., Stofan, J., Horn, M.K. & Eddy, D. (1999) A comparison of the gastric emptying characteristics of selected sports drinks. *International Journal of Sport Nutrition and Exercise Metabolism*, 9: 263–274.

Myburgh, K.H., Hutchins, J., Fataar, A.B., Hough, S.F. & Noakes, T.D. (1990) Low bone density is an etiologic factor for stress fractures in athletes. *Annals of Internal Medicine*, 113(10): 754–759.

Nadel, E.R., Mack, G.W. & Nose, H. (1990) Influence of fluid replacement beverages on body fluid homeostasis during exercise and recovery. *Perspectives in Exercise Science and Sports Medicine, Fluid Homeostasis During Exercise*, Vol. 3, C.V. Gisolfi & D.R. Lamb (eds). Carmel, IN: Benchmark Press, pp. 181–206.

National Audit Office (2001) *Tackling Obesity in England*. London: The Stationery Office.

National Task Force on the Prevention and Treatment of Obesity (1993) Very low calorie diets. *Journal of the American Medical Association*, 270(8): 967–974.

Nevill, M.E., Boobis, L.H., Brooks, S. & Williams, C. (1989) Effect of timing on muscle metabolism during treadmill sprinting. *Journal of Applied Physiology*, 67: 2376–2382.

Newhouse, I.J., Clement, D.B., Taunton, J.E. & McKenzie, D.C. (1989) The effects of prelatent/latent iron deficiency on physical work capacity. *Medicine in Science in Sports and Exercise*, 21: 263–268.

Newhouse, I.J. & Finstad, E.W. (2000) The effects of magnesium supplementation on exercise performance. *Clinical Journal of Sports Medicine*, 10(3): 195–200.

Newsholme, E.A. & Leech (1983) *The Runner: Energy and Endurance. Fitness Books*. Oxford, England: Walter L. Meagher.

Nichols, J.F., Palmer, J.E. & Levy, S.S. (2003) Low bone mineral density in highly trained male master cyclists. *Osteoporosis International*, 14(8): 644–649.

Nichols, P.E., Jonnalagadda, S.S., Rosenbloom, C.A. & Trinkaus, M. (2005) Knowledge, attitudes and behaviours regarding hydration of collegiate athletes. *International Journal of Sport Nutrition and Exercise Metabolism*, 15: 515–527.

Noakes, T.D. (1985) *Lore of Running*. Cape Town, South Africa: Oxford University Press.

Noakes, T. (1992) *Lore of Running*. Cape Town, South Africa: Oxford University Press.

Noakes, T.D. (1993) Fluid replacement during exercise. *Exercise and Sport Sciences Reviews*, 21: 297–330.

Noakes, T.D. (1995) Dehydration during exercise: what are the real dangers? *Clinical Journal of Sports Medicine*, 5: 123–128.

Noakes, T. (2001) *Lore of Running*, 4th edn. Cape Town, South Africa: Oxford University Press.

Noakes, T.D. (2002) IMMDA advisory statement on guideleines for fluid replacement during marathon running. *New Studies in Athletics: The IAAF Technical Quarterly*, 17(1): 15–24.

Noakes, T.D. (2003a) Fluid replacement during marathon running. *Clinical Journal of Sports Medicine*, 13: 309–318.

Noakes, T.D. (2003b) Overconsumption of fluids by athletes. *British Medical Journal*, 327: 113–114.

Noakes, T.D. (2007) Drinking guidelines for exercise: What evidence is there that athletes should drink "as much as tolerable", "to replace the weight lost during exercise" or "*ad libitum*"? *Journal of Sports Sciences*, 25(7): 781–796.

Noakes, T.D. (2010) Is drinking to thirst optimum? *Annals of Nutrition and Metabolism*, 57(Suppl. 2): 9–17.

Noakes, T.D., Goodwin, N., Rayner, B.L., Brankin, T. & Taylor, R.K.N. (1985) Water intoxication: a possible complication of endurance exercise. *Medicine and Science Sports and Exercise*, 17: 370–375.

Noakes, T.D., Myburgh, K.H., Du Plessis, J., Lang, L., Lambert, M.I., Van Der Riet, C. & Schall, R. (1991) Metabolic rate, not percent dehydration, predicts rectal temperature in marathon runners. *Medicine and Science in Sports and Exercise*, 23: 443–449.

Noakes, T.D., Sharwood, K., Sppedy, D., Hew, T., Reid, S., Dugas, J., Almond, S., Wharam, P. & Weschier, L. (2005) Three independent biological mechanisms cause exercise-associated hyponatremia: Evidence from 2,135 weighed competitive athletic performances. *Proceedings of the National Academy of Sciences*, 102(51): 18550–18555.

Noakes, T.D. & Speedy, D.B. (2006) Case proven: exercise associated hyponatremia is due to overdrinking. So why did it take 20 years before the original evidence was accepted? *British Journal of Sports Medicine*, 40: 567–572.

Nogueira, J.A.D. & Da Costa, T.H.M. (2004) Nutrition intake and eating habits if triathletes on a Brazilian diet. *International Journal of Sport Nutrition and Exercise Metabolism*, 14(6): 684–697.

Nose, H., Mack, G.W., Shi, X. & Nadel, E.R. (1988a) Shift in body fluid compartments after dehydration in man. *Journal of Applied Physiology*, 65: 318–324.

Nose, H., Mack, G.W., Shi, X. & Nadel, E.R. (1988b) Role of osmolality and plasma volume during rehydration in humans. *Journal of Applied Physiology*, 65: 325–336.

Nose, H., Mack, G.W., Shi, X. & Nadel, E.R. (1988c) Involvement of sodium retention hormones during rehydration in humans. *Journal of Applied Physiology*, 65: 332–336.

Onywera, V.O., Kiplamai, F.K., Tuitoek, P.J., Boit, M.K. & Pitsiladis, Y.P. (2004) Food and macronutrient intake of elite Kenyan distance runners. *International Journal of Sport Nutrition and Exercise Metabolism*, 14: 709–719.

Oopik, V., Saaremets, I., Medijainen, L., Karelson, K., Janson, T. & Timpmann, S. (2003) Effects of sodium citrate ingestion before exercise on endurance performance in well-trained runners. *British Journal of Sports Medicine*, 37: 485–489.

Op't Eijnde, B., Vergauwen, L. & Hespel, P. (2001) Creatine loading does not impact on stroke performance in tennis. *International Journal of Sports Medicine*, 22(1): 76–80.

Ostojic, S.M. (2004) Creatine supplementation in young soccer players. *International Journal of Sport Nutrition and Exercise Metabolism*, 14: 95–103.

Ostojic, S.M. & Ahmetovic, Z. (2008) Gastrointestinal distress after creatine supplementation in athletes: are side effects dose dependent? *Research in Sports Medicine*, 16(1): 15–22.

Pasman, W.J., van Baak, M.A., Jeukendrup, A.E. & de Haan, A. (1995) The effect of different dosages of caffeine on endurance performance time. *International Journal of Sports Medicine*, 16: 225–230.

Pastene, J., Germain, M., Allevard, A.M., Gharib, C. & Lacour, J.R. (1996) Water balance during and after marathon running. *European Journal of Applied Physiology*, 73(1–2): 49–55.

Peeling, P., Dawson, B., Goodman, C., Landers, G. & Trinder, G. (2008) Athletic induced iron deficiency: new insights into the role of inflammation, cytokines and hormones. *European Journal of Applied Physiology*, 103(4): 381–391.

Petroczi, A. & Naughton, D.P. (2008) The age-gender-status profile of high performing athletes in the UK taking nutritional supplements: lessons for the future. *Journal of the International Society of Sports Nutrition*, 10(5): 2.

Peyreburne, M.C., Nevill, M.E., Donaldson, F.J. & Cosford, D.J. (1998) The effects of oral creatine supplementation on performance in single and repeated sprint swimming. *Journal of Sport Science*, 16: 271–279.

Phillips, S.M. (2009) Physiologic and molecular bases of muscle hypertrophy and atrophy: impact of resistance exercise on human skeletal muscle (protein and exercise dose effects). *Applied Physiology, Nutrition, and Metabolism*, 34: 403–410.

Phillips, S.M., Green, H.J., Tarnopolsky, M.A., Heigenhauser, G.J.F., Hill, R.E. & Grant, S.M. (1996) Effects of training duration on substrate turnover and oxidation during exercise. *Journal of Applied Physiology*, 81: 2182–2191.

Pitts, G.C., Johnson, R.E. & Consolazio, F.C. (1944) Working in the heat as affected by intake of water, salt and glucose. *American Journal of Physiology*, 142: 253–259.

Pluim, B.M., Ferrauti, A., Broekhof, F., Deutekom, M., Gotzmann, A., Kuipers, H. & Weber, K. (2006) The effects of creatine supplementation on selected factors of tennis specific training. *British Journal of Sports Medicine*, 40(6): 507–511.

Plunkett, B.T. & Hopkins, W.G. (1999) Investigation of the side pain "stitch" induced by running after fluid ingestion. *Medicine and Science in Sports and Exercise*, 31(8): 1169–1175.

Poortmans, J.R. & Francaux, M. (2000) Adverse effects of creatine supplementation: fact or fiction? *Sports Medicine*, 30(3): 155–170.

Potteiger, J.A., Nickel, G.L., Webster, M.J., Haub, M.D. & Palmer, R.J. (1996) Sodium citrate ingestion enhances 30 km cycling performance. *International Journal of Sports Medicine*, 17: 7–11.

Price, M., Moss, P. & Rance, S. (2003) Effect of sodium bicarbonate on prolonged intermittent exercise. *Medicine and Science in Sports and Exercise*, 35: 1303–1308.

Pruscino, C.L., Ross, M.L., Gregory, J.R., Savage, B. & Flanagan, T.R. (2008) Effects of sodium bicarbonate, caffeine, and their combination on repeated 200-m freestyle performance. *International Journal of Sport Nutrition and Exercise Metabolism*, 18(2): 116–130.

Pugh, I.G.C.E., Corbett, J.L. & Johnson, R.H. (1967) Rectal temperatures, weight losses, and sweat rates in marathon running. *Journal of Applied Physiology*, 23: 347–352.

Raatz, S.K., Torkelson, C.J., Redmon, J.B., Reck, K.P., Kwong, C.A., Swanson, J.E., Liu, C., Thomas, W. & Bantle, J.P. (2005) Reduced glycemic index and glycemic load diets do not increase the effects of energy restriction on weight loss and insulin sensitivity in obese men and women. *Journal of Nutrition*, 135(10): 2387–2391.

Rash, C.L., Malinauskas, B.M., Duffrin, M.W., Barber-Heidal, K. & Overton, R.F. (2008) Nutrition-related knowledge, attitude, and dietary intake of college track athletes. *The Sport Journal*, 11(1): 48–54.

Rasmussen, B.B., Tipton, K.D., Miller, S.L., Wolf, S.E. & Wolfe, R.R. (2000) An oral essential amino acid-carbohydrate supplement enhances muscle protein anabolism after resistance exercise. *Journal of Applied Physiology*, 88: 386–392.

Raymond-Barker, P., Petroczi, A. & Quested, E. (2007) Assessment of nutritional knowledge in female athletes susceptible to the female athlete triad syndrome. *Journal of Occupational Medicine and Toxicology (London, England)*, 2: 10.

Reilly, T. & Ekblom, B. (2005) The use of recovery methods post-exercise. *Journal of Sport Sciences*, 23(6): 619–627.

Reilly, T., George, K., Marfell-Jones, M., Scott, M., Sutton, L. & Wallace, J.A. (2009) How well do skinfold equations predict percent body fat in elite soccer players? *International Journal of Sports Medicine*, 30(8): 607–613.

Renner, E. (1983) *Milk and Dairy Products in Human Nutrition*. Munich, Germany: Volkswirtschaftlicher Verlag.

Requena, B., Zabala, M. Padial, P. & Feriche, B. (2005) Sodium bicarbonate and sodium citrate: ergogenic aids? *Journal of Strength and Conditioning Research*, 19(1): 213–224.

Richter, E.A., Mikines, K.J., Galbo, H. & Kiens, B. (1988) Effects of exercise on insulin action in human skeletal muscle. *Journal of Applied Physiology*, 66: 876–885.

Robins, A. & Hetherington, M.M. (2005) A comparison of pre-competition eating patterns in a group of non-elite triathletes. *International Journal of Sport Nutrition and Exercise Metabolism*, 15: 442–457.

Robinson, C.H., Lawler, M.R., Chenoweth, W.L. & Garwick, A.E. (1986) *Normal and therapeutic nutrition*, 17th edn. London: Collier Macmillan Publishers.

Robinson, T.A., Hawley, J.A., Palmer, G.S., Wilson, G.R., Gray, D.A., Noakes, T.D. & Dennis, S.C. (1995a) Water ingestion does not improve 1-h cycling performance in moderate ambient temperatures. *European Journal of Applied Physiology*, 71: 153–160.

Robinson, T.L., Snow-Harter, C., Taafe, D.R., Gillis, D., Shaw, J. & Marcus, R. (1995b) Gymnasts exhibit higher bone mass than runners despite similar prevalence of amenorrhea and oligomenorrhea. *Journal of Bone Mineral Research*, 10: 26–35.

Rodriguez, N.R., Di Marco, N.M. and Langley, S.; American Dietetic Association, Dietitians of Canada, American College of Sports Medicine (2009) American College of Sports Medicine position stand. Nutrition and athletic performance. *Medicine and Science in Sports and Exercise*, 41: 709–731.

Romer, L.M., Barrington, J.P. & Jeukendrup, A.E. (2001) Effects of oral creatine supplementation on high intensity, intermittent exercise per-formance in competitive squash players. *International Journal of Sports Medicine*, 22(8): 546–552.

Romero, V.E., Ruiz, J.R., Ortega, F.B., Artero, E.G., Vicente-Rodríguez, G., Moreno, L.A., Castillo, M.J. & Gutierrez, A. (2009) Body fat measurement in elite sport climbers: comparison of skinfold thickness equations with dual energy X-ray absorptiometry. *Journal of Sports Sciences*, 27(5): 469–477.

Rosenbloom, C.A., Jonnalagadda, S.S. & Skinner, R. (2002) Nutrition knowledge of collegiate athletes in a Division I National Collegiate Athletic Association institution. *Journal of the American Dietetic Association*, 102(3): 418–420.

Ross, R., et al (2000) Reduction in obesity and related comorbid conditions after diet-induced weight loss or exercise-induced weight loss in men: a randomized, controlled trial. *Annals of Internal Medicine*, 133: 92–103.

Rothstein, A., Adolph, E.F. & Wills, J.H. (1947) Voluntary dehydration. In: *Physiology of Man in the Desert*, E.F. Adolph (ed). New York: Interscience, pp. 254–270.

Ryan, A.J., Lambert, G.P., Shi, X., Chang, R.T., Summers, R.W. & Gisolfi, C.V. (1984) Effect of hypohydraton on gastric emptying and intestinal absorption during exercise. *Journal of Applied Physiology*, 84: 2581–2588.

Ryan, A.J., Lambert, G.P., Shi, X., Chang, R.T., Summers, R.W. & Gisolfi, C.V. (1998) Effect of hypohydration on gastric emptying and intestinal absorption during exercise. *Journal of Applied Physiology*, 84: 1581–1588.

Saltin, B. (1973) Metabolic fundamentals in exercise. *Medicine and Science in Sports*, 5: 137–146.

Sawka, M.N., Burke, L.M., Eichner, E.R., Maughan, R.J., Montain, S.J. & Stachenfeld, N.S. (2007) American College of Sports Medicine position stand: exercise and fluid replacement. *Medicine and Science in Sports and Exercise*, 39: 377–390.

Sawka, M.N. & Pandolf, K.B. (1990) Effects of body water loss on physiological function and exercise performance. In: *Perspectives in Exercise Science and Sports Medicine, Fluid Homeostasis During Exercise*, Vol. 3, C.V. Gisolfi & D.R. Lamb (eds). Carmel, IN: Benchmark Press, pp. 1–38.

Schabort, E.J., Bosch, A.N., Wetman, S.M. & Noakes, T.D. (1999) The effect of a pre-exercise meal on time to fatigue during prolonged cycling exercise. *Medicine and Science in Sports and Exercise*, 31: 464–471.

Schobersberger, W., Tschann, M., Hasibeder, W., Steidl, M., Herold, M., Nachbauer, W. & Koller, A. (1990) Consequences of 6 weeks of strength training on red cell O_2 transport and iron status. *European Journal of Applied Physiology and Occupational Physiology*, 60(3): 163–168.

Schumacher, Y.O., Schmid, A., Grathwohl, D., Bültermann, D. & Berg, A. (2002) Haematological indices and iron status in athletes of various sports and performances. *Medicine and Science in Sports and Exercise*, 34(5): 869–875.

Seidell, J.C., et al (1987) Assessment of intra-abdominal and subcutaneous abdominal fat: relation between anthropometry and computed tomography. *American Journal of Clinical Nutrition*, 45: 7–13.

Seifert, J., Harmon, J. & DeClercq, P. (2006) Protein added to a sports drink improves fluid retention. *International Journal of Sport Nutrition and Exercise Metabolism*, 16: 420–429.

Servan-Schreiber, D. (2004) *Healing without Freud or Prozac*. London: Rodale International.

Sharwood, K.A., Collins, M., Goedecke, J.H., Wilson, G. & Noakes, T.D. (2004) Weight changes, medical complications, and performance during an Ironman triathlon. *British Journal of Sports Medicine*, 38: 718–724.

Shaskey, D.J. & Green, G.A. (2000) Sport haematology. *Sports Medicine*, 29: 27–38.

Shave, R., Whyte, G., Siemann, A. & Doggart, L. (2001) The effects of sodium citrate ingestion on 3,000-metre time-trial performance. *Journal of Strength and Conditioning Research*, 15: 230–234.

Shaw, K., Gennat, H., O'Rourke, P. & Del Mar, C. (2006) Exercise for overweight or obesity. *Cochrane Database of Systematic Reviews*, Issue 4: CD003817.

Shaw, K., O'Rourke, P., Del Mar, C. & Kenardy, J. (2005) Psychological interventions for overweight or obesity. *Cochrane Database of Systematic Reviews*, Issue 2: CD003818.

Sherman, A.R. (1992) Zinc, copper and iron nutriture and immunity. *Journal of Nutrition,* 122: 604–609.

Sherman, W.M., Costill, D.L., Fink, W.J. & Miller, J.M. (1981) Effect of exercise and diet manipulation on muscle glycogen and its subsequent use during performance. *International Journal of Sports Medicine,* 2: 114–118.

Shi, X., Horn, M.K., Osterberg, K.L., Stofan, J.R., Zachwieja, J.J., Horswill, C.A., Passe, D.H. & Murray, R. (2004) Gastrointestinal discomfort during intermittent high-intensity exercise: effect of carbohydrate-electrolyte beverage. *International Journal of Sport Nutrition and exercise Metabolism,* 14(6): 673–683.

Shirreffs, S.M., Aragon-Vargas, L.F., Chamorro, M., Maughan, R.J., Serratosa, L. & Zachwieja, J.J. (2005) The sweating response of elite professional soccer players to training in the heat. *International Journal of Sports Medicine,* 26: 90–95.

Sichieri, R., Moura, A.S., Genelhu, V., Hu, F. & Willett, W.C. (2007) An 18-mo randomized trial of a low glycemic-index diet and weight change in Brazilian women. *American Journal of Clinical Nutrition,* 86(3): 707–713.

Silva, A.J., Machado Reis, V., Guidetti, L., Bessone Alves, F., Mota, P., Freitas, J. & Baldari, C. (2007) Effect of creatine on swimming velocity, body composition and hydrodynamic variables. *Journal of Sports Medicine and Physical Fitness,* 47(1): 58–64.

Silva, A.M., Fields, D.A., Quitério, A.L. & Sardinha, L. (2009) Are skinfold-based models accurate and suitable for assessing changes in body composition in highly trained athletes? *Journal of Strength and Conditioning Research,* 23(6): 1688–1696.

Singh, A. Evans, P. Gallagher, K.L. & Deuster, P.A. (1993) Dietary intakes and biochemical profiles of nutritional status of ultramarathoners. *Medicine and Science in Sports and Exercise,* 25: 328–334.

Sloth, B., et al (2004) No difference in body weight decrease between a low-glycemic-index and a high-glycemic-index diet but reduced LDL cholesterol after 10-wk ad libitum intake of the low-glycemic-index diet. *American Journal of Clinical Nutrition,* 80(2): 337–347.

Sport England (2006) *Active People Survey.* London: Sport England.

Spriet, L.L. & Gibala, M.J. (2004) Nutritional strategies to influence adaptations to training. *Journal of Sport Sciences,* 22: 127–141.

Stear, S.J., Castell, L.M., Burke, L.M. & Spriet, L.L. (2010) BJSM reviews: A–Z of nutritional supplements: dietary supplements, sport nutrition foods and ergogenic aids for health and performance Part 6. *British Journal of Sports Medicine,* 44: 297–298.

Stellingwerff, T., Boit, M.K. & Res, P.T. (2007) Nutritional strategies to optimize training and racing in middle-distance athletes. *Journal of Sports Sciences,* 25(Suppl. 1): S17–S28.

Stepto, L.M., Carey, A.L., Staudacher, H.M., Cummings, N.K., Burke, L.M. & Hawley, J.A. (2002) Effect of short-term fat adaptation on high-intensity training. *Medicine Science Sports Exercise,* 34: 449–455.

Stevenson, E., Willaims, C., Nute, M., Swaile, P. & Tsui, M. (2005) The effect of the glycemic index of an evening meal on the metabolic responses to a standard high glycemic index breakfast and subsequent exercise in men. *International Journal of Sport Nutrition and Exercise Metabolism,* 15: 308–322.

Stout, J.R., Echerson, J., Noonan, D., Moore, G. & Cullen, D. (1999) Effects of creatine supplementation on exercise performance and fat-free weight in football players during training. *Nutrition Research,* 19: 217–225.

Stuart, G.R., Hopkins, W.G., Cook, C. & Cairns, S.P. (2005) Multiple effects of caffeine on simulated high-intensity team-sport performance. *Medicine and Science in Sports and Exercise,* 37: 1998–2005.

Stubbs, R.J., et al (2002) The effect of graded levels of exercise on energy intake and balance of free-living men, consuming their normal diet. *European Journal of Clinical Nutrition*, 56(2): 129–140.

Stubbs, R.J., et al (2004) Rate and extent of compensatory changes in energy intake and expenditure in response to altered exercise and diet composition in humans. *American Journal of Physiology Regulatory: Integrative and Comparative Physiology*, 286: R350–R358.

Suominen, H. (1993) Bone mineral density and long term exercise. An overview of cross-sectional athlete studies. *Sports Medicine*, 16(5): 316–330.

Swinburn, B. & Ravussin, E. (1993) Energy balance or fat balance? *American Journal of Clinical Nutrition*, 57(Suppl. 5): 766S–771S.

Szlyk, P.C., Sils, I.V., Francesconi, R.P., Hubbard, R.W. & Matthew, W.T. (1989) Variability in intake and dehydration in young men during a simulated desert walk. *Aviation, Space and Environmental Medicine*, 60: 422–427.

Talbott, J.H., Edwards, H.T., Dill, D.B. & Drastich, L. (1933) Physiological responses to high environment and temperature. *Journal of Tropical Medicine and Hygiene*, 13: 381–397.

Tarnopolsky, M. (1999) Protein metabolism in strength and endurance activities. In: *The Metabolic Basis of Performance in Exercise and Sport: Perspectives in Exercise Science and Sports Medicine*, Vol. 12, D.R. Lamb & R. Murray (eds). Carmel, IN: Cooper, pp. 125–157.

Tarnopolsky, M. (2004) Protein requirements for endurance athletes. *Nutrition*, 25(7–8): 662–668.

Tarnopolsky, M.A. (2010) Caffeine and creatine use in sport. *Annuals of Nutrition and Metabolism*, 57(Suppl. 2): 1–8.

Terjung, R.L. Clarkson, P., Eichner, E.R., Greenhaff, P.L., Hespel, P.J., Israel, R.G., Kraemer, W.J., Meyer, R.A., Spriet, L.L., Tarnopolsky, M.A., Wagenmakers, A.J. & Williams, M.H. (2000) American College of Sports Medicine roundtable. The physiological and health effects of oral creatine supplementation. *Medicine and Science in Sports and Exercise*, 32(3): 706–717.

Thomas, B. (ed) & BDA (2001) *Manual of Dietetic Practice*, 3rd edn. Oxford: Blackwell Science Ltd.

Thomas, B. & Bishop, J. (2007) *Manual of Dietric Practice*, 4th edn. Oxford, England: Blackwell Publishers.

Thomas, D.E., Brotherhood, J.R. & Brand, J.C. (1991) Carbohydrate feeding before exercise: effect of glycemic index. *International Journal of Sports Medicine*, 12: 180–186.

Thomas, D.E., Elliot, E.J. & Baur, L. (2007). Low glycaemic index or low glycaemic load diets for overweight and obesity. *Cochrane Database of Systematic Reviews, Issue 3*.

Thompson, F.E. & Byers, T. (1994) Dietary assessment resource manual. *American Institute of Nutrition. Journal of Nutrition*, 124: 2245S–2317S.

Tilgner, S.A. & Schiller, M.R. (1989). Dietary intakes of female college athletes: The need for nutrition education. *Journal of the American Dietetic Association*, 89 (7): 967–969.

Tipton, K.D. (2010) Nutrition for acute exercise-induced injuries. *Annals of Nutrition and Metabolism*, 57(Suppl. 2): 43–53.

Tipton, K.D., Elliot, T.A., Ferrando, A.A., Aarsland, A.A. & Wolfe, R.R. (2009) Stimulation of muscle anabolism by resistance exercise and ingestion of leucine plus protein. *Applied Physiology, Nutrition and Metabolism*, 34(2): 151–161.

Tipton, K.D., Rasmussen, B.B., Miller, S.L., Wolf, S.E., Owens-Stovall, S.K., Petrini, B.E. & Wolfe, R.R. (2001) Timing of amino acid-carbohydrate ingestion alters anabolic response of muscle to resistance exercise. *American Journal of Physiology*, 281: E197–E206.

Tipton, K.D. & Wolfe, R.R. (2004) Protein and amino acids for athletes. *Journal of Sports Sciences*, 22: 65–79.

Todd, K.S., Butterfield, G.E. & Calloway, D.H. (1984) Nitrogen balance in men with adequate and deficient energy intake at three levels of work. *Journal of Nutrition*, 114: 2107–2118.

Todorovic, W.E. & Micklewright, A. (2000) *A Pocket Guide to Clinical Nutrition*, 2nd edn, revised. Birmingham, England: The British Dietetic Association.

Van der Berrie, F., Van den Eynde, B.M., Van den Berghe, K. & Hespel, P. (1998) Effect of creatine on endurance capacity and sprint power in cyclists. *International Journal of Sports Medicine*, 8: 2055–2063.

Van Erp-Baart, A.M.J., Saris, W.H.M., Binkhorst, R.A., Vos, J.A. & Elvers, J.W.H. (1989) Nationwide survey on nutritional habits of elite athletes. Part II: mineral and vitamin intake. *International Journal of Sports Medicine*, 10(Suppl. 1): 3–10.

van Hamont, D., Harvey, C.R., Massicotte, D., Frew, R., Peronnet, F. & Rehrer, N.J. (2005) Reduction in muscle glycogen and protein utilization with glucose feeding during exercise. *International Journal of Sport Nutrition and Exercise Metabolism*, 15: 350–365.

van Loon, L.J.C. & Saris, W.H.M. (2005) Dietary considerations for sport and exercise. In: *Human Nutrition*, 11th edn, C.A. Geissler & H.J. Powers (eds). Edinburgh: Elsevier Churchill Livingstone.

van Nieuwenhoven, M.A., Brouns, F. & Kovacs, E.M. (2005) The effect of two sports drinks and water on GI complaints and performance during an 18 km run. *International Journal of Sports Medicine*, 26(4): 281–285.

Volek, J.S., et al (1997) Creatine supplementation enhances muscular performance during high-intensity resistance exercise. *Journal of the American Dietetic Association*, 97: 765–770.

Walsh, R.M., Noakes, T.D., Dennis, S.C. & Hawley, J.A. (1994) Impaired high intensity cycling performance times at low levels of dehydration. *International Journal of Sports Medicine*, 15: 392–398.

Walton, P. & Rhodes, E.C. (1997) Glycemic index and optimal performance. *Sports Medicine*, 23: 164–172.

Wardlaw, G.M., Hampl, J.S. & DiSilvestro, R.A. (2004) *Perspectives in Nutrition*, 6th edn. Boston: McGraw-Hill.

Warren, J.A., Jenkins, R.R., Packer, L., Witt, E.H., Armstrong, R.B. (1992) Elevated muscle vitamin E does not attenuate eccentric exercise-induced muscle injury. *Journal of Applied Physiology*, 72: 2168–2175.

Waterhouse, J., Reilly, T. & Edwards, B. (2004) The stress of travel. *Journal of Sport Sciences*, 22: 946–966.

Watt, K.K.O., Graham, A.P. & Snow, R.J. (2004) Skeletal muscle total creatine content and creatine transporter gene expression in vegetarians prior to following creatine supplementation. *International Journal of Sports Nutrition and Exercise Metabolism*, 14(5): 517–531.

Wee, S.L., Williams, C., Gray, S. & Horabin, J. (1999) Influence of high and low glycemic index meals on endurance running capacity. *Medicine and Science in Sports and Exercise*, 31: 393–399.

Weinstein, A.R. (2004) Relationship of physical activity vs body mass index with type 2 diabetes in women. *Journal of the American Medical Association*, 292: 1198–1194.

Weir, J., Noakes, T.D., Myburgh, K. & Adams, B. (1987) A high carbohydrate diet negates the metabolic effects of caffeine. *Medicine and Science in Sports and Exercise*, 19: 100–105.

Westererp-Plantenga, M.S., Rolland, V., Wilson, S.A. & Westererp, K.R. (1999) Satiety related to 24 h diet-induced thermogenesis during high protein/carbohydrate vs high fat diets measured in a respiration chamber. *European Journal of Clinical Nutrition*, 53: 495–502.

Wharam, P. & Weschler, L. (2005) Three independent biological mechanisms cause exercise-associated hyponatremia: evidence from 2,135 weighed competitive athletic performances. *Proceedings of the National Academy of Sciences*, 102(51): 18550–18555.

White, A., et al (1991) *Health Survey for England*. London: HMSO.

Wiles, J.D., Bird, S.R., Hopkins, J. & Riley, M. (1992) Effect of caffeinated coffee on running speed, respiratory factors, blood lactate and perceived exertion during 1500 m treadmill running. *British Journal of Sports Medicine*, 26: 116–120.

Wilkes, D., Geldhill, N. & Smyth, R. (1983) Effect of acute induced metabolic alkalosis on 800-m racing time. *Medicine and Science in Sports and Exercise*, 15: 277–280.

Wilkinson, J.G., Martin, D.T., Adams, A.A. & Liebman, M. (2002) Iron status in cyclists during high-intensity interval training and recovery. *International Journal of Sport Medicine*, 23(8): 544–548.

Williams, M.H. & Branch, J.D. (1998) Creatine supplementation and exercise performance: an update. *Journal of American College of Nutrition*, 17(3): 205–206.

Williams, M.H., Kreider, R.B. & Branch, J.D. (1999) *Creatine: The Power Supplement*. Champaign, IL: Human Kinetics.

Willis, K.S., Petersen, N.J. & Larsen-Meyer, D.E. (2008) Should we be concerned about the vitamin D status of athletes? *International Journal of Sports Nutrition and Exercise Metabolism*, 18(2): 204–224.

Wilmore, J.H. (1996) Increasing physical activity: alterations in body mass and composition. *American Journal of Clinical Nutrition*, 63: 456S–460S.

Wilmore, J.H. & Costill, D.L. (2004) *Physiology of Sport and Exercise*, 3rd edn. Champaign, IL: Human Kinetics.

Winger, J.M., Dugas, J.P. & Dugas, L.R. (2011) Beliefs about hydration and physiology drive drinking behaviours in runners. *British Journal of Sports Medicine*, 45: 646–649.

Winters-Stone, K.M. & Snow, C.M. (2004) One year of oral calcium supplementation maintains cortical bone density in young adults female distance runners. *International Journal of Sports Nutrition and Exercise Metabolism*, 14: 7–17.

Wojtaszewski, J.P.F., Nielson, P., Kiens, B. & Richter, E.A. (2001) Regulation of glycogen synthase kinase-3 in human skeletal muscle: effects of food intake and bicycle exercise. *Diabetes*, 50: 265–269.

Wolever, T.M.S. (2006) *The Glycemic Index*. Wallingford, England: CABI Publishers.

Wolever, T.M.S, Jenkins, D.J., Jenkins, A.L. & Josse, R.G. (1991) The glycemic index: methodology and clinical implications. *American Journal of Clinical Nutrition*, 54: 846–854.

Wong, J.M.W., Josse, A.R., Augustin, L., Esfahani, A., Banach, M.S., Kendall, C.W.C. and Jenkins, D.J.A. (2009) Glycemic index and glycemic load: effects on glucose, insulin, and lipid regulation. In: *Nutraceuticals, Glycemic Health and Type 2 Diabetes*, V.K. Pasupuleti & J.W. Anderson (eds). Oxford, England: Wiley-Blackwell.

World Health Organization (2003) *Global Strategy on Diet, Physical Activity and Health. Report of a WHO consultation*. Geneva, Switzerland: WHO.

Worme, J.D., Doubt, T.J., Singh, A., Ryan, C.J., Moses, F.M. & Deuster, P.A. (1990) Dietary patterns, gastrointestinal complaints, and nutrition knowledge of recreational triathletes. *American Journal of Clinical Nutrition*, 51: 690–697.

Wu, C.L. & Williams, C. (2006) A low glycemic index meal before exercise improves endurance running capacity in men. *International Journal of Sport Nutrition and Exercise Metabolism*, 16: 510–527.

Wyndham, C.H. (1977) Heatstroke and hyperthermia in marathon runners. *Annals of the New York Academy of Sciences*, 301: 128–138.

Wyndham, C.H. & Strydom, N.B. (1969) The danger of an inadequate water intake during marathon running. *South African Medical Journal*, 43: 893–896.

Wyndham, C.H., Strydom, N.B., Van Rensburg, A.J., Benade, A.J.S. & Heyns, A.J. (1970) Relation between VO2 max and body temperature in hot humid air conditions. *Journal of Applied Physiology*, 29: 45–50.

Yannakoulia, M., Keramompoulos, A. & Matalas, A. (2004) Bone mineral density in young active females: the case of dancers. *International Journal of Sport Nutrition and Exercise Metabolism*, 14: 285–297.

Yeo, W.K., Carey, A.L., Burke, L., Spriet, L.L. & Hawley, J.A. (2011) Fat adaptation in well-trained athletes: effects on cell metabolism. *Applied Physiology, Nutrition and Metabolism*, 36(1): 12–22.

Zawila, L.G., Steib, C.M. & Hoogenboom, B. (2003) The female collegiate cross-country runner: nutritional knowledge and attitudes. *Journal of Athletic Training*, 38(1): 67–74.

Zelasko, C.J. (1995) Exercise for weight loss: what are the facts? *Journal of the American Dietetic Association*, 95(12): 1414–1417.

Zilva, J.F., Pannall, P.R. & Mayne, P.D. (1988) *Clinical Chemistry in Diagnosis and Treatment*, 5th edn. London: Hodder & Stoughton.

Zouhal, H., Groussard, C., Vincent, S., Jacob, C., Abderrahman, A.B., Delamarche, P. & Gratas-Delamarche, A. (2009) Athletic performance and weight changes during the 'Marathon of Sands' in athletes well-trained in endurance. *International Journal of Sports Medicine*, 30: 516–521.

Further reading

Food Standards Agency (2002) *McCance and Widdowson's The Composition of Foods*, 6th summary edn. Cambridge, England: Royal Sciety of Chemistry.

Internet Resources

The British Olympic Association (BOA), www.olympics.org.uk

UK Sport, www.uksport.gov.uk

Sport England, www.sportengland.org

Sport Wales, www.sportwales.org.uk

Sport Scotland, www.sportscotland.org.uk

Sport Northern Ireland, www.sportni.net

The British Dietetic Association, www.bda.uk.com

British Nutrition Foundation, www.nutrition.org.uk

The Nutrition Society, www.nutsoc.org.uk

Food Standards Agency, www.foodstandards.gov.uk

The National Health Service/Healthy Eating, www.nhs.uk/livewell
www.eatwell.gov.uk

The Dairy Council, www.milk.co.uk

The British Association of Sport and Exercise Medicine (BASEM), www.basem.co.uk

The British Association of Sport and Exercise Sciences (BASES), www.bases.co.uk

English Institute of Sport (EIS), www.eis2win.co.uk

Association of Dietetics in South Africa, www.adsa.org.za

New Zealand Dietetic Association, www.dietitians.org.nz

Dietitians Association of Australia, www.daa.asn.au

American Dietetic Association, www.eatright.org

Dietitians of Canada, www.dietitians.ca

World Anti-doping Association, www.wada-ama.org

UK Anti-doping, www.ukad.org.uk

Sports Coach UK, www.sportscoachUK.org

Nutrition for Sport and Exercise: A Practical Guide, First Edition. Hayley Daries.
© 2012 Blackwell Publishing Ltd. Published 2012 by Blackwell Publishing Ltd.

Index

Note: Page numbers with italicised *f*'s and *t*'s refer to figures and tables, respectively.

Nutrition for Sport and Exercise: A Practical Guide, First Edition. Hayley Daries.
© 2012 Blackwell Publishing Ltd. Published 2012 by Blackwell Publishing Ltd.